....
Controversies in Neuro-Oncology

Frontiers of Radiation Therapy and Oncology

Vol. 33

Series Editors   *John L. Meyer*, San Francisco, Calif.
W. Hinkelbein, Berlin

KARGER

Basel · Freiburg · Paris · London · New York ·
New Delhi · Bangkok · Singapore · Tokyo · Sydney

3rd International Symposium on Special Aspects of Radiotherapy,
Berlin, Germany, April 30 – May 2, 1998

···························

Controversies in Neuro-Oncology

Volume Editors   *T. Wiegel*, Berlin
                                          W. Hinkelbein, Berlin
                                          M. Brock, Berlin
                                          T. Hoell, Berlin

92 figures, 3 in color, and 65 tables, 1999

KARGER   Basel · Freiburg · Paris · London · New York ·
New Delhi · Bangkok · Singapore · Tokyo · Sydney

Frontiers of Radiation Therapy and Oncology

Founded 1968 by J.M. Vaeth, San Francisco, Calif.

••••••••••••••••••••

Dr. T. Wiegel
Prof. Dr. W. Hinkelbein
Dr. M. Brock
Dr. T. Hoell

Freie Universität Berlin
Radiologische Klinik und Poliklinik
Abteilung für Strahlentherapie
Universitätsklinikum Benjamin Franklin
Hindenburgdamm 30
D–12200 Berlin

Library of Congress Cataloging-in-Publication Data
International Symposium on Special Aspects of Radiotherapy (3rd:1998: Berlin, Germany)
(Controversies in neuro-oncology / 3rd International Symposium on Special Aspects of Radiotherapy,
Berlin, Germany, April 30–May 2, 1998; volume editors, T. Wiegel ... [et al.].
Frontiers of radiation therapy and oncology; vol. 33)
Includes bibliographical references and indexes.
1. Brain – Cancer – Radiotherapy Congresses.   2. Metastasis – Treatment Congresses.   I. Wiegel, T.
II. Title.   III. Series.
[DNLM: 1. Brain Neoplasms – radiotherapy Congresses.   2. Brain Neoplasms – surgery Congresses.
3. Radiotherapy – methods Congresses. W3 FR935 v.33 1999 / WL 358 I606c 1999]
RC280.B7.I556 1999
616.99′4810642–dc21
ISSN 0071–9676
ISBN 3–8055–6834–7 (hardcover : alk. paper)

Bibliographic Indices. This publication is listed in bibliographic services, including Current Contents® and Index Medicus.

© Copyright 1999 by S. Karger AG, P.O. Box, CH–4009 Basel (Switzerland)
www.karger.com
Printed in Switzerland on acid-free paper by Reinhardt Druck, Basel
ISBN 3–8055–6834–7

Contents

Glioblastoma: New Perspectives and Experimental Therapy

Radiation Tolerance and Re-Irradiation of the CNS

Preface

The meeting on 'Controversies in Neuro-Oncology' in Berlin as the 'Third Meeting on Special Aspects of Radiotherapy', organized by the Departments of Radiotherapy and Neurosurgery of the University Hospital Benjamin Franklin and the Department of Radiotherapy of the Charité, focused on the treatment of brain tumors.

Major advances have been made in recent years in surgical techniques including neuronavigation, chemotherapy, knowledge of pathology, diagnostic techniques and experience with radiotherapy for brain tumors. The development of sophisticated methods, as for example neuronavigation, three-dimensional treatment planning and stereotactic radiotherapy, represents the technical and medical standards of both cooperating disciplines in an extremely specialized field of oncology and neurosurgery.

We hope this textbook will update currently available information, thus providing valuable reading for the community of radiation oncologists, neuropathologists and neurosurgeons and hopefully help further improve the radiotherapy and surgery of brain tumors.

T. Wiegel, T. Hoell
M. Brock, W. Hinkelbein

Introduction

Wiegel T, Hinkelbein W, Brock M, Hoell T (eds): Controversies in Neuro-Oncology.
Front Radiat Ther Oncol. Basel, Karger, 1999, vol 33, pp 1–8

····················

Controversies in Neuro-Oncology – Overview

R. Sauer

Department of Radiation Oncology, University of Erlangen-Nürnberg, Erlangen
(Germany)

Diagnosis and management, including surgery, radiotherapy and chemotherapy for primary and metastatic intracranial malignancies require an interdisciplinary approach and a close cooperation between representatives of the
different specialities. Only with this combined effort can treatment modalities
be optimized for the benefit of our patients. An autistic attitude of the physician
as a kind of overestimation of his or her abilities is completely inadequate in
this situation. This present book highlights some of the issues which require
most urgently innovation and cooperation. We owe our gratitude to Prof. Dr.
W. Hinkelbein, who prepared this edition. A summary and comment on the
main conclusions of the articles of the book is given below.

Technical Innovations in Neuro-Oncology

Presently positron emission tomography (PET) using the glucose analogue
2-^{18}F-fluorodeoxyglucose (FDG), is becoming available on a wider clinical
scale. It is helpful for tumor grading, prediction of prognosis and diagnosis
of tumor recurrence. The domain of amino acids appears to be the definition
of tumor extent, the evaluation of tumor recurrence and response to therapy.
Amino acids are not yet available for routine diagnostics, but ^{18}F-labeled amino
acids for PET may be introduced in the near future. Amino acid imaging of
brain tumors at slightly lower spatial resolution, however, can already be
performed with amino acid analogue L-3 (^{123}I)iodo-α-methyltyrosine (IMT).
Recently it was shown that the results of IMT SPECT are similar to those of
MET PET (Langen et al.). The combination of cerebral activation studies

with the superior imaging of tumor extent by amino acids is a promising new approach to improve treatment planning of brain tumors (Feldmann et al.).

For planning neurosurgical procedures, a precise localization of the sensorimotor strip as well as of eloquent brain areas is of outmost importance. Motor functional magnetic resonance imaging (fMRI) and echo planar imaging (EPI) allow to locate precisely the rolandic fissure in patients harboring astrocytomas in or around the motor strip (Conesa et al.). Also, intraoperative mapping is a reliable and proven tool to identify cognitive functions such as language and speech intraoperatively (Eisner et al.). Ebmeier and co-workers established a preoperative MEG mapping for the same intention. Hoell et al. introduced a MRI technique to obtain a high level 3D navigation for surgery as well as for radiation planning.

During recent years the development of commercially available add-on devices for medical linear accelerators have offered new possibilities for Linac-based stereotactic radiosurgery and conformal radiotherapy of small intracranial targets. Two working groups, one from Vienna (Georg et al.) and the other from Berlin (Wurm et al.), have tested the m3 computer-controlled micro-MLC (m3), a joint development project of Brain LAB GmbH, Germany, and Varian Inc., USA, and found that the target volume could be accurately irradiated to the precision demanded by radiosurgery applications. Significant normal tissues sparing in the region treated to more than 50% of the prescribed dose can be achieved.

On the other hand, the introduction of the boron neutron capture treatment protocol by the EORTC BNCT study group (Pignol et al.) and the intraoperative radiotherapy protocol by Rübe et al. concern a more experimental field for treating malignant gliomas which are not completely removable.

Craniopharyngioma

A retrospective review of the files of 46 children and adolescents operated in three institutions during a 23-year period was performed by Rilliet et al. They found that transsphenoidal surgery enables a unique radical surgical approach with an excellent visual outcome and a small percentage of complications due to a less aggressive surgery. Long-term outcome with no mortality and morbidity and excellent quality of life compares very favorably with the primary intracranial approach. Therefore, the group of patients who may benefit from transsphenoidal surgery should be identified and selected.

Becker and co-workers pointed out the role of radiotherapy in managing craniopharyngiomas. They compared the controversial therapeutic strategies for craniopharyngioma in respect to recurrence rate, survival, salvageability if recurrence does occur, side effects and quality of life after therapy in an outstanding review of the present literature. The authors conclude that radiotherapy combined with a limited surgical procedure minimizes the potential morbidity (10%) and the recurrence rate to 21%, improves the survival (10 years 77%, 20 years 66%), whereas the acute complications are moderate with 14%, mostly due to cystic enlargement of the tumor. The quality of life after limited surgery and radiotherapy is good in more than 80% and poor in only 11% of the patients. These results led to the recommendation to prefer radical surgery in young children (e.g. <5 years of age), small tumors and favorable localization. Limited surgery followed by irradiation is indicated in older children, large tumors and tumors in a critical location.

Glioblastoma – Clinical Treatment Strategies

Wiestler and co-workers discuss new developments and controversies in the neuropathology of malignant gliomas in an excellent overview. They debate the major areas of pitfalls and deficits in the surgical neuropathology: (1) the issue of grading and assessment of the risk for malignant progression in individual patients; (2) significant interindividual variations in the clinical course of histopathological entities, and (3) the reliable identification of chemotherapy-responsive gliomas. The authors point out that the application of molecular tools promises advances in all three areas, especially for the classification and grading of gliomas.

Four clinical groups report current approaches to radiation therapy for malignant gliomas (Brada, Nieder et al., Papsdorf et al., Schleicher et al.). They conclude that despite the fact that radiotherapy is an effective treatment modality, there has been no real progress either in terms of reduction in treatment toxicity or improvement in survival. There is a plethora of positive and encouraging phase II trials which have all to date failed to yield positive phase III trials, which must remain the gold standard in assessing new forms of therapy. And concerning the role of chemotherapy in adult malignant glioma, van den Brent comes to the conclusion that until better agents become available, the present increase in survival with adjuvant chemotherapy in newly diagnosed gliomas is of only minor clinical significance. In the same context, Grabenbauer and colleagues report first promising results in a phase II trial by Topotecan as a 21-day continuous infusion with accelerated 3D-conformal radiotherapy. Also Mühling et al. found that in case of repeated surgery of glioblastoma, the patients had the longest survival if they underwent a combination of radiotherapy and BCNU following the first operation compared with either radiotherapy or BCNU alone.

Glioblastoma: New Perspectives and Experimental Therapy

The concept of locoregional application has been undertaken in the context of intravascular, intracavitary and interstitial application of effective agents of which there are only few with nitrosoureas and platinum compounds as most widely used substances. In 1997/98, Westphal and Giese started a study with intracavitary application of drugs which are encapsulated in slow-release biodegradable polymers beginning with carmustine BCNU (Gliadel®) in patients with recurrent malignant glioma. There was an efficacy shown as measured as 6 months' survival of 56% in the treatment group compared to 36% in the placebo group. A very attractive concept which has been introduced into the treatment of gliomas and is also based on the attempt of local control is gene therapy. Virus and nonvirus vectors can be effectively targeted to experimental brain tumors (Rainov et al.). Maybe this is the beginning of a long-term anti-invasive concept. Weber et al. evaluated MRI characteristics and histological changes in glioblastoma after intracerebral injection of vector producer cells (VPC). They found that this administration of VPC is a safe procedure.

In the present situation with rather poor systemic options, local control appears the most important treatment assignment in high-grade gliomas. Therefore, an attempt was made by the EORTC (22972) and the MRC (BR10) to improve the local control of glioma with increased dose of radiation using focal fractionated conformal stereotactic boost following conventional radiotherapy. With the modern immobilization techniques in this ongoing phase III protocol it has become possible to fractionate stereotactic radiotherapy, exploiting the potential benefit of fractionation in terms of further sparing of normal tissue (Baumert and Brada). It is estimated that only 10–20% of patients with malignant glioma will be eligible for this study that is based on the assumption of a 10% difference in a 2-year survival.

Radiation Tolerance and Re-Irradiation of the CNS

The chapter written by Kian Ang summarizes the general clinical and pathological features of iatrogenic neurotoxicity. Potential clinical applications of radiobiological concepts and experimental data, generated from radiation myelopathy models, in these settings are discussed. Although the clinical material on radiation myelopathy is limited, the dose-incidence relationship is reasonably well established in adults. A realistic estimate of the 5% complications risk for 2-Gy fractions is between 57 and 61 Gy. This dose-response relationship, based on clinical data, is now reasonably well established from rhesus monkey data along with relatively large series of reported human myelopathy cases. The radiation doses inducing 50 and 1% incidence of myelopathy in rhesus monkeys are 76.1 ± 1.9 and 59.1 ± 5.5 Gy, respectively, delivered in ~ 2-Gy fractions. Based on the dose-response data, it is sensible to deliver a dose of 50 Gy in 25 fractions to the spinal cord in an otherwise healthy patient when necessary for better coverage of tumor since it has an extremely low risk of inducing myelopathy. In addition, the importance of intervals between fractions has recently drawn much interest because of the occurrence of an unexpectedly high incidence of radiation myelopathy associated with the use of accelerated radiation regimen, referred to as CHART, delivering 3 irradiations per day. The time between fractions was kept at a minimum of 6 h based on the initial results of a rodent study showing a half-time ($T_{1/2}$) of repair of ~ 1.5 h. A subsequent experimental study on repair kinetics in adult rat spinal cord showed that cellular repair of sublethal lesions proceeds at a slower than anticipated rate. It was found that a biexponential model fits the data better than a monoexponential model. Analysis with a biexponential model revealed a $T_{1/2}$ of 0.7 h for the faster component and $T_{1/2}$ of 3.8 h for the slower component. The higher than expected incidence of myelopathy after 3 fractions a day can at least partly be attributed to compounding incomplete repair between fractions. Therefore, it is prudent to allow at least 6 h, preferably 8 h, interfraction interval to minimize the risk for neurotoxicity. More recently, larger animal models were undertaken to evaluate the relationship between commonly used clinical radiation volume and spinal cord tolerance. It was found that an increase in the treatment volume reduces the threshold level and steepens the slope of the sigmoid dose-response curve for myelopathy. The influence of volume on the tolerance dose is less pronounced at low incidence level than at high incidence level.

As the length of survival of cancer patients increases, radiation oncologists are more frequently faced with the problem of treatment of second tumors situated within or close to a previously treated site or occasionally late recurrences. Limited clinical experiences on retreatment of recurrent brain tumors and nasopharyngeal cancers suggests the existence of long-term recovery in the CNS. Unfortunately, until recently data on tolerance of previously irradiated spinal cord to reirradiation have not been available. A study on neonatal guinea pigs showed that as the interval increased, higher doses were needed to induce the same effect. The magnitude of the dose increment also depended on the size of the dose given in the first radiation course. Studies in rats also provided convincing evidence that the spinal cord has a large capacity to recover occult radiation injury. The data obtained with rhesus monkeys indicate that about 75% of occult injury induced by the initial 44 Gy is recovered within 2 years. Further studies are underway.

Niewald et al. investigated radiomyelopathy after conventionally fractionated and hyperfractionated radiotherapy. 276 healthy female Wistar rats were included in the animal experiments. These resulted in the significant probability that by using hyperfractionation, a 28% higher dose (at the 50% level of damage) or a 39% higher dose (at the 5% level of damage) could be applied compared to using conventional fractionation. The α/β value was 1.54 Gy at the 50% level of damage and 0.17 Gy at the 5% level of damage. The authors conclude that based on own clinical experience, a total dose of 50 Gy in daily single doses of 2.0 or 64.8 Gy in twice-daily single doses of 1.2 Gy seems to be safely applicable in human cervical spinal cord.

Debus et al. analyzed the volume of the brainstem at certain dose levels with protons and high-energy X-rays. The conclusion was that tolerance to fractionated radiotherapy appears to depend not only on maximum doses of the brainstem but is also a function of brainstem volume included in high-dose regions. Rauhut et al. also found that in patients with pituitary adenomas the risk of encephalopathy was associated with the irradiated brain volume.

Focal brain necrosis has rarely been observed at radiation doses < 60 Gy for conventionally fractionated external beam irradiation given as a single modality treatment. A threshold of 57.6 Gy has been reported for daily irradiation with fraction sizes < 2 Gy. The incidence is highly dependent upon fraction size. Hopewell and van der Kogel presented results indicating that there is both direct and indirect evidence that the vasculature is a primary target, damage to which results in a cascade of changes leading to the development of white matter necrosis. This cascade does involve an interaction with parenchymal elements. The indirect evidence for vasculature involvement is also encouraging since it suggests that intervention after irradiation can influence the incidence of early delayed lesions. Since it seems reasonable to suggest that this indifference in the tissue's response to injury may be normal tissue-specific, it offers a possible opportunity for a safe escalation of the radiation dose with the potential for an improvement in the therapeutic ratio for radiotherapy treatment.

Winkler et al. presented clinical results which confirm the expectance of Kian Ang that reirradiation of recurrent brain tumors after primary curative radiotherapy is feasible; 30–70 Gy were given in 5 fractions of 1.5, 1.8 or 2.0 Gy/week. Alheit et al. from the same department investigated the effects of high dose radiotherapy to tumors of the pituitary on the optic chiasm. Their long-term observations after radiation therapy of pituitary tumors with unusual high doses between 60 and 80 Gy are not in contrast to the results reported by others, indicating the TD5/5 of the optic chiasm is higher than 50 Gy at 2-Gy fractions. Considering the grave consequences of radiation-induced damage to the chiasm, it is needless to say that in most clinical situations 'safe doses' well below the TD5/5 would be chosen.

Treatment of Brain Metastases

Five papers concern the treatment of brain metastases. Over the last two decades the number of patients with diagnosed brain metastases has increased clearly. Responsible for the increased frequency are, among others, improved radiological imaging, effective therapeutical control of primary cancer with the prolongation in median survival time as well as changes in the age pyramid resulting in increasing affection to tumor disease (Engenhart-Cabillic). Patients undergoing surgery and radiotherapy have significantly fewer recurrences at the initial metastatic sight compared to those receiving radiotherapy alone. They also have significantly increased survival and improved quality of life. The biological and physical characteristics of metastases, the lack of invasion, <3 cm in diameter and spherical, appear to make them ideal radiosurgery targets. Stereotactic radiosurgery (SRS) is now an established treatment modality for solitary brain metastases. In general, SRS is not recommended as first-line treatment of multiple brain metastases, but may represent a reasonable option for recurrent metastases. Potential advantages of SRS over surgery are reduced morbidity and reduced health-care costs. Without compromising survival and local control it is reasonable to postulate that SRS may be able to replace neurosurgical resection as the treatment of choice in most patients with solitary brain metastases.

In order to approximate answers to questions regarding criteria of optimal individualized treatment strategies in brain metastases, Meyer et al. started a prospective study with patients eligible for radical microsurgical resection. They conclude that only a randomized prospective multicenter trial, comparing microsurgery and radiosurgery, will definitively solve the problems and will most likely show that both forms of treatment are complementary and not exclusive.

Höcht et al. deal with their experiences with irradiation for recurrent brain metastases. In properly selected patients, reirradiation of brain metastases with whole-brain irradiation is a valuable therapeutic strategy, and when given with single doses of 1.8–2.0 Gy and a total dose of 20–25 Gy, the beneficial effect outweighs potential future hazards in the form of late complications by far.

The use of systemic chemotherapy for treatment of brain metastases is limited by the inability of most chemotherapeutic agents to cross the intact blood-brain barrier (Korfel and Thiel). But, the major advantage of chemotherapy in the treatment of brain metastases is the simultaneous therapy of extracranial disease. Thus, chemotherapy can be considered a treatment option in patients with brain metastases of chemosensitive tumors and advanced systemic disease. It can be optimized by knowledge of a drug's kinetics. Although the results of the few clinical studies performed so far are encouraging, the role of chemotherapy in the treatment of brain metastases has still to be proven in prospective randomized trials. The efficacy of Topotecan in lung cancer and its ability to pass the blood-brain barrier suggests that it is particularly interesting for first-line protocols. 93% response rates in first-line SCLC patients were reported. Topotecan may be the drug of choice in induction regimens because it may also prevent brain metastases seen in patients with SCLC under effective chemotherapy. In addition, the radiosensitizing effect of Topotecan may be a drive to combine this drug with radiation therapy.

Thiel, Korfel and Hinkelbein introduced a new randomized multicentric study for primary CNS lymphoma (PCNSL). Whole-brain radiotherapy has been the standard treatment for PCNSL in the last 20 years. The result was an increase in survival from 3 to 4 months without any treatment to 12–16 months with whole-brain irradiation. The 92% local failure rate shows the limit of radiation alone for treatment of PCNSL. After the combined treatment of whole-brain irradiation with chemotherapeutic drugs, the survival of patients increased. But the incidence of leukoencephalopathy in long-term survivors was estimated to be 26–37%. The aim of the proposed multicenter trial is to compare the median survival and the late neurotoxicity after chemotherapy alone versus chemotherapy with subsequent whole-brain irradiation. The protocol is based exclusively on brain-blood barrier-penetrating drugs. All complete responders should be randomized into subsequent whole-brain irradiation with 45 Gy or an additional course of the effective chemotherapy regimen.

In summary, the new addition in hand gives an excellent survey of technical innovations, the clinical treatment strategies, new perspectives and experimental therapy in neuro-oncology. It is recommended for all physicians involved in neuropathology, neurosurgery, radio-oncology and chemotherapy of primary and secondary brain tumors.

Prof. Dr. Rolf Sauer, Klinik für Strahlentherapie,
Universitätsstrasse 27, D–91054 Erlangen (Germany)
Tel. +49 9131 8533 405, Fax +49 9131 8539 335

Wiegel T, Hinkelbein W, Brock M, Hoell T (eds): Controversies in Neuro-Oncology.
Front Radiat Ther Oncol. Basel, Karger, 1999, vol 33, pp 9–22

....

Recent Advances of PET in the Diagnosis of Brain Tumors

Karl-Josef Langen, Matthias Weckesser

Institute of Medicine, Research Center Jülich, Germany

Introduction

Positron emission tomography (PET) has been available for nearly two decades but it is only recently that it has been introduced on a wider clinical scale. Advantages of PET are the high spatial resolution in relation to conventional nuclear medicine techniques and the physiological positron-emitting radionuclides which can readily be incorporated into metabolically important substrates, physiologically important compounds or therapeutic agents. Furthermore, PET offers the possibilty to quantify tracer concentration and kinetics in organs and thus to apply physiological models in order to calculate physiological reactions. This potential has attracted the attention of nearly all clinical specialities and the number of scientific publications using PET is enormous. A major problem of the method, however, are the high costs. The majority of interesting radiopharmaceuticals for PET can only be labeled with the short-lived positron emitter ^{11}C (20 min half-life) which is restricted to centers with an on-site cyclotron unit and a laboratory for nuclear chemistry. These necessities make the technique extremely expensive. Nevertherless, two important developments have induced a spread out of the method into clinical routine within the last years: (1) the development of an effective radiosynthesis of ^{18}F-fluorodeoxyglucose (FDG, ^{18}F = 2 h half-life) which can now be delivered in large amounts to any nuclear medicine department and the outstanding results of FDG-PET for the detection of unknown neoplastic lesions, recurrences and metastases in peripheral tumors [for reviews, see 1, 2]. Therefore, PET is becoming more and more clinically available.

Neurooncology is a clinical field which may particularly profit from this development. Cranial computer-assisted tomography (CT) and magnetic resonance imaging (MRI) are unsurpassed diagnostic modalities for the detection of cerebral space-occupying lesions. Their spatial resolution in the range of 1–2 mm is clearly superior to that of PET which ranges from 4 to 8 mm depending of the scanner type and scanning protocol. Nevertheless, using CT and MRI the differentiation of tumor tissue from edematous, necrotic and fibromatous tissue is sometimes not optimal and PET with its capacity to investigate biochemical and physiological parameters adds relevant information to improve tumor diagnosis.

In order to optimize patients' management a number of questions have to be answered where MRI and CT are still unsatisfactory. After detection of a brain tumor, information on grade of malignancy is essential to determine the aggressiveness of therapeutic intervention. A method to target biopsies is advantageous since tumors may be histologically heterogeneous and may have necrotic parts. Another challenge is the visualization of the degree of intracerbral infiltration by gliomas which is insufficient with MRI or CT scanning. In the follow-up of treated patients, a differentiation of scarring and tumor recurrence may provide difficulties. Moreover it is difficult to predict the reponse of an individual tumor to radiation therapy or chemotherapy and methods are needed to decide at an early stage whether the tumor is responding to therapy or not. Since these therapies may induce tumor swelling even in case of a good response, morphological imaging may fail at an early stage to predict outcome of the therapy. Beside the definition of the tumor itself, it is important to define the relationship of cortical function in the area surrounding the tumor correctly. Especially in tumors in the proximity of the motor or language area, operation-induced damage may lead to major handicaps and may reduce quality of life considerably. The known distribution of normal brain function fails to clearly predict postoperative functional deficits because of the displacement of function by tumor growth.

Many basic studies in brain tumors have been undertaken with PET to evaluate physiological parameters like blood flow, oxygen consumption, blood volume, metabolic parameters and uptake of chemotherapeutic drugs. In this report we will focus on recent advances of PET and on applications that might become clinically relevant in the near future.

Methods

Glucose Metabolism

The most widely applied radiopharmaceutical for the investigation of tumor metabolism is the glucose analogue FDG. Following intravenous injection, FDG initially follows the same metabolic pathway as glucose. It is carried into the cell by means of endothelial glucose transporter proteins where it is phosphorylated by hexokinase to ^{18}F-fluoroeoxyglucose-6-

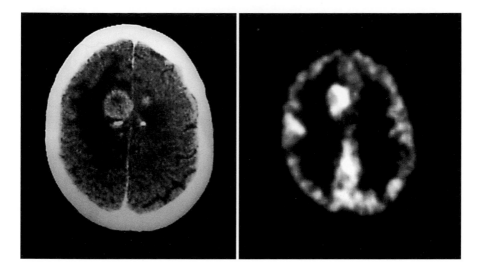

Fig. 1. High uptake of FDG in a glioblastoma which indicates a poor prognosis. On the left is shown the CT scan with contrast enhancement in the tumor.

phosphatase. Unlike glucose, there is little further metabolism and the molecule remains essentially trapped in the cell, with the rate of accumulation proportional to glucose utilization. A number of experimental studies have been undertaken in order to evaluate the mechanisms and meaning of increased FDG uptake in tumor cells [for review, see 3]. It has been found that the enhanced utilization of glucose by tumors is a consequence of upregulation of hexokinase and decreased glucose-6-phosphatase acitivity as well as changes in the expression of glucose membrane transporters, especially Glut-1. There is presently no consensus regarding which step is most important in determining the accumulation of FDG. Uptake of FDG by tumors has been related to both grade and proliferative status – generally low-grade/slowly proliferating tumors take up less FDG than poorly differentiated/rapidly growing tumors. These relationships between tumor characteristics and glucose utilization correspond to differences in hexokinase, glucose-6-phosphatase and expression of glucose membrane transporters.

A number of small studies have examined the effect of therapy-induced changes on FDG uptake [3]. Decreased uptake of FDG after chemotherapy and/or radiotherapy, compared with pretreatment, is generally considered to be an early indicator of tumor response. Although exceptions have been reported, unchanged or increased FDG uptake suggests a nonresponse. Some studies, however, have shown that the presence of inflammatory cells after therapy may result in persistent high FDG uptake despite tumor response to therapy.

The application of FDG in brain tumors is partly complicated by the high glucose metabolism of the surrounding gray matter. Unlike other organs, the brain covers energy metabolism mainly with glucose and it is the organ with the highest glucose consumption in the body. This leads to the observation that brain tumors may have a lower glucose consumption than the surrounding normal cortical tissue. Nevertheless, high-grade gliomas usually have a higher FDG accumulation than the corresponding cortex. An example of an FDG PET scan in a patient with a glioblastoma is shown in figure 1.

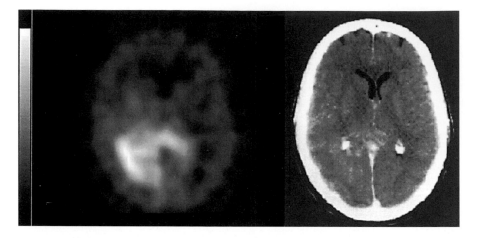

Fig. 2. PET with MET (left) and contrast enhanced CT (right) in a patient with an astrocytoma grade II. There is a large area with increased tracer uptake in the occipital lobe while CT showed no major abnormality. MRI (not shown) showed diffuse unspecific changes.

Amino Acids

A number of amino acids have been labeled with positron-emitting isotopes mainly with ^{11}C. Among these, *L*-[methyl-^{11}C]methionine (MET) is widely used for PET studies because it has high blood-brain barrier permeability and ^{11}C labeling is not too complicated. It was suggested that the significance of this tracer is its application to measuring protein synthesis rates. Experiments in mice, however, have shown that an inhibition of protein synthesis did not influence the uptake of MET in tumors and brain [4] suggesting that alterations of amino acid transport rather than increased protein synthesis may cause increased uptake in tumors. A PET study in glioma patients with *L*-[2-^{18}F]fluorotyrosine demonstrated that the difference of uptake between gliomas and normal brain was due to an increase of the rate constant of tracer transport k_1. In that study the rate constant k_3 describing binding to the metabolic compartment was not altered or even decreased in gliomas [5]. These studies indicate that changes of transport are an important factor for increased uptake of amino acids in brain tumors.

Although disturbance of the blood-brain barrier may partly account for the tumoral accumulation of MET [6], several studies indicate that MET uptake mainly occurs independent of its disruption. Concordantly, numerous clinical studies have shown the tumoral distribution of MET to be different to the pattern of contrast enhancement in CT or MRI [7, 8]. An example of a MET PET scan in a patient with an astrocytoma is shown in figure 2.

Since most amino acids have been labeled with the short-lived ^{11}C, these studies are limited to the few PET centers with an on site cyclotron facility and not available for routine clinical practice. There are attempts to label amino acids with the longer-lived ^{18}F that can be delivered to other PET centers like FDG but until today the radiosynthesis of these amino acids is rather ineffective [9, 10].

The introduction of the amino acid analogue *L*-3[^{123}I]iodo-α-methyltyrosine (IMT) which can be used with single-photon emission computed tomography (SPECT) has offered a widespread application of amino acid imaging of brain tumors [11]. Recently it was shown that the results of IMT SPECT are similar to those of MET PET [12]. Initial clinical investigations have indicated the potential of SPECT with IMT for tumor grading, diagnosis of recurrence and therapeutic response [13, 14].

The specificity of increased amino acid uptake in tumors needs further evaluation. High MET uptake in two cases of cerebral abscesses was reported [15]. Kuwert et al. [13] found that IMT uptake in abscesses was low.

Nucleic Acid Metabolism

Another approach to measure the proliferative activity of a tumor is the investigation of nucleic acid metabolism. Since neurons in the adult brain do not show proliferation this approach can be expected to be sensitive and specific for neoplastic lesions. Furthermore, this approach should be useful to evaluate the effects of therapy. The investigation of nucleic acid metabolism has not yet been applied to a large series of patients. Tjuvajev et al. [16] used ^{131}I-iododeoxyuridine to investigate 6 patients with gliomas. Uptake was compared to that of FDG and thallium and correlated to gadolinium enhancement in MRI. Specific uptake of the tracer was found only on late images and only a small proportion of the tracer was accumulated in the brain. Count rates were thus extremely low and not suitable for delineating the tumor. Vander Borght et al. [17] studied 20 patients with PET by using 2-[^{11}C]thymidine (Tdr), and the results were compared with FDG-PET data. They found that the tumor lesions were better visualized with Tdr than with FDG, the specificity of Tdr accumulation, however, remained unclear. Tracers for nucleic acid metabolism are not yet clinically established and not available on a clinical basis.

Cerebral Activation (Blood Flow)

In recent years a multitude of papers have been published on the investigation of brain function with PET. In these studies regional cerebral blood flow is measured using ^{15}O-labeled water or ^{15}O-labeled butanol during specific tasks and during reference conditions. The blood flow increases during the activation period and the brain structures involved in processing the task can be localized. In higher brain function it may be necessary to investigate a group of normals to gain statistically valid results. It is however easy to localize a certain motor function or to a lesser extent the position of language processing. In patients with gliomas adjacent to motor or speech areas, the putative benefit of resection is counterbalanced by possible postoperative deficits. Although it is possible to assess function to a certain extent by intraoperative cortical stimulation, the technique of functional mapping of brain function promises a further improvement of preoperative evaluation. An example of cerebral activation study in a patient with an astrocytoma grade II is shown in figure 3.

Clinical Application

Grading of Primary Brain Tumors and Prediction of Prognosis

Many studies have shown a relationship between FDG uptake and tumor grade and the value of this investigation for the prediction of prognosis [for review, see 18]. These results were confirmed by recent studies. Goldman et al.

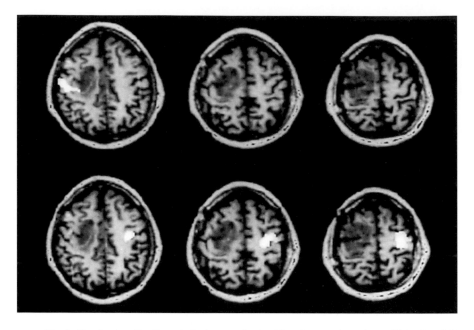

Fig. 3. Cerebral activation study in a patient with a large astrocytoma II in the right hemisphere. The rCBF increase (white areas) related to finger movements of the left symptomatic hand occurs ventrolaterally adjacent to the tumor (upper row). Activation of the left motor cortex (lower row) is loco typico [from 36].

[19] investigated 20 patients with high- and low-grade gliomas. A total of 161 biopsy samples was compared to regional glucose metabolism. They found a correlation of glucose metabolism and the presence of anaplastic cells in the sample. They concluded that regional inhomogeneity of FDG uptake is probably related to histological heterogeneity.

De Witte et al. [20] showed that increased glucose metabolism in low-grade tumor is a predictor of poor outcome. These results indicated that FDG may yield additional information on the prognosis in low-grade tumors which may be superior to histological grading based on biopsies. They concluded that patients with low-grade tumors but high glucose metabolism should be considered for a more aggressive therapeutic strategy.

Barker et al. [21] showed that the investigation of glucose metabolism is a predictor of a poor prognosis in recurrent high-grade gliomas.

The clinical experiences with amino acids for grading of gliomas and prediction of prognosis are still limited. Derlon et al. [22] reported higher MET uptake in high-grade gliomas than in low-grade gliomas, but MET uptake did not correlate to prognosis. In a series of 196 consecutive patients investigated for focal brain lesions, Herholz et al. [23] found high uptake of MET, which was independent of contrast enhancement in CT or MRI and which allowed differentiation of low-grade gliomas from nontumoral lesions in most cases. Furthermore, a difference in uptake between high-grade and low-grade gliomas was reported but the overlap of the two groups was too high to predict grading precisely in individual tumors.

Ogawa et al. [24] reported on the results of MET PET in 50 patients with cerebral gliomas. The rate of uptake of MET in high-grade glioma was significantly higher than in low-grade glioma but in individual cases it was difficult to evaluate the grade of malignancy only from the degree of MET accumulation. Also, IMT uptake tended to be higher in high-grade gliomas than in low-grade gliomas [11, 13].

Goldman et al. [25] compared regional MET and FDG uptake in high-grade gliomas to anaplasia by PET-guided stereotactic biopsy. They found that uptake of both tracers was significantly higher on the site of tumor samples showing anaplastic changes than in the rest of the tumor. Presence of necrosis in anaplastic areas of the tumor significantly reduced the uptake of MET. They concluded that anaplasia is a factor of increased uptake of both tracers, but microscopic necrosis in anaplastic areas influences their uptake differently.

Summarizing, the FDG method is presently more established and appears to have more promising results with respect to grading of brain tumors and the prediction of prognosis than the use of radiolabeled amino acids. Amino acids may be superior to FDG for the differentiation of low-grade gliomas from nontumoral lesions. The role of nucleic acids for these questions has not yet been sufficiently addressed.

Delineation of Brain Tumors

While FDG plays an important role to identify areas with increased metabolism within a brain tumor, the method is unsuited to define the extent of gliomas due to the high glucose metabolism in the surrounding brain tissue. This is also demonstrated by a double tracer autoradiographic study in a rat glioma model from our laboratory (fig 4). A number of studies have shown that amino acids are especially useful to image the true extent of cerebral gliomas. In 1983, Bergström et al. [7] investigated a patient with a cerebral glioma with PET using MET and CT. They found that the extent of the tumor in MET PET was much larger than area of contrast enhancement in the CT scan. Since this patient died a few days after these investigations, they could compare the anatomical brain slice of this patient to these studies and they found that MET exactly matched the tumor size while CT did not show the true extent of the tumor. These results were confirmed by further studies of

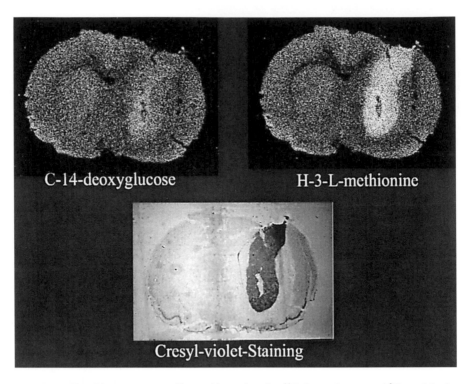

Fig. 4. Double tracer autoradiographic study using ^{14}C-deoxyglucose and ^{3}H-methionine in a rat glioma model. ^{14}C-deoxyglucose shows slightly increased uptake in the center of the tumor but only ^{3}H-methionine shows a clear delineation of the tumor versus the surrounding brain tissue compared to histopathological staining.

this group comparing MRI and CT imaging to MET PET with stereotactic serial biopsies as a reference. It was shown that MET is more reliable to image the cerebral extent of a glioma than CT and MRI [8]. These results were confirmed by recent clinical studies.

Ogawa et al. [24] examined 50 patients with cerebral gliomas with PET and MET to assess the grade of malignancy and tumor extent. MET was highly accumulated in the lesion in 31 of 32 patients with high-grade gliomas and 11 of 18 patients with low-grade gliomas. In most cases, the area of increased accumulation of MET did not correspond to the abnormalities seen at CT. Surgical intervention confirmed that MET delineated the extent of cerebral gliomas more clearly than did CT. The authors concluded that MET PET has greater utility in assessing the extent rather than the grade of malignancy of cerebral glioma.

In a recent study on 196 patients with focal brain lesions, MET PET enabled the differentiation of gliomas from nontumoral lesions in nearly all

Table 1. PET studies in neurooncology

Clinical indications
  Diagnosis of tumor recurrence in high-grade gliomas (FDG)
  Diagnosis of tumor recurrence in low-grade gliomas (MET)
  Diagnosis of tumor dedifferentiation (FDG)
  Targeting biopsies in gliomas (FDG, MET)
  Delineation of tumor extent (MET)
  Tumor grading (FDG)
  Prediction of prognosis (FDG)

Experimental state
  Prediction of therapy response (FDG, MET)
  Evaluation of peritumoral function

FDG = 2-^{18}F-fluorodeoxyglucose; MET = L-[methyl-^{11}C]methionine.

---

cases. Uptake of MET was independent from contrast enhancement in CT or MRI. Low-grade gliomas showed increased MET uptake in 28/31 cases which was useful for the location and delineation of the tumors [23].

Summarizing these results it is obvious that MET PET is a promising method to image intracerebral extent of gliomas.

Recognition of Tumor Recurrence

The clinical potential of FDG-PET for the detection of tumor recurrences has been proven by a number of studies [for review, see 18]. This application of FDG-PET appears to be one of the most useful from the clinical point of view (table 1). Recently, Barker et al. [26] investigated 55 patients in whom MRI or CT scan after surgery or radiation therapy demonstrated enlarging lesions. While morphological imaging was not able to differentiate radiation necrosis from tumor progression, FDG-PET was an independent predictor of outcome. In this study patients with high-grade gliomas were included.

Clinical studies using amino acids for the detection of tumor recurrences are still rare. Ogawa et al. [27] studied 15 patients clinically suspected to have recurrent brain tumor or radiation injury, using FDG and MET. MET clearly delineated the extent of recurrent brain tumor as focal areas of increased accumulation and was found to be useful for early detection of recurrent brain tumor. Low FDG uptake was observed in all patients with radiation injury, but was also found in 1 patient with recurrent malignant brain tumor. MET uptake was low in all patients with radiation injury. The authors recommended the combined use of MET and FDG to improve the accuracy of differentiation of recurrent brain tumor from radiation injury.

Viader et al. [28] reported on a recurrent oligodendroglioma in whom CT and MRI were normal and no means other than MET PET could demonstrate tumor recurrence and therefore lead to the correct therapeutic management.

Kuwert et al. [14] used IMT SPECT for the evaluation of 27 patients on follow-up after surgery for gliomas. They reported a sensitivity of 78% and a specificity of 100% of IMT SPECT to differentiate recurrence from nonneoplastic posttherapeutic tissue abnormalities. In summary, beside FDG-PET also amino acid studies using PET or SPECT are promising diagnostic tools for the recognition of tumor recurrence after therapy.

Prediction of Therapy Response
While for peripheral tumors there is a consensus that the early reduction of FDG uptake during radio- or chemotherapy can predict clinical outcome, the experiences on FDG-PET in the prediction of therapy response in brain tumors are still limited [29, 30]. A clear relationship of early changes in FDG uptake and therapy response could not be established. Derlon et al. [22] followed 8 patients with cerebral glioma with MET PET during intra-arterial chemotherapy but found no relationship to clinical response and survival time. Würker et al. [31] investigated the ability of FDG and MET PET to monitor effects of therapy in low-grade gliomas after the implantation of ^{125}I seeds. MET but not FDG showed a dose-dependent uptake reduction. The authors concluded that methionine is superior to investigate early effects of therapy in low-grade gliomas with the exception of tumors that do not show increased methionine uptake in the initial study.

Barker et al. [21] showed that a reduction of glucose metabolism in gliomas during therapy hints at a good response to the therapy although macrophage infiltration in the necrotic tissue may show glucose metabolism.

Ogawa et al. [32] investigated 10 patients with cerebral lymphomas with PET and MET during radiotherapy. PET clearly depicted the lymphomas before radiation therapy as an increased accumulation of MET. The extent of increased accumulation of the radiotracer in tumor tissue markedly decreased after radiation therapy. The area of increased uptake was larger than the enhancing lesions on CT or MR images in most cases. The authors concluded that MET PET is useful for the delineation of CNS lymphoma and for monitoring the therapeutic effect of irradiation.

Our experiences with IMT SPECT in the evaluation of an individualized chemotherapy in 12 patients with gliomas after in vitro testing of chemosensitivity are promising. An example of IMT SPECT in the follow-up of chemotherapy in a patient with an oligodendroglioma grade III is shown in figure 5. Patients with constant or decreasing IMT uptake showed a stable clinical

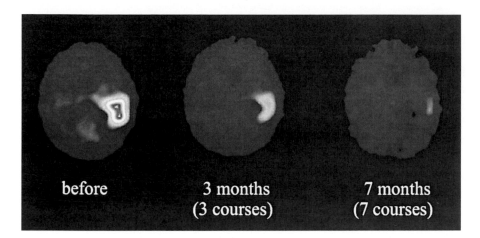

before   3 months   7 months
                    (3 courses)   (7 courses)

Fig. 5. Consecutive SPECT scans with the amino acid IMT during chemotherapy in a patient with an oligodendroglioma grade III. Reduced tracer uptake was accompanied by complete remission of the tumor.

course and later a reduction of tumor volume on MRI/CT scans while patients with increasing IMT uptake showed tumor progression.

Summarizing the limited clinical experiences, it appears that amino acid uptake in brain tumors is a more sensitive and specific parameter for the evaluation of early treatment response than FDG imaging.

Peritumoral Function

The combination of cerebral activation studies with tumor imaging is one of the latest developments using PET. Herholz et al. [33] investigated patients with brain tumors preoperatively using functional PET imaging with ^{15}O-water. Eight right-handed patients with astrocytomas in the dominant hemisphere close to language-related areas were chosen for this investigation. Significant blood flow increases during a word-generation task as compared to a control condition were delineated. As compared to intraoperative testing using cortical electric stimulation, a sensitivity of 73% and a specificity of 81% were found in the prediction of aphasic disturbance during intraoperative stimulation. The authors explain the differences between functional imaging and intraoperative stimulation by the limited resolution of functional PET imaging.

Wunderlich et al. [34] used PET and transcranial magnetic stimulation for presurgical monitoring of motor hand function in 6 patients with gliomas of the precentral gyrus. Movement-related increases of the regional cerebral blood flow occurred only outside the tumor in surrounding brain tissue. Compared with the contralateral side, these activations were shifted by 20 + 13 mm (standard deviation) within the dorsoventral dimension of the precentral gyrus. This shift of cortical hand representation could not be explained by the deformation of the central sulcus as determined from the spatially aligned magnetic resonance images but was closely related to the location of the maximal tumor growth. Dorsal tumor growth resulted in ventral displacement of motor hand representation, leaving the motor cortical output system unaffected, whereas ventral tumor growth leading to dorsal displacement of motor hand representation compromised the motor cortical output, as evident from transcranial magnetic stimulation. In 2 patients, additional activation of the supplementary motor area was present. They concluded that their PET data provided evidence for the reorganization of the human motor cortex to allow for preserved hand function in grade II astrocytomas.

Nariai et al. [35] combined the superior tumor delineation with MET and the possibility to map brain function with perfusion activation studies in 13 patients with tumors adjacent to language or motor cortex. They found the determination of functional anatomy particularly useful when the gyral anatomy was altered by tumor infiltration or tumor swelling. In a subgroup of 12 patients operated on, resection could be done without major neurological deterioration. Although it is reasonable to assume that this technique improves outcome, comparison of postoperative deficits in patients in whom functional anatomy is unknown would be needed to prove the superiority of this approach.

In summary: Presently PET using FDG is becoming available on a wider clinical scale. It is a helpful technique for tumor grading, prediction of prognosis and diagnosis of tumor recurrence. The domain of amino acids appears to be the definition of tumor extent, the evaluation of tumor recurrence and response to therapy. Amino acids are not yet available for routine diagnostics but ^{18}F-labeled amino acids for PET may be introduced in the near future. Amino acid imaging of brain tumors at slightly lower spatial resolution, however, can already be performed with amino acid analogue IMT. The results of IMT SPECT are similar to those of MET PET. The combination of cerebral activation studies with the superior imaging of tumor extent by amino acids is a promising new approach to improve treatment planning of brain tumors.

References

1   Brock CS, Meikle SR, Price P: Does fluorine-18 fluorodeoxyglucose metabolic imaging of tumours benefit oncology? Eur J Nucl Med 1997;24:691–705.
2   Conti PS, Lilien DL, Hawley K, Keppler J, Grafton ST, Bading JR: PET and [^{18}F]-FDG in oncology: A clinical update. Nucl Med Biol 1996;23:717–735.
3   Smith TA: FDG uptake, tumour characteristics and response to therapy: A review. Nucl Med Commun 1998;19:97–105.

4   Ishiwata K, Kubota K, Murakami M, Kubota R, Sasaki T, Ishii S, Senda M: Re-evaluation of amino acid PET studies: Can the protein synthesis rates in brain and tumor tissues be measured in vivo? J Nucl Med 1993;34:1936–1943.

5   Wienhard K, Herholz K, Coenen HH, Rudolf J, Kling P, Stöcklin G, Heiss WD: Increased amino acid transport into brain tumors measured by PET of L-[2-^{18}F]fluorotyrosine. J Nucl Med 1991; 32:1338–1346.

6   Bergström M, Ericson K, Hagenfeldt L, Mosskin M, von Holst H, Noren G, Eriksson L, Ehrin E, Johnstrom P: PET study of methionine accumulation in glioma and normal brain tissue: Competition with branched chain amino acids. J Comput Assist Tomogr 1987;11:208–213.

7   Bergström M, Collins VP, Ehrin E, Ericson K, Eriksson L, Greitz T, Halldin C, von Holst H, Langström B, Lilja A: Discrepancies in brain tumor extent as shown by computed tomography and positron emission tomography using [^{68}Ga]EDTA, [^{11}C]glucose, and [^{11}C]methionine. J Comput Assist Tomogr 1983;7:1062–1066.

8   Mosskin M, Ericson K, Hindmarsh T, von Holst H, Collins VP, Bergström M, Eriksson L, Johnstrom P: Positron emission tomography compared with magnetic resonance imaging and computed tomography in supratentorial gliomas using multiple stereotactic biopsies as reference. Acta Radiol 1989; 30:225–232.

9   Coenen HH, Kling P, Stöcklin G: Cerebral metabolism of L-2-^{18}F]fluorotyrosine, a new PET tracer of protein synthesis. J Nucl Med 1989;30:1367–1372.

10   Ogawa T, Miura S, Murakami M, Iida H, Hatazawa J, Inugami A, Kanno I, Yasui N, Sasajima T, Uemura K: Quantitative evaluation of neutral amino acid transport in cerebral gliomas using positron emission tomography and fluorine-18 fluorophenylalanine. Eur J Nucl Med 1996;23:889–895.

11   Langen KJ, Coenen HH, Roosen N, Kling P, Muzik O, Herzog H, Kuwert T, Stöcklin G, Feinendegen LE: SPECT studies of brain tumors with L-3-[^{123}I]iodo-α-methyltyrosine: Comparison with PET, ^{124}IMT and first clinical results. J Nucl Med 1990;31:281–286.

12   Langen KJ, Ziemons K, Kiwit JCW, Herzog H, Kuwert T, Bock WJ, Stöcklin G, Feinendegen LE, Müller-Gärtner HW: [^{123}I]-iodo-α-methyltyrosine SPECT and [^{11}C]-L-methionine uptake in cerebral gliomas: A comparative study using SPECT and PET. J Nucl Med 1997;38:517–522.

13   Kuwert T, Morgenroth C, Woesler B, Matheja P, Palkovic S, Vollet B, Samnick S, Maasjosthusmann U, Lerch H, Gildehaus FJ, Wassmann H, Schober O: Uptake of iodine-123-α-methyltyrosine by gliomas and non-neoplastic brain lesions. Eur J Nucl Med 1996;23:1345–1353.

14   Kuwert T, Woesler B, Morgenroth C, Lerch H, Schafers M, Palkovic S, Matheja P, Brandau W, Wassmann H, Schober O: Diagnosis of recurrent glioma with SPECT and iodine-123-alpha-methyltyrosine. J Nucl Med 1998;39:23–27.

15   Ishii K, Ogawa T, Hatazawa J, Kanno I, Inugami A, Fujita H, Shimosegawa E, Murakami M, Okudera T, Uemura K: High L-methyl-[^{11}C]methionine uptake in brain abscess: A PET study. J Comput Assist Tomogr 1993;17:660–661.

16   Tjuvajev J, Macapinlac H, Daghighian F, Scott A, Ginos J, Finn R, Kothari P, Desai R, Zhang J, Beattie B, Graham M, Larson St, Blasberg R: Imaging of brain tumor proliferative activity with iodine-131-iododeoxyuridine. J Nucl Med 1994;35:1407–1417.

17   Vander Borght T, Pauwels S, Lambotte L, Labar D, De Maeght S, Stroobandt G, Laterre C: Brain tumor imaging with PET and 2-[carbon-11]thymidine. J Nucl Med 1994;35:974–982.

18   Coleman RE, Hoffman JM, Hanson MW, Sostman HD, Schold SC: Clinical application of PET for the evaluation of brain tumors. J Nucl Med 1991;32:616–622.

19   Goldman S, Levivier M, Pirotte B, Brucher JM, Wikler D, Damhaut P, Stanus E, Brotchi J, Hildebrand J: Regional glucose metabolism and histopathology of gliomas. A study based on positron emission tomography-guided stereotactic biopsy. Cancer 1996;78:1098–1106.

20   De Witte O, Levivier M, Violon P, Salmon I, Damhaut P, Wikler D, Hildebrand J, Brotchi J, Goldman S: Prognostic value positron emission tomography with [^{18}F]fluoro-2-deoxy-D-glucose in the low-grade glioma. Neurosurgery 1996;39:470–476.

21   Barker FG Jr, Chang SM, Valk PE, Pounds TR, Prados MD: 18-Fluorodeoxyglucose uptake and survival of patients with suspected recurrent malignant gliomas. Cancer 1997;79:115–126.

22   Derlon JM, Bourdet C, Bustany P, Chatel M, Theron J, Darcel F, Syrota A: [^{11}C]L-methionine uptake in gliomas. Neurosurgery 1989;25:720–728.

23 Herholz K, Hölzer T, Bauer B, Schröder R, Voges J, Ernestus RI, Mendoza G, Weber-Luxemburger G, Löttgen J, Thiel A, Wienhard K, Heiss WD: ^{11}C-methionine PET for differential diagnosis of low-grade gliomas. Neurology 1998;50:1316–1322.

24 Ogawa T, Shishido F, Kanno I, Inugami A, Fujita H, Murakami M, Shimosegawa E, Ito H, Hatazawa J, Okudera T, Uemura K, Yasui N, Mineura K: Cerebral glioma: Evaluation with methionine PET. Radiology 1993;186:45–53.

25 Goldman S, Levivier M, Pirotte B, Brucher JM, Wikler D, Damhaut P, Dethy S, Brotchi J, Hildebrand J: Regional methionine and glucose uptake in high-grade gliomas: A comparative study on PET-guided stereotactic biopsy. J Nucl Med 1997;38:1459–1462.

26 Barker FG, Chang SM, Volk PE, Pounds TR, Prados MD: 18-Fluorodeoxyglucose uptake and survival of patients with suspected recurrent malignant glioma. Cancer 1997;79:115–126.

27 Ogawa T, Kanno I, Shishido F, Inugami A, Higano S, Fujita H, Murakami M, Uemura K, Yasui N, Mineura K, Kowada M: Clinical values of PET with ^{18}F-fluorodeoxyglucose and L-methyl-^{11}C-methionine for diagnosis of recurrent brain tumor and radiation injury. Acta Radiol 1991;31: 197–202.

28 Viader F, Derlon JM, Petit-Taboue MC, Shishido F, Hubert P, Houtteville JP, Courtheoux P, Chapon F: Recurrent oligodendroglioma diagnosed with ^{11}C-L-methionine and PET: A case report. Eur Neurol 1993;33:248–251.

29 Blasberg RG: Prediction of brain tumor therapy response by PET. J Neurooncol 1994;22:281–286.

30 Langen KJ, Roosen N, Kuwert T, Herzog H, Kiwit JC, Rota Kops E, Muzik O, Bock WJ, Feinendegen LE: Early effects of intra-arterial chemotherapy in patients with brain tumours studied with PET: Preliminary results. Nucl Med Common 1989;10:779–790.

31 Würker M, Herholz K, Voges J, Pietrzyk U, Treuer H, Bauer B, Sturm V, Heiss WD: Glucose consumption and methionine uptake in low-grade gliomas after iodine-125 brachytherapy. Eur J Nucl Med 1996;23:583–586.

32 Ogawa T, Kanno I, Hatazawa J, Inugami A, Fujita H, Shimosegawa E, Murakami M, Okudera T, Uemura K, Yasui N: Methionine PET for follow-up of radiation therapy of primary lymphoma of the brain. Radiographics 1994;14:101–110.

33 Herholz K, Reulen JH, von Stockhausen HM, Thiel A, Ilmberger J, Kessler J, Eisner W, Yousry T, Heiss WD: Preoperative activation and intraoperative stimulation of language-related areas in patients with glioma. Neurosurgery 1997;41:1253–1262.

34 Wunderlich G, Knorr U, Herzog H, Kiwit JC, Freund HJ, Seitz RJ: Precentral glioma location determines the displacement of cortical hand representation. Neurosurgery 1998;42:18–26.

35 Nariai T, Senda M, Ishii K, Machara T, Wakabayashi S, Toyama H, Ishiwata K, Hirakawa K: Three-dimensional imaging of cortical structure, function and glioma for tumor resection. J Nucl Med 1997;38:1563–1568.

36 Seitz RJ, Huang Y, Knorr U, Tellmann L, Herzog H, Freund HJ: Large-scale plasticity of the human motor cortex. Neuroreport 1995;6:742–744.

Karl-Josef Langen, MD, Institute of Medicine, Research Center Jülich,
PO Box 1913, D–52425 Jülich (Germany)
Tel. +49 2461 61 6347, Fax +49 2461 61 2990, E-Mail k.j.langen@fz-juelich.de

Wiegel T, Hinkelbein W, Brock M, Hoell T (eds): Controversies in Neuro-Oncology.
Front Radiat Ther Oncol. Basel, Karger, 1999, vol 33, pp 23–27

....

EPI Functional MRI: A Useful Tool for Preoperative Rolandic Fissure Localization

G. Conesa[a], *J. Pujol*[b], *J. Deus*[b], *L. López-Obarrio*[a], *A. Gabarrós*[a],
A. Marnov[a], *R. Rodriguez*[a], *R. Navarro*[a], *A. Capdevila*[b], *F. Isamat*[a]

[a] Department of Neurosurgery of the Ciutat Sanitaria I Universaria de Bellvitge and
[b] Magnetic Resonance Center of Pedralbes, University of Barcelona, Spain

A precise localization of the sensorimotor strip is of outmost importance in the management of lesions involving these areas. A distortion of the anatomy because of mass effect or difficulty in visualizing the sulci because of brain edema can sometimes be factors affecting the identification of the rolandic fissure. Functional magnetic resonance imaging (fMRI) has progressively been gaining credit in the present decade as a useful tool for visualizing brain activity in vivo. A lot of information has been gathered in recent years regarding the feasibility of this method for accurately locating sensory and motor areas in healthy volunteers. More scarce have been papers trying to evaluate applicability of the method in the clinical setting as well as its validation correlating it with intraoperative sensorimotor mappings.

After initial research in volunteers as previously reported [1], we established a protocol for motor fMRI, which was used consecutively in a series of 50 patients, all of them bearing a lesion near the central sulcus [2]. Twenty-two of these patients afterwards underwent a surgical resection in which the sensorimotor regions were defined intraoperatively by means of an electrical cortical stimulation. This group was used for validation of the fMRI study.

Afterwards we started using echo planar imaging (EPI), and also introduced subtle changes in the fMRI acquisition sequence. We report our experience with 4 new patients in whom this new EPI sequence has been experienced. In all 4 patients a validation study was done comparing intraoperative mapping for sensorimotor cortex with the fMRI findings. Pathological results in this group were 3 low-grade and 1 anaplastic astrocytoma. Two of these patients had a mild paresis of the hand. A selective area of hand motor activation was found in each case.

Patients were required to make repetitive self-paced opening and closing movements of the hand. Instructions were given to force both the flexion and extension phases of the cyclic movement at an approximate rate of 1/s. The use of a similar task previously proved to produce notable sensorimotor activation with little propagation of motion to the subject's head [1, 2].

Each patient was positioned supine in the MRI system and motion was minimized by using two standard cervical collars as head-holders. One of them was placed around the patient's neck without pressure and the forehead and fixed to the coil with a Velcro band.

An activation trial consisted of six 30-second periods in which the patients alternatively performed the specified motor task with their left or right hand (three 30-second periods per hand) without a rest condition. Patients began the trial by moving the hand corresponding to the lesion side. The order to change the active hand was given at the end of each period via the system intercom.

A 1.5-Tesla Signa system (GE Medical Systems, Milwaukee, Wisc., USA) with a multisection EPI was used. The functional sequence consisted of a spoiled Grass (TR/TE/pulse angel = 3.000/60/60) with a 96×64 pixel matrix, within a field of view of 24 cm, with a section of thickness of 5 mm and an interslice gap of 2 mm. Scan included 3 oblique-axia intersleeved slices centered at the hand level of sensorimotor cortex, selected from a t1-weighted sagittal view. Field homogeneity was adjusted in each subject at the level of the central slice. Each functional time series consisted of 60 consecutive sets of 3 images obtained in 3 min.

As in previous studies a 'cross-hand' (left vs. right) comparison was done. A pixel-by-pixel comparison using a t-statistical method was made using specific analysis softward (FuncTool; GE Medical Systems, Buc, France). We considered only activity above a statistical threshold with clusters > 13 pixels with t values > 2, or clusters > 3 pixels with a t value > 4. Besides, we only accounted an activation focus when it was both selective and reproducible. We established that an activation focus was selective when activity around the sulcus was at least twice the activation in other areas. We accounted a focus as reproducible when it activated in at least two different functional sequences. In order to minimize the exploration time, a practical online analysis was done on an auxiliary workstation connected to the main unit (SPARC Station 20; SUN Microsystems, Mountain View, Calif., USA).

For validation studies, the relative position of the tumor and the rolandic sulcus was compared intraoperatively using 3D models with a surface rendering and a craniotomy simulation (Version 1.2; GE Advantage Windows, GE Medical Systems).

Intraoperative cortical mapping during an awake craniotomy procedure was performed [3], using a commercially available constant current electrical cortical stimulator (OCS, Radionics, Burlington, Mass., USA) that produces a train of biphasic square pulses. We used a 50-Hz current with 0.3 ms single-phase duration and an increasing intensity that was started at 2 mA level, with a train duration of 3 s or stopped when a positive response was adverted. The correlation between the motor fMRI and the cortical stimulation was made using the tumor as the landmark, considering the case as validated when the relative location of the motor cortex was coincidental within the same gyrus with both methods.

In these 4 patients a selective and reproducible focal activity was found. In 2 patients a mild hand paresis was noted that did not interfere with a successful motor fMRI. Perilesional edema was not important even in the anaplastic astrocytoma patient (fig. 1). The tumor in this case was in the motor strip itself, showing clearly how an anaplastic astrocytoma can grossly invade a gyrus but still work as a fully functional area. The preoperative history in this case was of a single partial motor seizure and no deficit was found preoperatively. In all 4 patients the validation study correlated well with the findings of both methods.

Discussion

Several different methodologies with different activation tasks, different analysis methods and different fMRI protocols have been used for localization of the central sulcus. This makes analysis of the different methodologies very difficult. Furthermore, motor fMRI has been used extensively in healthy volunteers. This group tends to be very cooperative, more homogeneous and younger, and of course do not have brain edema, mass effect, abnormal vasculature or paresis that can interfere with the acquisition of the functional image.

Several groups [2, 4, 5] have already reported on the clinical application of this technique, especially in brain tumor patient. In spite of the methodology, there seem to be an agreement in all papers, pointing at the paresis as the major problem for finding a selective activation. In our previously reported experience with 50 patients, the central sulcus was considered as identified in 41 cases (82%), and the most important clinical factor in relation with a poor result was a moderate to severe paresis (no movement against resistance). All 5 patients included in that group and 2 patients with a mild paresis but a severe sensory loss were included in the failure group (78%). Other factors related to failure were older patients, lack of cooperation, excessive movement an the presence of abnormal vessels (AVM) with lack of selectivity.

The use of an EPI sequence has made the procedure faster, being the usual time spent in the hand motor fMRI of 6 min (tow sequences of 3 min).

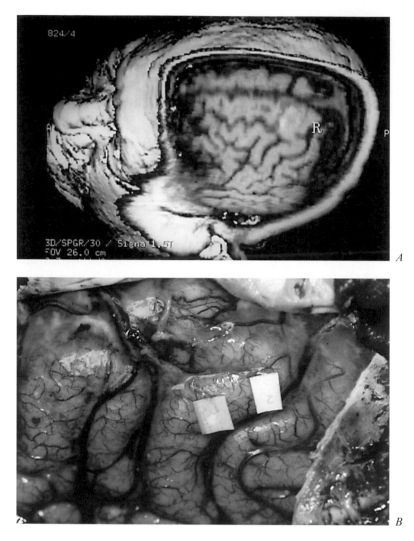

Fig. 1. A 3D reconstruction with surface rendering and craniotomy simulation of a patient with an anaplastic astrocytoma in the motor strip. *B* Intraoperative cortical mapping of the same patient.

In this preliminary experience it also seems to be more sensitive to changes in oxyhemoglobin. All 4 patients had a successful fMRI but none of them had a severe motor deficit. Also all 4 patients' fMRI results were considered as validated when comparing with the intraoperative electrical cortical stimulation. When adding this small group to the 22 previously reported validated patients, we have a 100% specificity in a total of 26 patients, when with either protocol we have considered a fMRI as successful.

We have to acknowledge our results with the EPI protocol as still very preliminary because of the few cases included. Nevertheless, the experience with similar protocols in other groups allow us to think that the degree of paresis will play a similar role as the major problem for localizing the motor strip.

Conclusions

Motor fMRI is a valuable technique for presurgical planning. The worldwide availability of MR machines allows a great many centers to perform these studies. EPI hand motor fMRI allows to precisely locate the rolandic fissure in patients harboring astrocytomas in or around the motor strip, and without or with moderate motor deficit. Further experience with this protocol will allow us to compare both fMRI methodologies.

Acknowledgment

This study was supported in part by grant No. 98/0289 from the Fondo de Investigaciones Sanitarias (FIS).

References

1   Pujol J, Conesa G, Deus J, et al: Presurgical identification of the sensorimotor cortex by functional magnetic resonance imaging. J Neurosurg 1996;84:7–13.
2   Pujol J, Conesa G, Deus J, et al: Clinical application of functional magnetic resonance imaging in presurgical identification of the central sulcus. J Neurosurg 1998;88:863–869.
3   Berger MS, Ojemann GA: Techniques of functional localization during removal of tumours involving the cerebral hemispheres; in Loftus CM, Traynelis VC (eds): Intraoperative Monitoring Techniques in Neurosurgery. New York, McGraw-Hill, 1994, pp 113–127.
4   Atlas SW, Howard RS II, Maldjian J, et al: Functional magnetic resonance imaging of regional brain activity in patients with intracerebral gliomas: Findings and implications for clinical management. Neurosurgery 1996;38:329–338.
5   Yousry TA, Schmid UD, Jassoy AJ, et al: The central sulcal vein: A landmark for identification of the central sulcus using functional magnetic resonance imaging. J Neurosurg 1996;85:608–617.

G. Conesa, Neurogroup, Clinica Sagrada Familia, Neurocirurgía,
Torras y Pujalt, 1, E–08022 Barcelona (Spain)

Wiegel T, Hinkelbein W, Brock M, Hoell T (eds): Controversies in Neuro-Oncology.
Front Radiat Ther Oncol. Basel, Karger, 1999, vol 33, pp 28–36

....

Intraoperative Mapping of Eloquent Brain Areas

W. Eisner [a], *H.-J. Reulen* [a], *J. Ilmberger* [b], *U. Swozil* [c], *K. Bise* [d]

[a] Neurosurgical Department and Departments of [b] Physical Medicine,
[c] Neuroanesthesia and [d] Neuropathology, Ludwig Maximilians University Munich,
  Klinikum Grosshadern, Germany

Introduction

Mapping of cortical functions by electrical stimulation has been possible for more than 125 years. During cortical stimulation contractions of muscle groups of the contralateral extremity can be observed or tingling paresthesia may be evoked in awake patients. Stimulation at other cortical areas remains without visible or sensory effect. Penfield and Roberts [1959] were able to disturb higher cognitive functions such as language, speech or short-time memory by electrical stimulation. Patients had to execute special tasks like picture naming. If simultaneously the brain is stimulated electrically, resulting disorders can be observed in cortical language areas. The disorder is transient and function recovers immediately if the stimulation period is not followed by epileptic afterdischarge. Ojemann and Whitaker [1978] and few others have been using the technique of cortical mapping to avoid postoperative language deficits in epilepsy surgery. The studies of Ojemann and co-workers revealed that the cortical language/speech areas are smaller than estimated. They consist of mosaic-like structures with individual sites having an average size of 1–2 cm². A high interindividual variability regarding cortical distribution of higher cognitive functions such as language or short-time memory were found. We adapted Ojemann's technique of intraoperative language monitoring to tumor surgery. Until the end of the 1980s tumor surgery in or next to cortical language areas contained a high risk of postoperative deficits. Three possible strategies were used. The first strategy was not to operate and 'wait and see'. The second strategy was to take a biopsy or to stay within the tumor borders to gain histopathology, followed by radiation therapy. The third strategy was to try to remove the tumor radically.

The last strategy contained a high risk of postoperative deficit for the patient. We wanted to minimize this risk by improving surgical strategies and results as well as life quality in our tumor patients.

Patients and Methods

From 1991 to 1997 we treated 80 patients with space-occupying lesions in the language-dominant hemisphere using a prospective protocol. Preoperatively all patients were evaluated neuroradiologically with MRI. Standardized T1- and T2-weighted imaging was performed, T1 without and with contrast amplification. Postoperatively the same sequences were used within 32 h after surgery. The handedness of the patients gives a rough estimate of the language dominance. Handedness was examined by Oldfield's questionnaire [1971]. If the score indicated bimanual or left handedness, a Wada test was performed [Wada and Rasmussen, 1960]. Pre- and postoperatively the patients were tested neuropsychologically with a German aphasia battery [Huber et al., 1983] and a German version of the Californian Verbal Learning and Memory Test. As paradigm for intraoperative language monitoring, we chose a picture-naming task, as Benson [1988] was able to show that all aphasic syndromes correlate with naming disturbances. Huber et al. [1989] could demonstrate that counting and recalling the days of the week is often not disturbed in patients with aphasia and thus is not suitable for intraoperative testing. 50 concrete drawings of objects including a carrier phrase like 'this is a ...' were developed. The patient always had to read the carrier phrase and to name the object shown (e.g. 'This is a ... bird'). The material was also shown to the patient preoperatively; only material that could preoperatively be named 100% correct was used. The patient was informed extensively on awake surgery and intraoperative monitoring. In the surgical theater the patient's head and shoulders were comfortably positioned on a vacuum pillow molded around the head and shoulders and topped by cotton. The skull was partly shaved. The skin incision and the tumor were drawn on the patient's skin. Local infiltration anesthesia was performed by Bupivacain hydrochloride 0.25% combined with Ornipressin, the strongest physiological vasoconstrictor. For sedation analgesia, Alfentanil hydrochloride and Disoprivan, later Remifentanil hydrochloride and Disoprivan, were used. The sedation analgesia allowed us to keep the patient in a precise state of consciousness. After opening the skull, the dura was anesthetized by local anesthesia given on a cotton layer before opening. Before intraoperative mapping was performed, the patient had to name pictures in order to identify the intraoperative baseline condition. All stimulation sites were marked by sterile numbers, their location was documented in a drawing and slide (fig. 1).

The time course of intraoperative language and speech monitoring was as follows: The stimulation period is 4 s. During that time the cortex is stimulated electrically and the patient is shown the drawing of an object as described above, which has to be named within the 4 s. Picture-naming without cortical stimulation is performed after a language or speech error in order to clinically detect epileptic afterdischarge. All stimulation sites are stimulated consecutively with the same intensity followed by a second or third course with the same or another intensity. Electrical cortical stimulation is performed bipolar using an isolated coagulation forceps. Bipolar stimulation defines the stimulation area between the two tips of the coagulation forceps in contrast to monopolar stimulation, which has a stimulation area circularly around the stimulation instrument. The distance between the two tips of the

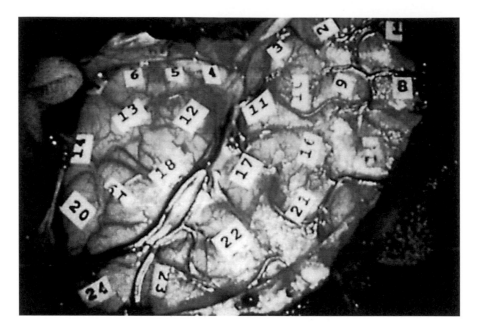

Fig. 1. Intraoperative stimulation site.

forceps is about 5 mm. We use a square wave impulse with a 0.2-ms duration and 50 stimuli/s. The stimulation intensity ranges from 7 to 35 mA; mostly 7 to 15 mA are used. For electrophysiological detection of epileptic afterdischarge we use a direct cortical EEG recording performed by a 6-channel array electrode. As stimulation device we use a Nicolet Viking II. Our stimulation setup is fully digitized, which means that the stimulating machine and the displayed pictures on an LCD display are triggered by a personal computer. All the proceedings and the patient's utterances are registered by DAT recordings and by handwritten protocol. Before and after tumor resection, a photograph is taken and a video of the operation procedure is recorded. Typical disorders of language and speech may be described as follows: an aphasic arrest describes a situation where the carrier phrase is produced correctly but the object name is missing. Aphasic disturbance means a correctly given carrier phrase followed by wrong object naming. Often semantic paraphasias are observed. Aphasic arrest and aphasic disturbances thus are naming disturbances and therefore disturbances of language function. A dysarthric or an unrecognizable utterance is called speech disturbance. A completely missing utterance is classified as speech arrest. Speech disturbance and speech arrest are based on a disturbance or inhibition of the articulating organs. In case of a speech arrest we tell the patient to move his tongue to the left and right side outside the mouth while we stimulate the cortex. Very often the movement is stopped in this condition. Stimulation sites where aphasic arrest or aphasic disturbances could be evoked are therefore called language sites and stimulation sites with speech arrest or speech disturbance are called speech sites (fig. 2).

In the last 6 years we have operated on 80 patients, 37 male and 43 women, with an average age of 38 ± 9.8 years. The youngest patient was 17 years and the oldest patient was

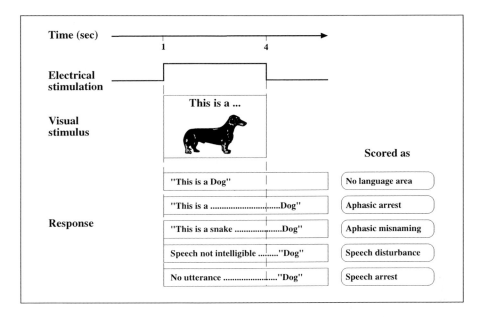

Fig. 2. Scheme of intraoperative stimulation and examples of neuropsychological findings.

60 years. The initial symptoms were seizures in 64 patients (80%), very often followed by a postictal dysphasia. Eleven patients (14%) showed an isolated aphasic disturbance. In 5 patients a slowly progressing hemiparesis led to a neurological examination.

Results

In 56 patients (70%) a gross total tumor resection could be achieved. In 34 patients (30%) a subtotal tumor resection was performed. In most cases the neuropathologist was directly assisting surgery. Smear preparation as neuropathological examination guided us through the tumor borders or tumor resection near to positive stimulation sites. There we performed resection under permanent functional control. The patient had to name pictures or to move extremities throughout resection next to functional areas. Seven patients had a cavernous malformation (8.8%), 1 a tumor-like lesion (1.3%), 1 an ictogenous scar (1.3%), 1 a gliosarcoma (1.3%), 45 astrocytoma WHO grade II (56.3%), 7 oligodendrogliomas WHO grade II (8.8%), 16 astrocytomas WHO grade III (18.8%), and 2 astrocytomas WHO grade IV (2.6%). The locations of the space-occupying lesions in the left cerebral hemisphere were 27 times fronto-precentral, 2 central, 35 temporal, 11 temporo-parietal and 5 times temporo-occipital. In 5 patients we had a surgical complication, no patient died. In 2 patients (2.5%) we discovered as reason for a postoperative deterioration of the neurological and neuropsychological examination a rebleeding in the resection cavity, 1 patient required reoperation. One patient (1.3%) suffered from a bleeding because of venous stasis due to closure of a dominant Labbé vein, and hence required surgery. Another patient showed an arterial opercular infarction (1.3%). One patient postoperatively developed a meningitis (1.3%). No wound healing disturbances or lethal complication occurred. Comparing the preoperative to the postoperative neuropsychological examination, we had an increase of language disturbances from 7 to 10%. Disorders of speech function decreased from 12 to 10%. Preoperatively 6% of the patients had a hemiparesis. Postoperatively in 10% of the patients a deterioration of motor function was present. When examined 6 months after surgery, all patients were able to work. Of the 8 patients with persisting aphasia, 4 showed a slight disturbance and another 4 medium disturbance of language functions. In 12% of our patients we discovered function within the tumor borders. As resection margin to functional cortical areas we found in a distance of more than 1.5 cm no higher incidence of postoperative deficits. Resections closer than 1.5 cm showed a 45% risk of postoperative deficits for the first 12 days after surgery. If one language site was resected, in 66% of the cases postoperative deficits were seen during the first 12 days after surgery. It has to be mentioned that all patients had multiple positive language sites. As a result of our intraoperative language and speech mapping we found cortical language and speech representations to be distributed beyond Wernicke and Broca areas. Sites were distributed in a mosaic-like fashion. The size of a single positive stimulation site was 1–2 cm^2. 50% of positive stimulation sites were separated by non-language functional cortical areas. We could identify language function in all three temporal gyri and in all three frontal gyri.

Conclusions

Our method is a reliable and proven tool to intraoperatively identify higher cognitive functions such as language and speech. It enables the surgeon to recognize the individual distribution of cortical functions despite the loss of anatomical landmarks caused by the space-occupying effect of the tumor. Even in critical moments of surgery next to cortical functional areas, the intraoperative stimulation gives clear information on the particular anatomical structure. In comparison to noninvasive methods such as PET or fMRI, our method identifies the absolutely essential cortical areas. We could prove that it is possible to resect tumors in or next to cortical language functional areas without higher risk of postoperative deficits.

References and Suggested Reading

Ammirati M, Galicich JH, Arbit E, Liao Y: Reoperations in the treatment of recurrent intracranial malignant gliomas. Neurosurgery 1987;21:607–614.

Ammirati M, Vick N, Liao Y, Ciric I, Mikhael M: Effect of the extent of surgical resection on survival and quality of life in patients with supratentorial glioblastomas and anaplastic astrocytomas. Neurosurgery 1987;21:201–216.

Archibald YM, Wepman JM, Jones LV: Nonverbal cognitive performance in aphasic and nonaphasic brain-damaged patients. Cortex 1967;3:275–294.

Bartholow R: Experimental investigations into functions of the human brain. Am J Med Sci 1874;67: 305–313.

Basso A, Faglioni P, Spinnler H: Non-verbal colour impairment of aphasics. Neuropsychologia 1976;14: 183–193.

Benke T, Andree B, Wagner M, Schelowsky L: Sprache bei linkshirnigen Tumoren: Ein prä- und postoperativer Vergleich. 19. Jahrestagung der Aphasieforschung und -Behandlung, Wien, 5–7. November 1992.

Benson DF: Classical syndromes of aphasia; in Boller F, Grafmann J (eds): Handbook of Neuropsychology. Amsterdam, Elsevier, 1988, vol 1.

Berger MS, Ghatan S, Haglund MM, Dobbins J, Ojemann GA: Low-grade gliomas associated with intractable epilepsy: Seizure outcome utilizing electrocorticography during tumor resection. J Neurosurg 1993;79:62–69.

Berger MS, Ojemann GA: Cortical mapping techniques used to maximise tumor resection and safety in children with brain tumors. Ann Neurol 1988;24:361.

Berger MS, Ojemann GA, Lettich E: Brain mapping techniques to maximize resection, safety, and seizure control in children with brain tumors. Neurosurgery 1989;25:786–792.

Berger MS, Ojemann GA, Lettich E: Neurophysiological monitoring during astrocytoma surgery. Neurosurg Clin North Am 1990;1:65–80.

Black P, Ronner SF: Cortical mapping for defining the limits of tumor resection. Neurosurgery 1987;20: 914–919.

Bogen J, Bogen G: Wernicke's region – Where is it? Ann NY Acad Sci 1975;280:834–843.

Böcher W: Erfahrungen mit dem Wechslerschen Gedächtnistest (Wechsler Memory Scale) bei einer deutschen Versuchsgruppe von 200 normalen Versuchspersonen. Diagnostica 1963;9:56–68.

Broca P: Remarques sur le siège de la faculté du language articulé, survie d'une observation d'aphémie (perte de la parole). Bull Soc Anat Paris 1861;36:330–357.

Burchiel KJ, Clark H, Ojemann G: Use of stimulation mapping and corticography in the excision of arteriovenous malformations in sensorimotor and language-related neocortex. Neurosurgery 1989; 24:323–327.

Cawthon D, Lettich E, Ojemann G: Human temporal lobe neuronal activity: Inhibition during naming in only one of two languages. Soc Neurosci 1987;13:839.

Ciric I, Ammirati M, Vick N, Mikhael M: Supratentorial gliomas: Surgical considerations and immediate postoperative results. Neurosurgery 1987;21:21–26.

Cushing H: A note upon the faradic stimulation of the postcentral gyrus in conscious patients. Brain 1909;32:44–54.

Damasio A: Concluding remarks: Neurosciences and cognitive science in the study of language of the brain; in Blum F (ed): Language, Communication and the Brain. New York, Blum, 1988, pp 275–282.

Damasio AR: Aphasia. N Engl J Med 1992;326:531–539.

Damasio H: Neuroimaging contributions to the understanding of aphasia; in Boller F, Grafmann J (eds): Handbook of Neuropsychology. Amsterdam, Elsevier, 1989, vol 2.

Ebeling U, Schmid U, Reulen HJ: Tumor surgery within the central motor strip: Surgical results with the aid of electrical motor cortex stimulation. Acta Neurochir 1990;101:100–107.

Ebeling U, Schmid U, Ying Z: Mapping bei Tumorpatienten in der Zentralregion. Schweiz Rundsch Med Prax 1991;47:1318–1323.

Ebeling U, Steinmetz H, Huang Y, Kahn T: Topography and identification of the precentral sulcus in MR-imaging. Am J Neuroradiol 1989;10:937–942.

Eisner W, Ilmberger J, Schmid UD, Ebeling U, Gutbrod K, Reulen H.-J.: Intraoperative speech and language monitoring in patients with space occupying lesions in the language-dominant hemisphere. Zentralbl Neurochir (Suppl) 1996:12–13.

Eisner W, Ilmberger J, Schmid UD, Reulen HJ: Intraoperative language and speech monitoring as guidance for neurosurgical strategies in removing tumors in the language-dominant cerebral hemisphere; in Hütter BO, Gilsbach JM (eds): Neuropsychology in Neurosurgery, Psychiatry and Neurology. Aachen, Verlag der Augustinus Buchhandlung, 1997.

Eisner W, Schmid UD, Ilmberger J, Reulen HJ: Tumor surgery in the language-dominant cerebral hemisphere: Intraoperative language/speech monitoring. Electroencephalogr Clin Electrophysiol 1996; 99:343.

Eisner W, Schmid UD, Reulen HJ, et al: The mapping and continuous monitoring of the intrinsic motor nuclei during brain stem surgery. Neurosurgery 1995;37:255–265.

Eisner W, Steude U, Waidhauser E, Bise K, Schmid UD: Surgery of subcortical lesions in the motor strip combining a stereotactically guided mini-craniotomy with electrophysiological mapping of the motor cortex; in Siegenthaler W., Haas R. (eds): The Decade of the Brain. Stuttgart, Thieme, 1995, p 70.

Fedio P, Van Buren J: Memory deficits during electrical stimulation of the speech cortex in conscious man. Brain Lang 1974;1:29–42.

Foerster O: The cerebral cortex of man. Lancet 1931;109:309–312.

Fried I, Ojemann GA, Fetz EE: Language-related potentials specific to human language cortex. Science 1981;212:353–356.

Fritsch G: Über die elektrische Erregbarkeit des Grosshirns. Arch Anat Physiol Wiss Med. 1870;37: 300–332.

Galaburda AM, Sanides F, Geschwind N: Human brain. Cytoarchitectonic left-right asymmetries in the temporal speech region. Arch Neurol 1978;35:812–817.

Geschwind N: The varieties of naming errors. Cortex 1967;3:97–112.

Goldman-Rakic PS: Topography of cognition: Parallel distributed networks in primate association cortex. Annu Rev Neurosci 1988;11.

Goodglass H: Understanding Aphasia. San Diego, Academic Press, 1993.

Haas J, Vogt G, Schiemann M, Patzold U: Aphasia and non-verbal intelligence in brain tumor patients. Neurology 1982;227:209–218.

Heilman KM, Wilder BJ, Malzone WF: Anomic aphasia following anterior temporal lobectomy. Trans Am Neurol Assoc 1972;97:291–293.

Herholz K, Reulen HJ, Stockhausen von HM, Thiel A, Ilmberger J, Kessler J, Eisner W, Yousry T, Heiss WD: Preoperative activation and intraoperative stimulation of language-related areas in patients with glioma. Neurosurgery 1997;41:1253–1262.

Huber W, Poeck K, Weniger D, Wilmes D: Der Aachener Aphasie Test. Hogrefe-Verlag für Psychologie, Göttingen, 1983.

Huber W, Poeck K, Weniger D, Willmes D: Aphasie; in Poeck K (ed): Klinische Neuropsychologie. Stuttgart, Thieme Verlag, 1989.

Ilmberger J, Werani A, Eisner W, Schmid UD, Reulen HJ: Intraoperative language mapping: Naming latency data. Exp Brain Res 1997;117:47–48.

Ilmberger J, Werani A, Kessler J, Eisner W, Schmid UD, Reulen HJ: Naming and semantic discrimination in intraoperative language mapping; in Hütter BO, Gilsbach JM (eds): Neuropsychology in Neurosurgery, Psychiatry and Neurology. Aachen, Verlag der Augustinus Buchhandlung, 1997.

Kertesz A: Localisation of lesions in Wernicke's aphasia; in Kertesz A (ed): Localisation in Neuropsychologia. Orlando USA, Harcourt Brace, Academic Press (London), 1983.

King RB, Schell GR: Cortical localisation and monitoring during cerebral operations. J Neurosurg 1987; 67:210–219.

Kohn SE, Goodglas H: Picture-naming in aphasia. Brain Lang 1985;24:266–283.

Laws ER, Taylor WF, Clifton MB, Okazaki H: Neurosurgical management of low-grade astrocytoma of the cerebral hemispheres. J Neurosurg 1984;61:665–673.

Le Roux PD, Berger MS, Haglund MM, Pilcher WH, Ojemann GA: Resection of intrinsic tumors from nondominant face motor cortex using stimulation mapping. Report of two cases. Surg Neurol 1991; 36:44–48.

Lesser RP, Hahn J, Lueders H, Rothner AD, Ehrenberg G: The use of chronic subdural electrodes for cortical mapping of speech. Epilepsia 1981;22:240.

Lesser RP, Lueders H, Dinner DS, et al: The location of speech and writing functions in the frontal language area. Results of extraoperative cortical stimulation. Brain 1984;107:275–291.

Lesser RP, Lueders H, Hahn J, Dinner DS, Morris HH, Klem G: Afterdischarge and functional alteration thresholds in the frontal and temporal lobes: Extraoperative testing. Epilepsia 1983;24:518–519.

Levesque MF, Sutherland WW, Risinger M, Becker DP, Crandall PH: Variability of speech cortex during functional localisation – Implication for plasticity. J Neurosurg 1989;70:329–330.

Levine DN, Sweet E: Localisation of lesions in Broca's motor aphasia; in Kertesz A (ed): Localisation in Neuropsychology. Orlando USA, Harcourt Brace, Academic Press, London, 1983.

Lueders H, Lesser RP, Dinner DS, et al: Inhibition of motor activity by elicited electrical stimulation of the human cortex. Epilepsia 1983;24:519.

Lueders H, Lesser RP, Hahn J, et al: Basal temporal language area demonstrated by electrical stimulation. Neurology 1986;36:505–510.

Luria A: Differences between disturbances of speech and writing in Russian and French. Int J Slavic Ling Poet 1960;3:13–22.

Luria AR: Das Gehirn in Aktion. Hamburg, Rowohlt, 1977.

Mateer CA, Cameron PA: Electrophysiological correlates of language: Stimulation mapping and evoked potentials; in Grafmann FB, Boller F (eds): Handbook of Neuropsychology. Amsterdam, Elsevier, 1989.

Mohr JP: Broca's area and Broca's aphasia; in Whitaker H, Whitaker HA (eds): Studies in Neuroliguistics. Vol 1. New York, Academic Press, 1976, pp 201–236.

Obane WG, Laxer KD, Cogen PH, Walker JA, Davis RL, Barbaro NH: Resection of dominant gliosis in refractory partial epilepsia. J Neurosurg 1992;77:632–639.

Ojemann GA: Language and the thalamus: Object naming and recall during and after thalamic stimulation. Brain Lang 1975;2:101–120.

Ojemann GA: Individual variability in cortical localisation of language. Brain Lang 1979;6:239–260.

Ojemann GA: Electrical stimulation and the neurobiology of language. Behav Brain Sci 1983a;6:221–230.

Ojemann GA: Brain organisation for language from the perspective of electrical stimulation mapping. Behav Brain Sci 1983b;6:189–206.

Ojemann GA: Effect of cortical and subcortical stimulation in human language and verbal memory; in Plum F (ed): Language Communication and the Brain. New York, 1988, pp 101–115.

Ojemann GA: Some brain mechanisms for reading; in Euler C (ed): Brain and Reading. New York, 1989, pp 47–59.

Ojemann GA, Creutzfeld O, Lettich E, et al: Neuronal activity in human lateral temporal cortex related to short-term verbal memory, naming and reading. Brain 1988;111:1383–1403.

Ojemann GA, Dodrill CB: Verbal memory deficits after left temporal lobectomy for epilepsy. Mechanism and intraoperative prediction. J Neurosurg 1985;62:101–107.

Ojemann GA, Fried I, Lettich E: Electrocorticographic correlates of language. 1. Desynchronisation in temporal language cortex during object naming. EEG Clin Neurophysiol 1989;73:453–463.

Ojemann GA, Ojemann J, Lettich E, Berger MS: Cortical language localisation in left, dominant hemisphere. An electrical stimulation mapping investigation in 117 patients. J Neurosurg 1989;71:316–326.

Ojemann GA, Whitaker HA: Language localisation and variability. Brain Lang 1978a;6:239–260.

Ojemann GA, Whitaker HA: The bilingual brain. Arch Neurol 1978b;35:409–412.

Oldfield RC: The assessment and analysis of handedness: The Edinburgh Inventory. Neuropsychologia 1971;7:97–113.

Otto H, Kubik S, Abernathey CD: Atlas of Cerebral Sulci. New York, 1990.

Penfield W, Jasper HH: Epilepsy and the Functional Anatomy of the Human Brain. Boston, Penfield, 1954.

Penfield W, Roberts L: Speech and Brain Mechanism. Princeton, University Press, 1959.

Rank JBJ: Which elements are excited in electrical stimulation of mammalian central nervous system. Brain Res 1975;98:417–440.

Reulen HJ, Schmid UD, Ilmberger J, Eisner W, Bise K: Tumorchirurgie im Sprachkortex in Lokalanästhesie. Nervenarzt 1997;68:813–824.

Rostomily RC, Berger MS, Ojemann GA, Lettich E: Postoperative deficits and functional recovery following removals of tumors involving the dominant hemisphere supplementary motor area. J Neurosurg 1991;75:62–68.

Schmid UD, Eisner W, Reulen HJ, et al: Funktionskontrollierte Neurochirurgie. Nervenarzt 1995;66: 582–595.

Schuri U: Lernen und Gedächtnis; in Von Cramon D, Zihl J (eds): Neuropsychologische Rehabilitation. Berlin, Springer Verlag, 1988.

Van Buren JM, Fedio P, Frederick GC: Mechanism and localisation of speech in parietotemporal cortex. Neurosurgery 1978;2:233–239.

Wada J, Rasmussen T: Intracarotid injection of sodium amytal for the lateralisation of speech dominance. J Neurosurg 1960;17:266–282.

Weingart J, Olivi A, Brem H: Supratentorial low-grade astrocytomas in adults. Neurosurg Q 1991;1: 141–159.

Wernicke C: Der aphasische Symptomenkomplex. Breslau, Universitätsschrift, 1874.

Whitaker H, Selnes O: Anatomic variations in the cortex: Individual differences and the problem of the location of language functions. Ann NY Acad Sci 1975;280:844–854.

Whitaker HH, Ojemann GA: Graded localisation of naming from electrical stimulation mapping of left cerebral cortex. Nature 1978;270:50–51.

Willmes K: An approach to analyzing a single subject's scores obtained in a standardized test with application to the Aachen Aphasia Test. J Clin Exp Neuropsychol 1985;7:331–352.

Woods RP, Dodrill CB, Ojemann GA: Brain injury, handedness, and speech lateralisation in a series of amobarbital studies. Ann Neurol 1988;23:510–518.

Wygotski LS: Denken und Sprechen. Frankfurt am Main, Fischer Wissenschaft, 1986.

Yasargil MG, von Ammon K, Cavazos E, Doczi T, Reeves JD, Roth R: Tumors of the limbic and paralimbic systems. Acta Neurochir 1992;118:50–52.

Yousry TA, Schmid UD, Jassoy AG, Schmid D, Eisner WE, Reulen HJ, Reiser MF, Lissner J: Topography of the cortical motor hand area: Prospective study with functional MR imaging and direct motor mapping at surgery. Radiology 1995;195:23–29.

Yousry TA, Schmid UD, Schmid D, Heiss D, Jassoy AG, Eisner WE, Reulen HJ, Reiser MF: The motor hand area. Noninvasive detection with functional MRI and surgical validation with cortical stimulation. Radiologe 1995;35:252–255.

Dr. W. Eisner, Universitätsklinik für Neurochirurgie, A.Ö. Landeskrankenhaus Innsbruck, Anichstrasse 35, A–6020 Innsbruck (Austria)

Wiegel T, Hinkelbein W, Brock M, Hoell T (eds): Controversies in Neuro-Oncology.
Front Radiat Ther Oncol. Basel, Karger, 1999, vol 33, pp 37–42

....

The Value of Iodine-123-Alpha-Methyl-L-Tyrosine Single-Photon Emission Tomography for the Treatment Planning of Malignant Gliomas

H.J. Feldmann [a], *A.L. Grosu* [a], *W. Weber* [b], *P. Bartenstein* [b], *M. Gross* [a], *M. Schwaiger* [b], *M. Molls* [a]

Departments of [a] Radiation Oncology and [b] Nuclear Medicine, Klinikum rechts der Isar, Technical University Munich, Germany

Introduction

The management of malignant gliomas requires aggressive treatment including neurosurgery and radiotherapy. Nevertheless, the prognosis of these tumors remains poor. There are some improvements in radiation therapy of these tumors with the incorporation of computer tomography (CT) and magnetic resonance imaging (MRI) as well as three-dimensional (3-D) treatment planning approaches.

The accurate identification of viable tumor margins has been improved using MRI in comparison to CT. In a study of Thornton et al. [1] the additional information of the MRI contrast-enhanced volume leads to a 1.5-fold increase of the macroscopical tumor volume in comparison to CT alone. However, several studies have demonstrated that CT and MRI cannot reliably differentiate viable tumor tissue from tumor-associated edema, postoperative changes or radiation necrosis [2].

Metabolic parameters, which are independent of morphological changes, could improve the accurate and reliable identification of viable tumor margins. F-18-fluorodeoxyglucose (FDG) has been the most widely used radiopharmaceutical for differentiating necrotic tissue from viable tumor cells [3]. In contrast, due to the high uptake of FDG in normal brain tissue, this radiopharmaceutical provides only in a minority of patients additional information for target delineation of brain tumors [4]. As an alternative, the use of iodine-

123-alpha-methyl-*L*-tyrosine (IMT) has been proposed for imaging of brain tumors [4, 5]. IMT tumor uptake reflects amino acid transport rather than protein synthesis rate [6]. This tracer has been shown to accumulate intensively in brain tumors of different histologic types and grading, while the uptake in normal brain is low.

The aim of this study was firstly to determine the tumor volumes obtained with different imaging modalities and secondly to evaluate the additionally functional information of IMT single-photon emission tomography (SPECT) in comparison to MRI in the delineation of the target volume using 3-D radiation treatment planning.

Materials and Methods

Patients

We prospectively investigated 30 patients with residual macroscopic tumor masses after biopsy or surgery (15 males and 15 females). Age ranged from 18 to 80 years with a mean of 52 years. Tumors were graded as anaplastic astrocytoma (n = 14), anaplastic mixed glioma (n = 3) or glioblastoma multiforme (n = 13).

MRI

MRI was performed with a Philips 1.5-Tesla scanner (Gyroscan ACS II). Patient's heads were immobilized using the mask system. MRI studies were obtained using the standard body coil. Transaxial T1- and T2-weighted slices were required without inclination of the gantry. Slice thickness was 7 mm with a gap of 0.7 mm. In addition, T1-weighted axial, sagittal and coronal images were obtained after intravenous administration of Gd-DTPA (0.1 mmol/kg body weight).

IMT-SPECT Imaging

Patients were examined by IMT-SPECT after fasting for at least 4 h. The patients received 900 mg sodium perchlorate before the IMT injection to minimize radioactive iodide uptake by the thyroid. Data acquisition was started 30 min after intravenous injection of 185–370 MBq IMT. Images of 45 s duration were acquired with a triple-head camera equipped with a dedicated ^{123}I collimator [7].

Image Correlation

During MRI the patients were scanned in supine position. The patients' heads were fixed in the customized thermoplastic masks that were used during the course of radiotherapy. The IMT-SPECT investigation was performed without masks. A computer program was developed which allowed the reorientation of the SPECT images based on internal landmarks. After reorientation, fusion images were generated.

3-D Treatment Planning

Target volume and critical structures such as eyes, optic nerves, chiasms, brainstem and spinal cord were defined on each slice using a commercial 3-D radiotherapy planning

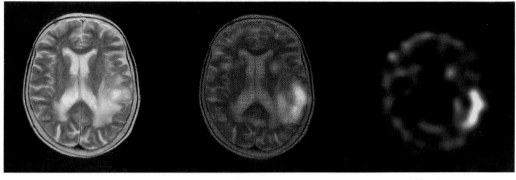

| T2-weighted MIR | Fusion image | 123I-IMT |

Fig. 1. Tumor volumes obtained by T2-weighted images and IMT-SPECT as well as the fusion image for a patient with an astrocytoma III. There is a significant uptake of IMT outside the T2-weighted scans.

system (Helax TMS). Following SPECT and MRI acquisition, treatment planning was performed using the additional information for defining the target volume which was covered by the 95% isodose according to the ICRU 50 conventions. The technique of 3-D treatment planning and conformal radiotherapy with noncoplanar beam arrangements and irregular-shaped portals has been described earlier [8].

Results

Twenty-six of 30 tumors showed contrast enhancement after administration of Gd-DTPA. Mean tumor volume in MRI T1-weighted images was 19 ± 18.5 ml with a range from 0 to 87 ml (table 1). All tumors with their edema were clearly detectable as hyperintense lesions in the T2-weighted scans with a mean volume of 76 ± 50.7 ml. The mean tumor volume defined in IMT-SPECT was 44 ± 35 ml.

In 19 from 30 tumors the area of IMT uptake was larger than the area of contrast enhancement, in 3 patients nearly identical volumes could be visualized in both investigations (T1 Gd and SPECT), 5 patients showed hot spots inside the area of contrast enhancement, and in 3 patients the macroscopic tumor was only visualized with IMT-SPECT (table 2). In addition, in 4 from 30 tumors the area of IMT uptake was larger than the hyperintensive area in T2-weighted images. 22 patients showed hot spots inside the T2 regions and in 4 patients nearly identical volumes were visualized in both investigations (T2 and SPECT).

Table 1. Tumor volumes (ml) obtained with the different imaging modalities

Imaging modality	Mean, ml	SD	Range, ml
MRI T1 Gd	19	18.5	0–87
MRI T2	76	50.7	12.5–225
IMT-SPECT	44	35.0	6.8–134
MRI T1 Gd + IMT	51	36.0	3.6–145
MRI T2 + IMT	93	55.0	16.5–225

Table 2. Qualitative analysis of tumor volumes with different methods

Comparison of tumor volumes	n
IMT-SPECT volume larger than contrast-enhanced T1 area	19
IMT-SPECT volume smaller than contrast-enhanced T1 area	5
Nearly identical volumes in both investigations	3
Visualization of the tumor only in IMT-SPECT	3
IMT-SPECT volume larger than hyperintensive T2 area	4
IMT-SPECT volume smaller than hyperintensive T2 area	22
Nearly identical volumes in both investigations	4

Calculations of the composite volumes showed an increase in the tumor volume by the SPECT information in 29 of 30 patients (T1 Gd and IMT) and in 4 of 30 patients (T2 and IMT). Figure 1 shows the tumor volumes obtained by T2-weighted images and IMT-SPECT as well as the fusion image for a patient with an astrocytoma III. There is significant IMT uptake outside the T2 region. Therefore, the composite showed an increase of the tumor volume by the SPECT information.

Discussion

In a former study [4] it could be demonstrated that IMT-SPECT was clearly superior to FDG-PET in the detection and delineation of tumor tissue despite the lower resolution and lower sensitivity of SPECT compared with PET. This study was designed to investigate whether the functional imaging modality IMT-SPECT provides additional information on the viable tumor mass in comparison to MRI. The results show that in a significant number of patients the regions of IMT uptake are different from the findings in MRI. All tumors could be detected by IMT-SPECT. Therefore, it is of great interest whether the additional information derived from IMT-SPECT will be of value for radiation treatment planning.

It is well known that the area of contrast enhancement underestimates the extension of malignant gliomas. In clinical practice, the planning target volume is primarily based on the MRI T2 hyperintensity plus a safety margin of about 2 cm [9]. In most cases, recurrences of locally treated malignant gliomas are evident within 2 cm of pretreatment borders [8, 9]. This could be explained by the insufficient extent of the initially treated volume as well as the insufficient intensity of the initial treatment to obtain long-term tumor control.

An improved delineation of the tumor extension will be essential for dose-escalation trials using 3-D radiation therapy to increase local control. Therefore, prospective studies are necessary to evaluate the impact of an improved delineation of the tumor extension using IMT-SPECT on the clinical results.

A serious limitation in our study is that there exist no histopathologic evaluation in cases with different localizations obtained by IMT-SPECT and MRI. Therefore, the specificity of the method appears promising but requires detailed evaluation in a larger series of patients with benign diseases.

In conclusion, IMT is a potential important tracer for metabolic assessment in patients with brain tumors using SPECT. Further studies have to be conducted in order to validate its use in 3-D radiation treatment planning and conformal therapy.

References

1   Thornton AF Jr, Sandler HM, Ten Haken RK, McShan DL, Fraas BA, LaVigne ML, Yanke BR: The clinical utility of magnetic resonance imaging in 3-dimensional treatment planning of brain neoplasms. Int J Radiat Oncol Biol Phys 1992;24:767–774.
2   Sartor K: Tumors and related conditions; in Sartor K (ed): MR Imaging of the Skull and Brain: A Correlative Text Atlas, ed 1. Berlin, Springer, 1992, pp 249–493.
3   Glantz MJ, Hoffman JM, Coleman RE, Friedman AH, Hanson MW, Burger PC, Herndon JE, Meisler WJ, Schold SC Jr: Identification of early recurrence of primary central nervous system tumors by F-18-fluorodeoxyglucose positron emission tomography. Ann Neurol 1991;29:347–355.
4   Weber WA, Bartenstein P, Gross M, Daschner H, Feldmann HJ, Reidel G, Ziegler S, Lumenta C, Molls M, Schwaiger M: F-18-fluorodeoxyglucose PET and ^{123}I-alpha-methyl-tyrosine SPECT in the evaluation of brain tumors. J Nucl Med 1997;38:802–808.
5   Woesler B, Kuwert T, Morgenroth C: Non-invasive grading of primary brain tumors: Results of a comparative study between SPECT with ^{123}I-alpha-methyl-tyrosine and PET with 18F-deoxyglucose. Eur J Nucl Med 1997;24:428–434.
6   Langen KJ, Coenen H, Roosen N: SPECT studies of brain tumors with L-3-^{123}I-iodo-alpha-methyl-tyrosine: Comparison with PET, [124]I-IMT and first clinical results. J Nucl Med 1990;31:281–286.

7   Münzing W, Raithel E, Tatsch K, Hahn K: Entwurf eines speziellen Kollimators fpr ^{123}I und erste Erfahrungen bei der Anwendung (Abstract). Nuklearmedizin 1996;35:A48.

8   Grosu A, Feldmann HJ, Albrecht C, Kneschaurek P, Molls M: Drei-dimensionale Bestrahlungsplanung von Hirntumoren: Vorteile der Methode und klinische Ergebnisse. Strahlenther Oncol 1998;174:1–6.

9   Gross MW, Weber WA, Feldmann HJ, Bartenstein P, Schwaiger M, Molls M: The value of F-18-fluorodeoxyglucose PET for the 3-D radiation treatment planning of malignant gliomas. Int J Radiat Oncol Biol Phys 1998;41:989–995.

PD Dr. Horst J. Feldmann, Klinik und Poliklinik für Strahlentherapie und Radiologische Onkologie, Klinikum rechts der Isar, Technische Universität München, Ismaninger Strasse 22, D–81675 München (Germany) Tel. +49 4140 4512, Fax +49 4140 4587

Wiegel T, Hinkelbein W, Brock M, Hoell T (eds): Controversies in Neuro-Oncology.
Front Radiat Ther Oncol. Basel, Karger, 1999, vol 33, pp 43–50

....

Boron Neutron Capture Enhancement of Fast Neutron for *Nonremoved* Glioblastomas: Rationale of a Clinical Trial

J.P. Pignol [a], *P. Paquis* [b], *N. Breteau* [c], *P. Chauvel* [d], *W. Sauerwein* [e], *EORTC BNCT Study Group*

Departments of [a] Radiotherapy, Hôpital du Hasenrain, Mulhouse;
[b] Neurosurgery, Hôpital Pasteur, Nice; [c] Radiotherapy, Hôpital de la Source, Orléans;
[d] Biomedical Cyclotron, Center Antoine-Lacassagne, Nice, France, and
[e] Radiotherapy, Universitätsklinikum, Essen, Deutschland

High linear energy transfer (LET) irradiations with fast neutrons have been investigated since the 1970s to circumvent the high radioresistance of glioblastoma (GBM). Although more than 900 patients have been involved in phase I/II trails, no therapeutic window has been found [1]. Whereas tumor control was observed on autopsies for physical doses over 13 $Gy_{n,\gamma}$, white matter changes occurred for doses over 11 $Gy_{n,\gamma}$ [2–5]. Nevertheless, one of the major lessons from these trials is that high LET particles appear to be able to sterilize GBM cells from a brain. In order to create artificially a differential effect for fast neutrons, an enhancement with ^{10}B neutron capture reaction has been suggested [6–10]. This technique, called boron neutron capture enhancement of fast neutron (BNCEFN), uses the thermal neutrons generated after fast neutron diffusion in the tissues to yield $^{10}B(n, \alpha)^7Li$ reactions as a 'boost' dose achieved selectively within tumor cells. The nuclear reaction produces an α particle and a ^7Li ion which share an energy of 2.79 MeV. These particles have ranges in biological tissues of respectively 9 and 5 μm, i.e. close to tumor cell diameter [11, 12].

Two important requisites must be fulfilled in order to gain a significant enhancement: (1) To get high ^{10}B concentrations within tumor cells, and lower ones in the blood and in normal brain, using a boronated compound with a high tumor affinity. (2) To get a significant thermal neutron flux after diffusion of the primary beam.

The recent publications of Barth and co-workers [13, 14] suggest that the use of each one of the boronated compounds which are used in clinical trials, i.e. ^{10}B-boronophenylalanine (BPA) or borosulfhydryl (BSH), allows to obtain a ^{10}B concentration very close to 100 µg/g after intra-arterial (IA) administration with prior blood-brain barrier (BBB) disruption.

Concerning the thermal neutron flux, many authors have demonstrated that it is strongly dependent on the fast neutron irradiation field size and on the presence of a diffusing media surrounding the patient's head [6, 8, 15]. It is possible to demonstrate theoretically that the use of a 20-cm wide lead multileaf collimation placed in close contact to the patient's head, and of a graphite patient immobilization material, allows to make the thermal neutron flux independent of the field size and to yield a 20% physical dose enhancement provided that 100µg/g of ^{10}B can be loaded in the tumor, for the fast neutron beam of the cyclotron at Orleans (p34 MeV + Be) [pers. commun.[1]].

This article reviews the rationale and the technical aspects of a phase I clinical trial to be opened at the Orleans facility, within the frame of the EORTC BNCT Study Group, since all the feasibility studies will be achieved. This protocol aims at treating nonoperated GBM with fast neutron and after BSH IA administration. The feasibility of IA administrations, fast neutron dose prescription, fractionation and the dose escalation are discussed in order to define the safest treatment. On the other hand, the most important requisite for the enhancement optimization are specified in order to reach a certain level of efficiency.

Intra-Arterial Administration of Boronated Compound

Choice of Boronated Compound

While many boronated compounds have shown their ability to target selectively and efficaciously tumor cells, only two compounds are presently available for clinical purposes, i.e. they are registered as drugs by the health administrations. The first one, BPA, has been used in the USA (in Boston and Brookhaven) for two clinical trials of boron neutron capture therapy (BNCT) for adjuvant irradiation of GBM [16, 17]. The second one, BSH, has been used in Japan since 1968 [18, 19] and in Europe since 1997 for an EORTC clinical trial [20].

---

[1] Communication presented at the Third International Symposium: Controversies in Neuro-Oncology, Berlin, April 30–May 2, 1998.

Table 1. ^{10}B concentrations measured on F98 gliosarcoma-bearing rats after BPA or BSH IA administrations preceded by BBB mannitol disruption [13, 14]

	Dose mg/kg	Tumor ^{10}B content, μg/g	Tumor/ blood ratio	Tumor/ brain ratio
BPA	500	94	10.9	7.5
BSH	52	48	5	12.3

BPA ($BC_9H_{12}NO_4$) which is an amino-acid analog to tyrosine, shows active and passive incorporations within the tumor, with a ratio of roughly 3 between normal cells and tumor [21]. This molecule crosses the BBB, and ^{10}B is found in normal brain. The pharmacokinetic shows short half-lives within the blood and in the tissues after intravenous administration [22]. Although this molecule is remarkable nontoxic, its solubility is one of the major problems in clinical application. A complex of BPA-fructose, made just prior to its administration, seemed to avoid the perfusion of huge amounts of liquid [16].

BSH ($Na_2B_{12}H_{11}SH$) is a boron cage which does not cross the BBB unless in the tumor bed [19, 23]. No boron is found in the normal brain, and only a few parts after BBB disruption [13, 14]. Its pharmacokinetic shows very long half-lives for the blood and tissue clearances. Although no active incorporation has been detected, it is believed that it is the pharmacokinetic which explains the selective incorporation in various tumors seen 12 h after intravenous administration [23].

Table 1 summarizes the data published by Barth and co-workers [13, 14] of BPA or BSH injections to F98 gliosarcoma-bearing rats, with IA administration preceded by a mannitol bolus in order to disrupt the BBB. Concentrations close to 100 μg/g are found for BPA but not for BSH. Nevertheless, it must be noted that the BSH dose is only half the one used in the Petten trial [20]. While ^{10}B concentrations are believed to be strongly proportional to the administered dose, it is likely that a higher BSH dose could yield a higher ^{10}B concentrations within the tumor [21, 24].

In the BNCEFN protocol, BSH has been chosen for the following reasons: (1) This molecule has been used by Hatanaka and co-workers [19], with IA injections on 84 patients, without any mention of side effects related to this administration mode. (2) The slow pharmacokinetic allows to maintain a stable ^{10}B level in the irradiated organs during the fast neutron irradiation. (3) There is no solubility problem. (4) Less boron is found in the normal brain. This is important for a phase I protocol in which the dose to normal tissues is of major concern. (5) This molecule is registered as an experimental drug in Europe. (6) BSH is the molecule used in the Petten BNCT clinical trial. The use of the same molecule allows better comparison between the two protocols.

Safety of BSH Administration and ^{10}B Concentrations Expected

On animals, the LD_{50} has been found to be correlated both with the compound purity and the infusion rate [24]. For a pure product, the LD_{50} is over 1,000 mg/kg with an infusion rate of 33 mg/kg/min, of 300 mg/kg for an infusion rate of 200 mg/kg/min and of 215 mg/kg for an infusion rate of 1,200 mg/kg/min. It is thus expected that a dose of 100 mg/kg delivered in 40 min will be safe as the infusion rate is only 2.5 mg/kg/min.

The carotid arterial blood flow is around 250 ml/min [25], and the instantaneous ^{10}B blood concentration will be over 500 ppm. With a mean volume of 45 liters for the central compartment of distribution, a first clearance half-life of 4.6 h, the ^{10}B concentration in blood might be below 50 ppm after 2.5 h. The ^{10}B concentration within the tumor is expected to be over 100 μg/g at the same time.

Use of a Prior BBB Disruption

Barth et al. [13] have shown that the use of a prior disruption of the BBB with mannitol allows to increase the ^{10}B concentration within the tumor from 42.7 to 94 μg/g (+120%) with BPA, and from 30.8 to 48.6 μg/g for BSH (+58%). This BBB disruption does not change ^{10}B gradient versus blood or brain, as the tumor-to-blood ratio is found to be 5 and tumor-to-brain ratio is 12.3 after 2.5 h [14]. It is likely that the same phenomenon could be observed in humans and it was decided to perform a BBB disruption with a bolus injection of 100 ml of 20% mannitol prior to the BSH administration.

BBB disruption with mannitol weights down the treatment schedule: as the mannitol injection may cause acute pains in the facial region, a neuroleptanalgesia is mandatory. This means that patients must be deferred to the radiology department to receive an IA administration of BSH via retrofemoral catheterization before each irradiation fraction. Anesthesia is performed with Propofol® before mannitol administration, then BSH infusion is performed over 40 min. Finally, the patient is woken up and sent to the fast neutron facility to receive irradiation 2.5 h later.

Dose Prescription

Definition and Prescription

Because of the various biological efficiencies of each irradiation component, the reported dose cannot be simply the addition of each 'physical' dose. Dose modification factor (DMF) must be used in order to weigh each component.

In BNCEFN, the irradiation can be understood as a 'standard' fast neutron irradiation, to which is simply added $^{10}B(n, \alpha)^7Li$ reactions. Thus the simplest way to handle the dosimetry is to take into account only these two components: the 'standard' fast neutron dose and a ^{10}B dose to which a DMF must be applied.

Previously published data show that a DMF of 2 can be calculated for GBM cells irradiated under the Nice fast neutron beam with or without 100 µg/g of ^{10}B added to the growth medium under the form of 95% enriched boric acid which diffuses freely in all cellular compartments [26]. These results are in good agreement with other data which show that, comparatively to photon irradiation, the RBE of fast neutron is generally considered to be close to 3, while $^{10}B(n,\alpha)^7Li$ reactions have an RBE of 6–7 [27]. Nevertheless, while the RBE is strongly dependent on the microscopic ^{10}B localization at subcellular level [27–29], it is not possible to define a DMF for various clinical endpoints: the RBE will depend on the compound used and on the clinical effect specified.

The aim of an escalation dose phase I protocol is to define the therapeutic toxicity and the safest dose that could be delivered, which means that the prescription dose must predict the effects on the normal brain. It has been demonstrated that the normal brain contains less boron than the blood compartment [19, 23]. Moreover, while most of the side effects are related to vascular damage, it has been demonstrated that the endothelial cells do not retain firmly ^{10}B when BSH is used. Then, a DMF of 2 as defined above for a homogeneous ^{10}B distribution within the tissues is likely to overestimate the DMF to be applied for the normal brain dose.

Finally, a dose calculation method which sums the 'standard' fast neutron dose and twofold the ^{10}B physical dose, based on the ^{10}B blood concentration at the irradiation time, will be a safe and meaningful way to report the dose for a phase I trail. In summary, in BNCEFN, *the dose is prescribed to the normal brain.*

Fractionation

The necessity of BSH IA administration with prior BBB disruption dictates to decrease the number of fast neutron fractions. While the dose-response relationship of normal tissues after neutron irradiation is characterized by a relatively high α/β ratio, they are less protected by fractionation as they are with low LET radiations [30]. Clinical experience shows that the best tolerance is seen when fast neutrons are delivered over 2 weeks in 8–12 fractions, depending if it is only a boost or a full fast neutron treatment. It is proposed in the protocol to use less fractions over 2 weeks, in order to use only twice each femoral artery.

Except for the fraction number, the tolerance is also strongly dependent on the irradiated volume. Therefore, it is proposed to irradiate in the most 'conformal' manner the clinical target volume (CTV), which is defined as the tumor seen on T1-weighted RMI after gadolinium administration plus a 1.5-cm margin, using a lead multileaf collimator. Ideally, 6–8 irradiation fields must be used in order to decrease normal tissue dose. It is expected that the irradiated volume reduction will balance the fraction number reduction.

Finally, the central tumor necrosis which likely contains few ^{10}B will be irradiated essentially with fast neutron. The active part of the tumor will receive both fast neutron and BNCEFN, and, while thermal neutrons spread far away within the brain, it is expected that ^{10}B(n, α)^{7}Li reactions will touch 'guerilla' cells spreading out of the tumor bed.

Escalation of Dose

In previously published series, it can be seen that below 11 $Gy_{n, \gamma}$ of exclusive fast neutron irradiation, given sometime on the whole brain and with less quality beams, no serious side effects were noticed. The prescription dose as defined above will start at 10.5 Gy total dose, and will be increased, by 0.5-Gy steps to 12.5 Gy. Ten patients will be included in each step, and the escalation dose will be stopped if more than 2 patients present severe side effects like radionecrosis.

Discussion

Extensive data are available, however, concerning fast neutron irradiation for brain tumor; the introduction of a new component, here ^{10}B neutron capture reactions, yields a risk of serious adverse effects to the brain. It is therefore mandatory to perform a phase I trial in which all the treatment parameters are optimized to decrease the toxicity risks. To define the prescription dose to the normal brain, using the ^{10}B blood concentration at the irradiation time and a DMF of 2, to define the shortest CTV possible and to irradiate the tumor with 6–8 fields in a conformal manner using a multileaf collimation, are all choices which follow this aim.

The final objective of this dose escalation trial is to reach the theoretical point where there may exist a therapeutic window for GBM. It is not obvious that, even if GBM sterilizations without severe side effect to normal brain can be obtained, long survivors are awaited, but it is expected at least that the patients' survey median can be increased while a shorter treatment schedule is applied. This may be the main endpoint of a phase II trial, and only a strong enlargement of the survey median would justify to carry on the technique of phase III trial.

Acknowledgements

This work has been partly supported by grants from the European Union contract BMH4 CT96 0325, the Ligue Contre le Cancer du Loiret, and the Ligue Contre le Cancer des Alpes Maritimes.

References

1 Laramore GE: Neutron radiotherapy for high-grade gliomas: The search for the elusive therapeutic window. Int J Radiat Oncol Biol Phys 1990;19:493–495.

2 Caterall M, Bloom HJG, Ash DV, Walsh L, Richardson A, Uttley D, Gowing NFC, Lewis P, Chaucer B: Fast neutrons compared with megavoltage X-rays in the treatment of patients with supratentorial glioblastomas: A controlled pilot study. Int J Radiat Oncol Biol Phys 1980;6:261–266.

3 Duncan W, McLelland J, Jack WJL, Arnott SJ, Gordon A, Kerr GR, Williams JR: The results of a randomised trial of mixed-schedule (neutron/photon) irradiation in the treatment of supratentorial grade III and grade IV astrocytoma. Br J Radiol 1986;59:379–383.

4 Herskovic A, Ornitz RD, Shell M, Rodgers CC: Glioblastoma multiforme treated with 15 MeV fast neutrons. Cancer 1982;49:2463–2465.

5 Laramore GE, Griffin TW, Gerdes AJ, Parker RG: Fast neutron and mixed (neutron/photon) beam teletherapy for grade III and IV astrocytomas. Cancer 1978;42:96–106.

6 Buchholz TA, Laramore GE, Stelzer KJ, Risler R, Wooton P, Griffin TW: Boron neutron capture enhanced fast neutron radiotherapy for malignant gliomas and other tumors. J Neurooncol 1997; 33:171–178.

7 Lüdeman L, Matzen T, Matzke M, Schmidt R, Scobel W: Determination of the thermal neutron flux in a fast neutron beam by use of a boron-coated ionization chamber. Med Phys 1995;22: 1743–1747.

8 Pignol JP, Chauvel P, Paquis P, Courdi A, Iborra-Brassart N, Lonjon M, Lebrun-Frenay C, Frenay M, Grellier P, Chatel, M, Hérault J, Bensadoun RJ, Milano G, Nepveu F, Patau JP, Demard F, Breteau N: Boron neutron capture irradiation: Setting up a clinical programme in Nice. Bull Cancer Radiother 1996;83:201S–206S.

9 Sauerwein W, Zeigler W, Szypniewski H, Streffer C: Boron neutron capture therapy using fast neutrons: Effects in two human tumor cell lines. Strahlenther Onkol 1990;166:26–29.

10 Waterman M, Kuchnir FT, Skaggs LS, Bewley DK, Page BG, Attix FH: The use of ^{10}B to enhance the tumour dose in fast-neutron therapy. Phys Med Biol 1978;23:592–602.

11 Barth RF, Soloway AH, Fairchild RG, Brugger RM: Boron neutron capture therapy for cancer. Realities and prospects. Cancer 1992;70:2995–3007.

12 Pignol JP, Chauvel P: Irradiations par captures de neutrons: Principe, résultats actuels et perspectives. Bull Cancer Radiother 1995;82:283–297.

13 Barth RG, Yang G, Rotaru JH, Meschberger ML, Joel DD, Nawrocky MM, Goodman JH, Soloway AH: Boron neutron capture therapy of brain tumors: Enhanced survival following intracarotid injection of either sodium borocaptate or boronophenylalanine with or without blood-brain barrier disruption. Cancer Res 1997;57:1129–1136.

14 Yang W, Barth RF, Rotaru JH, Moeschberger ML, Joel DD, Nawrocky MM, Goodman JH, Soloway AH: Boron neutron capture therapy of brain tumors: Enhanced survival following intracarotid injection of sodium borocaptate with or without blood-brain barrier disruption. Int J Radiat Oncol Biol Phys 1997;37:663–672.

15 Pöller F, Sauerwein W, Rassow J: Dosimetry and fluence measurements with a new irradiation arrangement for neutron capture therapy of tumors in mice. Radiother Oncol 1991;21:179–182.

16 Busse PM, Zamenhof R, Madoc-Jones H, Solares G, Kiger S, Riley K, Chuang C, Rogers G, Harling O: Clinical follow-up of patients with melanoma of the extremity treated in a phase I boron neutron capture therapy protocol; in Larsson B et al (eds): Advances in Neutron Capture Therapy, vol I: Medicine and Physics. Amsterdam, Elsevier, 1997, pp 60–64.

17 Coderre JA, Elowitz EH, Chadha M, Bergland R, Capala J, Joel DD, Liu HB, Slatkin DN, Chanana AD: Boron neutron capture therapy for glioblastoma multiforme using *p*-boronophenylalanine and epithermal neutrons: Trial design and early clinical results. J Neurooncol 1997;33:141–152.

18 Hatanaka H, Nakagawa Y: Clinical results of long-surviving brain patients who underwent boron neutron capture therapy. Int J Radiat Oncol Biol Phys 1994;28:1061–1066.

19 Kageji T, Nakagawa Y, Kitamura K, Matsumoto K, Hatanaka H: Pharmacokinetics and boron uptake of BSH ($Na_2B_{12}H_{11}SH$) in patients with intracranial tumors. J Neurooncol 1997;33:117–130.

20 Sauerwein W: The clinical project at HFR Petten – A status report; in Larsson B et al (eds): Advances in Neutron Capture Therapy, vol I: Medicine and Physics. Amsterdam, Elsevier, 1997, pp 77–82.

21 Capala J, Makar MS, Coderre, JA: Accumulation of boron in malignant and normal cells incubated in vitro with boronophenylalanine, mercaptoborane or boric acid. Radiat Res 1996;146:554–560.

22 Coderre JA, Glass JD, Fairchild RG, Micca PL, Fand I, Joel DD: Selective delivery of boron by the melanin precursor analogue *p*-boronophenylalanine to tumors other than melanoma. Cancer Res 1990;50:138–141.

23 Gabel D, Preusse D, Haritz D, Grochulla F, Haselberger K, Frankhauser H, Ceberg C, Peters HD, Klotz U: Pharmacokinetics of $Na_2B_{12}H_{11}SH$ (BSH) in patients with malignant brain tumors as a prerequisite for a phase I clinical trial of boron neutron capture. Acta Neurochir 1997;139:606–612.

24 Peters HD, Gabel D: European Collaboration on Boron Neutron Capture Therapy: Compilation of Literature Data on Toxicity and Pharmacokinetics in Animals and Summary of the European Phase I toxicity and pharmacokinetic study. Bremen, European Collaboration on BNCT Editor, 1997, pp 1–14.

25 Ensminger WD: Intraarterial therapy; in Perry MC (ed): The Chemotherapy Source Book. Baltimore, Williams & Wilkins, 1992, pp 256–271.

26 Pignol JP, Courdi A, Paquis P, Iborra-Brassart N, Fares G, Hachem A, Lonjon M, Breteau N, Sauerwein W, Gabel D, Chauvel P: Potentialisation par captures de neutrons pour les gliblastomes inextirpables. J Chim Phys 1997;94:1827–1830.

27 Coderre JA, Makar MS, Micca PL, Nawrocky MM, Liu HB, Joel DD, Slatkin DN, Amols HI: Derivations of relative biological effectiveness for the high LET radiations produced during boron neutron capture irradiations of the 9L rat gliosarcoma in vitro and in vivo. Int J Radiat Oncol Biol Phys 1993;27:1121–1129.

28 Goodman JH, McGregor JM, Clendenon NR: Ultrastructural microvascular response to boron neutron capture therapy in an experimental model. Neurosurgery 1989;24:701–708.

29 Slatkin DN: A history of boron neutron capture therapy of brain tumors. Postulation of a brain radiation dose tolerance limit. Brain 1991;114:1609–1629.

30 Courdi A: Fractionation and therapeutic ratio with neutron therapy. Bull Cancer Radiother 1996; 83:64S–67S.

Jean Philippe Pignol, MD, Service de Radiotherapie, Hôpital du Hasenrain,
87, Avenue d'Altkirch, F–68051 Mulhouse Cedex (France)
Tel. +33 389 64 7520, Fax +33 389 64 7532, E-Mail: jp.pignol@infonie.fr

Wiegel T, Hinkelbein W, Brock M, Hoell T (eds): Controversies in Neuro-Oncology.
Front Radiat Ther Oncol. Basel, Karger, 1999, vol 33, pp 51–63

....

Commissioning of a Micro-Multileaf Collimator

D. Georg, U. Wolff, R.F.E. Hartl, J. Moitzi, U. Haverkamp, R. Pötter

Department of Radiotherapy and Radiobiology, University of Vienna, Austria

Introduction

During the last years the development of commercially available add-on devices for medical linear accelerators (linacs), circular collimators with small diameters and micro-multileaf collimators (mMLC), have offered new possibilities for linac-based stereotactic radiosurgery and/or conformal radiotherapy of small cranial targets.

The use of an mMLC offers several advantages compared to circular collimators, for example improved sparing of the normal tissue when treating nonspherical target volumes [Nedzi et al., 1993; Marks et al., 1995; Kubo et al., 1996]. Furthermore, the introduction of mMLC-based radiosurgery is expected to reduce the workload when nonspherical targets should be irradiated [Kubo et al., 1997].

An mMLC has been recently installed at our department (Clinic for Radiotherapy and Radiobiology, University of Vienna). Before new equipment can be used for clinical applications it is compulsory to check its performance and the quality of the intended treatment [Hartmann, 1995; Klein et al., 1995; Kutcher et al., 1995; Van Dyk et al., 1993]. The present work describes the measurements necessary for commissioning an mMLC. The paper reports on mechanical stability checks of the system linac plus mMLC and on the acquisition of basic disometric beam data. Additionally, preliminary results of the verification of the treatment planning system (TPS) are described, considering both calculations of relative dose distributions as well as monitor units calculations.

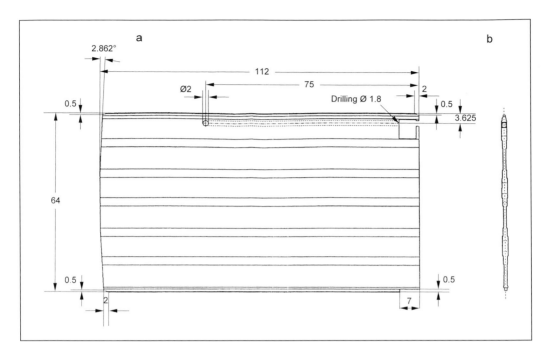

Fig. 1. a The three angled straight ends at the leaf tips to optimize beam penumbra (arc values in degrees, distance values in mm). *b* Display of the leaf cross-section showing the 'tongue and groove' design in order to keep interleaf leakage as small as possible.

Materials

mMLC System

The mMLC has two leaf banks, each consisting of 26 individually driven leaves (Brain-LAB, Germany). The leaf widths vary between 3 and 5.5 mm. Leaves are arranged symmetrically with respect to the collimator axis with the thinnest leaves closest to the collimator axis. With increasing distance from the collimator axis the leaf width increases. Each leaf can perform an overaxis travel of 5 cm, the maximum collimator opening of the mMLC is 10×10 cm^2 (at the isocenter).

The leaf edges have a special shape with three angled straight ends (fig. 1a) in order to reduce leaf penumbra, and a 'tongue and groove' design to reduce interleaf leakage (fig. 1b).

The mMLC is controlled by two computers: the first one runs the driver software while the second one permanently displays the actual mMLC field (leaf positions), acts as control console, and as the link to the TPS. The mMLC and the interface computer are connected by fiberoptics (two emitters and two receivers), the two computers by a parallel cable. Using the control console, different field shapes or the position of a single leaf can be set. The leaf settings (entered manually or prescribed via TPS) are converted into optoelectronical signals driving the individual leaf motors. The actual leaf position is verified against the indented one and displayed on the control console. The manufacturer states a 0.5-mm threshold for the primary as well as for the secondary leaf position readout. This value can be considered as the leaf positioning accuracy.

Using a special mounting system (trolley and adapter plate) the mMLC (which weighs approx. 31 kg) can be attached to the treatment head of a GE Saturne 43 linac. This mounting system allows a fast and easy set-up of the mMLC.

Treatment planning for conformal radiotherapy with the mMLC is carried out using a software (BrainSCAN, Version 3.5) provided by the mMLC manufacturer (BrainLAB, Germany). This software runs on a DEC Alpha workstation and performs calculations of relative dose distributions and monitor units.

Equipment for Mechanical and Dosimetrical Measurements

Mechanical accuracy checks are performed using either paper with a millimeter grid or Kodak X-OmatV films [e.g. Boyer et al., 1992; Mubata et al., 1995]. All films are processed in a microprocessor-controlled film-processing machine providing very stable conditions (especially with respect to temperature). Subsequently, films are digitized with a VIDAR VXR-12 scanner and evaluated with a film densitometry software, running on a PC (Poseidon from Precitron, Sweden). A sensitometric calibration curve is introduced in the software to translate optical densities into relative doses. A more detailed description of the film evaluation procedure has been described previously [Novotny et al., 1997; Georg et al., 1997].

All dosimetric measurements are performed for a 6-MV photon beam, since this is the energy used in clinics. Films are irradiated at 5 cm depth in a solid water phantom ($30 \times 30 \times 20$ cm^3), and 15 cm of solid water behind the film is used to ensure sufficient backscatter.

An ionization chamber (PTW 23323, 0.1 cm^3) and a silicon diode (Scanditronix EDP 10, sensitive volume 0.8 mm^3, 1.5 mm diameter of sensitive area) are used for output ratio measurements in a large full scatter water phantom (PTW, MP3 scanning system, Germany). The same ionization chamber and water phantom are used to measure cross-beam profiles and depth dose curves.

In order to check the TPS, absolute dose measurements are performed in a specially designed head-shaped water phantom. This phantom is a water-filled glass containing an adjustable positioning system. This system allows a precise positioning of different measuring systems, e.g. ionization chambers, silicon diodes and thermoluminescent dosimeters (TLDs).

The procedure to set up the head-shaped phantom is the same used for patient positioning in clinical routine. First a computer tomography-based three-dimensional (3D) treatment planning is performed, utilizing a special localizer providing 3D stereotactic localization of the patient's head. Treatment plans of simple circular or rectangular field shapes are verified using the different measurement systems in the head phantom. Treatment parameters (monitor units, table and gantry angle, position of the secondary collimator jaws, leaf position) are printed and the field shapes are exported via network to the control console. Besides calculations of relative dose distribution and monitor units, the planning software provides positioning charts. They can be fixed on a target-positioning device used for patient set-up. Thus the identical irregular treatment field, for a given gantry and table angle combination, can be visually checked against the actual field set-up.

Methods

Mechanical Checks

The first step of the commissioning procedure is the investigation of the mechanical performance of the system mMLC + linac. Initial tests are performed for a 10×10 cm^2 field size (at the isocenter plane) at gantry angle 0° and collimator angle 270°. This set-up will be referred to in the following as 'start position'.

The leaf positioning accuracy is checked at the 'start position' using a millimeter grid paper. Several square fields (side length: 18, 24, 30, 36, 42, 51, 60, 69, 80 and 91 mm) and circular fields (diameter: 18, 24, 30, 36, 42, 51, 60, 69, 80 and 91 mm) set by the mMLC control console are checked visually for geometrical accuracy against light field. The field diameters of circular fields are optimized in order to achieve the best beam shape taking into account the finite leaf width.

The light field-irradiation field congruence is checked with films for all field sizes described above. Films are irradiated at the isocenter plane at 5 cm depth in solid water with 30 monitor units (MU). 15 cm of solid water is placed behind the films as backscatter material.

In order to test the positioning reproducibility, i.e. the repositioning accuracy, an automatic routine supplied in the mMLC driving software is used. This routine adjusts automatically 100 different fields, where the last field set-up is the initial one.

The isocenter accuracy is checked with the so-called Winston-Lutz test using an 18-mm circular field shaped by the mMLC [Lutz et al., 1988]. A film is placed at a focus film distance of 140 cm on the electronic portal image device (EPID). For the Winston-Lutz test the secondary collimator of the linac is set to 10×10 cm^2. Additionally several spoke shots are performed at different gantry and table angles in order to determine the rotational accuracy of gantry and collimator. The films are analyzed using a paper with millimeter grid and templates with predefined circles ('inner and outer' circles diameter).

Basic Dosimeter Beam Data

The basic dosimetric data set is acquired in the 'start position' for all circular and square fields described above. Cross-beam profiles are measured in the water phantom with an ionization chamber at the depth of maximum dose (1.5 cm for 6 MV) as well as at 10 cm depth, in both X- and Y-direction at a constant SSD of 100 cm. Additionally, films are irradiated at the isocenter at a depth of 5 cm in the solid water phantom and evaluated with the film densitometry system.

Percentage depth dose (PDD) curves are measured along the central axis of the beam using the same experimental set-up (ionization chamber) as for cross-beam profile measurements.

In the present work, output ratios for the mMLC are defined as dose ratios without a tertiary collimator and with the added mMLC, for a given secondary collimator setting and the same number of MUs. Output ratios are measured at a depth of 5 cm. This definition is somewhat different as compared to conventionally used output factor definitions for mMLCs being a tertiary collimator system [Palta et al., 1994]. The relation between the nominal output of the linac (geometry used for beam calibration: 10×10 cm^2 secondary collimator setting, 100 MU, 10 cm depth) and the output of the system with mMLC is taken from PDD and output factor tables. Output ratios are measured for three different secondary collimator settings (3×3, 6×6 and 10×10 cm^2) in a full scatter phantom with a silicon diode as well as with an ionization chamber [Karlsson et al., 1997].

Verification of the TPS

Calculated monitor units are verified by ionization chamber measurements (at the isocenter) in the head-shaped radiosurgery phantom. The measured dose is compared with the dose stated by the TPS. Using the head phantom, a whole patient treatment is performed, containing all steps from treatment planning to treatment delivery (image acquisition, 3D planning, irradiation). Measurements are carried out for three square field sizes and three circular field sizes (dimensions: large –91 mm; medium –51 mm; small –30 mm) taking into account the mMLC capabilities for field definition. For these fields a $10 \times 10 \text{ cm}^2$ secondary collimator setting is used. Additionally irregular field shapes similar to clinically applied field shapes are investigated (secondary collimator setting $10 \times 10 \text{ cm}^2$).

Results

Mechanical Accuracy

As described previously, an automatic routine of the mMLC driver software is used to check the mechanical reproducibility. After a cycle of 100 different fields, none of the investigated fields showed a deviation larger than ± 0.4 mm from the initial leaf position.

Isocenter Deviation

The results of the Winston-Lutz test performed with the mMLC are comparable to those obtained with the circular collimators (mean value of the deviation at the isocenter level: 0.8 ± 0.35 mm). The collimator spoke shots showed a deviation of approximately ± 0.6 mm, while the gantry spoke shot showed a maximum deviation of ± 1.1 mm.

Basic Dosimetric Data Set
Beam Cross-Profiles

Beam penumbra (defined as the lateral distance between the 80% and the 20% isodose) obtained from the film dosimetry are of the same order of magnitude as the results of ionization chamber measurements. Beam penumbra obtained with films are about 4 mm for all field sizes. Those determined with the ionization chamber vary between 5 and 5.5 mm, dependent on field size. For field sizes smaller in diameter than 30 mm, penumbra acquired with ionization chamber are slightly larger (5.8 mm). This can be explained by the limited spatial resolution of the ionization chamber.

The agreement between the actual beam diameter and the intended one is found to be very good when checking the dimensions of the measured 50% isodose line. With both film measurements as well as with ionization chamber measurements, the agreement is found to be within 0.3 mm.

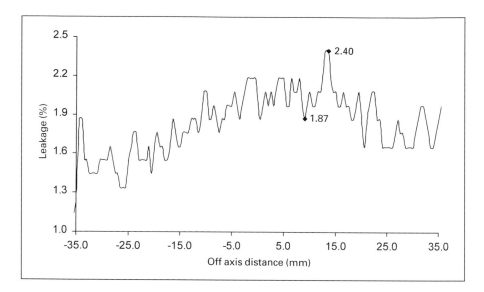

Fig. 2. Leakage scan performed with film dosimetry at a distance of 4.5 cm from the leaf tips at 5 cm depth (at the isocenter). The peak values represent interleaf leakage, the values between two peaks leaf transmission.

Leakage and transmission are determined using films irradiated at 5 cm depth in solid water. A profile at 4.5 cm distance from the leaf tip is shown in figure 2. The maximum peak value of such a scan represents the maximum interleaf leakage, the value between two peaks the leaf transmission. Leakage and transmission for this type of mMLC are determined as 2.4 and 1.9%, respectively (normalized to the dose at the central axis of a 10×10 cm^2 reference field without MLC). This is in good agreement with the results obtained by Cosgrove et al. [1997].

Figure 3 shows two profiles measured along the X- and Y-axis of a 30-mm circular field (secondary collimator setting 10×10 cm^2) where leaves are closed at the x = 0 position. Profile 1 is measured perpendicular to the direction of leaf movement along the x = 0 cm axis following the leaf junction line. From this profile the leaf tip transmission between fully closed opposed leaves is estimated. The transmission between two opposed abutting leaves reaches 12.5%. Profile 2 in figure 3 is acquired along the Y-direction parallel to the direction of leaf movement. Leaf transmission in this direction reaches only about 2%.

Figure 4 shows profiles of the same circular field measured with an ionization chamber, but leaves at 4.5 cm off axis position. The low-dose region of the upper curve (3) reflects an 'averaged' leakage and the transmission of

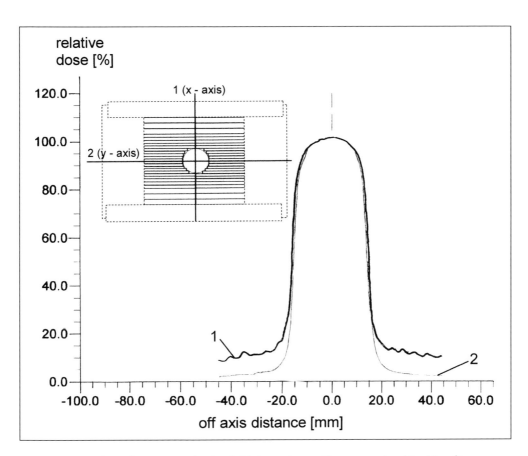

Fig. 3. Profiles of a 30-mm circular field (secondary collimator setting $10 \times 10 \text{ cm}^2$) measured with film dosimetry. The leaves are closed at on axis position. Curve 1 is acquired following the leaf junction line perpendicular to the direction of leaf movements, curve 2 in the direction parallel to the leaf movements following the $Y = 0$ axis.

about 3% in X-direction perpendicular to the direction of leaf movement. The lower curve (4) corresponds to curve 2 in figure 3.

The leaf tip transmission determined along the leaf junction line when leaves are closed at 4.5 cm off axis is only 7% (scan parallel to the X-axis 4.5 cm off axis in the set-up described with figure 4).

Percentage Depth Dose Curves

At larger depths, percentage depth dose curves show similar curve characteristics as without a tertiary collimator system. A detailed study of changes in the depth dose characteristics related to the added mMLC, e.g. the build-up region, is part of another study and will not be considered here.

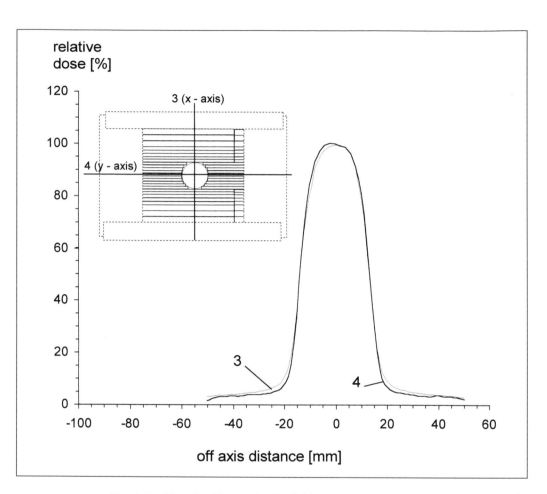

Fig. 4. Profiles of a 30-mm circular field (secondary collimator setting $10 \times 10 \text{ cm}^2$), measured with ionization chamber. Leaves are closed at 4.5 cm off axis position. Curve 3 is acquired in the central axis perpendicular to the direction of leaf movement, curve 4 corresponds to curve 2 in figure 3.

Output Ratios

For a fixed mMLC field size, output ratios depend on the secondary collimator setting. The output ratio variation with mMLC field size is shown in figure 5 as a function of secondary collimator setting. For a $3 \times 3 \text{ cm}^2$ field defined by the mMLC, with a fixed $10 \times 10 \text{ cm}^2$ secondary collimator setting, the output of the linac + mMLC decreases by about 10%.

Deviations between output ratios measured with an ionization chamber and those using diodes are observed for field sizes 30 mm in diameter. Deviations

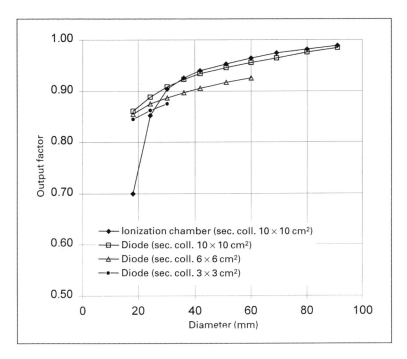

Fig. 5. Output ratio variation with field size as a function of mMLC setting and secondary collimator opening. The values are normalized to a 10×10 cm² secondary collimator opening without mMLC. Output ratios are determined with an ionization chamber as well as with a diode.

of 20% are observed for an 18-mm field size, and 5% for the 24-mm field. For larger field sizes both methods to determine output ratios agree within 2%.

Verification on the TPS

For small fields (e.g. 3 cm in diameter) an agreement of 3% between the calculated and measured dose values is found. This deviation increases with increasing diameter of the circular field (5 cm diameter resulted in 5% deviation) and reaches 9% for a field of 9 cm in diameter. The measured dose in the irregular field (about 2×3 cm outer field dimensions) shows a deviation of about 2% as compared to the dose stated by the TPS.

Discussion and Conclusion

The leaf positioning reproducibility (± 0.4 mm) fulfils the accuracy requirements to guarantee a reliable and reproducible mMLC field shaping.

The results of collimator and gantry spoke shots indicate no difference in geometrical accuracy as compared to the commonly used 'classical' stereotactic equipment. Hence it is concluded that a similar geometrical accuracy can be obtained with the mMLC as compared to the conventional circular collimator.

The combined results of leakage and transmission measurements and those of cross-beam profiles indicate the necessity of closing all leaves off axis which are not used to define the beam aperture. Even when leaves are not 'shielded' by the secondary collimator, transmission at the position of leaf junction line (in X-direction) is reduced from 12.5 to 7% by only closing leaves off axis instead of on axis.

The isodose evaluation of mMLC fields in planes perpendicular to the incident photon beam show the MLC inherent stair step effect. However, for most fields the 80% isodose line, which is used in our department as a reference to judge treatment plans, is rather smooth. However, the influence of the finite leaf width is not negligible. An example of an isodose evaluation is shown in figure 6. The investigation of the stair step effect at different depths, giving information about effective beam shape changes with increasing depth, will be considered in another study. These results will allow to draw conclusions concerning the dose to organs at risk (e.g. the optical nerve, or the lens for uveal melanoma treatments) related to the mMLC stair step effect.

For the same field size and larger depths, PDD values of mMLC-shaped fields show no significant differences as compared to the PDDs of fields defined by circular tungsten collimators. The changes in the build-up region, especially at depths close to the surface, have to be considered in a more detailed investigation. The different electron contamination of the two collimator systems may have an influence at shallow depths.

Output ratio measurements clearly indicate the necessity of a small volume detector when investigating small field sizes. The use of a fairly large ionization chamber is limited by its dimensions (3.5 mm diameter, 12 mm length). A diode or a diamond detector, if available, are considered to be superior for small field sizes. The length of the ionization chamber used in the present study limits the field size for which measurements can be carried out. Output ratios determined with the ionization chamber are underestimated by up to 20% for field sizes <30 mm in diameter (fig. 5). On the other hand, when measuring output ratios under full scatter conditions with diodes, special attention has to be paid for large field sizes [Karlsson et al., 1997]. At larger field sizes more low photon energies are present and the photoelectric interaction coefficient of Si relative to water can influence the results. The lower field size limit for output ratio measurements is given by the lateral distance necessary to ensure lateral electronic equilibrium for the detector volume. If electronic

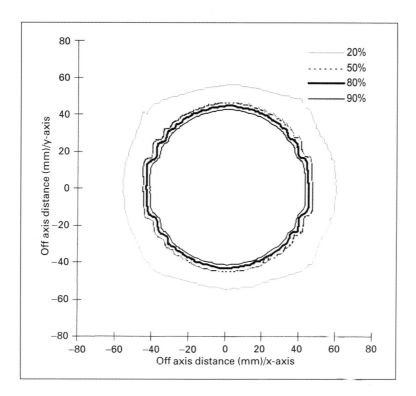

Fig. 6. Isodose display of a 91-mm circular field (secondary colliomator setting 10×10 cm^2) measured with film at 5 cm depth.

equilibrium is not fulfilled, absorbed dose cannot be directly obtained from measured ionization [Weber et al., 1997]. For 6-MV photon beams, results for fields < 18 mm in diameter or square field length have to be considered with caution [Li et al., 1995].

In order to keep the dose to healthy tissues as small as possible, the secondary collimator setting of the linac has to be optimized. Since the output ratio variation with field size is also determined by the secondary collimator setting, this effect can be easily accounted for in monitor unit calculations.

Large deviations are found between measured doses and the doses stated by the TPS for small mMLC fields as well as for large highly irregular fields. These large deviations might be explained by a fairly simple and coarse dose calculation algorithm of the planning system. Dosimetric quantities of irregular fields are approximated by those of a circular field encompassing the irregular field. For clinical routine this implies that special attention has to be paid for patients to be irradiated with small or highly irregular fields.

The results of cross-beam profiles obtained with film dosimetry are in good agreement with those obtained using an ionization chamber. However, films offer the advantage of giving two-dimensional information and a superior spatial resolution. These features make them an appropriate tool for isodose verification and for measurements of MLC inherent dosimetric characteristics, such as leakage and transmission, or the stair step effect due to finite leaf widths. When using films for such purposes, optical densities have to be carefully translated into relative dose values and the overresponse of films in low-dose regions must not be forgotten.

For absolute dose measurements, for determination of depth dose curves, and for output ratio measurements of large mMLC field sizes (>30 mm diameter) a small volume 'standard' ionization chamber can be used. But for small field dosimetry, smaller detectors (e.g. a diamond detector or a semiconductor detector) are required in order to ensure correct beam data acquisition. Accurate beam data acquisition and beam data implementation into the TPS is a prerequisite for accurate dose delivery to the patient. The clinical implementation of an mMLC requires special dosimetric tools with a high spatial resolution in order to achieve the necessary accuracy. 'Standard' dosimetric equipment generally used for dosimetry in external beam therapy has its inherent limitations when applied to stereotactic equipment.

Acknowledgments

The authors would like to thank the Department of Radiotherapy, U.Z. Leuven (Belgium), for making their film densitometry system available. Dr. Colotto is acknowledged for assisting in the preparation of the manuscript.

References

Boyer AL, Ochran TG, Nyerick CE, Waldron TJ, Huntzinger CJ: Clinical dosimetry for implementation of a multileaf collimator. Med Phys 1992;19:1255–1261.
Cosgrove V, Scheffler A, Mischel M, Bauer S, Budech V, Wurm R: Preliminary dosimetry and measurements with a computer-controlled micro-multileaf collimator (mMLC). Eighth Varian European Users Meeting, Vila Moura, Portugal, 1997.
Georg D, Julia F, Briot E, Huyskens D, Wolff U, Dutreix A: Dosimetric comparison of an integrated multileaf-collimator versus a conventional collimator. Phys Med Biol 1997;42:2285–2303.
Hartmann GH: Quality Assurance Program on Stereotactic Radiosurgery. Berlin, Springer, 1995.
Karlsson MG, Karlsson M, Sjögren R, Svensson H: Semi-conductor detectors in output factor measurements. Radiother Oncol 1997;42:293–296.
Klein EE, Harms WB, Low DA, Willcut V, Purdy JA: Clinical implementation of a commercial multileaf collimator: Dosimetry, networking, simulation and quality assurance. Int J Radiat Oncol Biol Phys 1995;33:1195–1208.
Kubo HD, Pappas CTE, Wilder RB: A comparison of arc-based and static mini-multileaf collimator-based radiosurgery treatments plans. Radiother Oncol 1997;45:89–93.

Kubo HD, Walder RB, Pappas C: Dose comparison of rotational multiarc vs static mini-MLC-based radiosurgery. Med Phys 1996;23:1052.

Kutcher GJ, Coia L, Gillin M, Hanson WF, Leibel S, Morton RJ, Palta JR, Purdy JA, Reinstein LE, Svensson GK, Weller M, Wingfield L: Comprehensive quality assurance for radiation oncology. Report of the AAPM Radiation Therapy Committee Task Group 40. Med Phys 1994;21: 581–618.

Li XA, Soubra M, Gerig LH: Lateral electronic equilibrium and electron contamination in measurements of head scatter factors using mini-phantoms and brass caps. Med Phys 1995;22:1167–1170.

Lutz W, Winston MD, Maleki N: A system for stereotactic radiosurgery with a linear accelerator. Int J Radiat Oncol Biol Phys 1988;14:373–381.

Marks LB, Sherouse WG, Das S, Bentel GC, Spencer DP, Turner D: Conformal radiation therapy with fixed shaped coplanar or noncoplanar radiation beam bouquets: A possible alternative to radiosurgery. Int J Radiat Oncol Biol Phys 1995;33:1209–1219.

Mubata CD, Childs P, Bidmead AM: A quality assurance procedure for a Varian multi-leaf collimator. Phys Med Biol 1995;42:423–431.

Nedzi LA, Kooy HM, Alexander E III, Svensons GK, Loeffler JS: Dynamic field shaping for stereotactic radiosurgery: Modelling study. Int J Radiat Oncol Biol Phys 1993;25:859–869.

Novotny J, Gomola I, Izewska J, Huyskens D, Dutreix A: External audit of photon beams by mailed film dosimetry: Feasibility study. Phys Med Biol 1997;42:1277–1288.

Palta JR, Yeung DK, Frouhar V: Dosimetric considerations for a multieaf collimator system. Med Phys 1994;23:1219–1224.

Van Dyk J, Bernett RB, Cygler JE, Shragge PC: Commissioning and quality assurance of treatment planning computers. Int J Radiat Oncol Biol Phys 1993;26:261–273.

Weber L, Nilsson P, Ahnesjö A: Build-up cap materials for measurement of photon head scatter factors. Phys Med Biol 1997;42:1875–1886.

Dr. U. Wolff, Department of Radiotherapy and Radiobiology, University of Vienna,
Währinger Gürtel 18–20, AH 1090 Vienna (Austria)
Tel. +43 1 40400 26 92, Fax +43 1 40400 26 93

Wiegel T, Hinkelbein W, Brock M, Hoell T (eds): Controversies in Neuro-Oncology.
Front Radiat Ther Oncol. Basel, Karger, 1999, vol 33, pp 64–77

....

Commissioning of a Micro-Multileaf Collimator for Conformal Stereotactic Radiosurgery and Radiotherapy

R.E. Wurm, V.P. Cosgrove, L. Schlenger, A. Kaiser, G. Zeunert, S. Dinges, J. Bohsung, J. Groll, M. Pfaender, S. Bauer, G. Leonhardt, U. Jahn, M. Stuschke, V. Budach

Klinik für Strahlentherapie, Charité, Humboldt University, Berlin, Germany

Introduction

Stereotactic radiosurgery (SRS) and radiotherapy (SRT) seeks to maximize the radiation dose to damage or destroy an intracranial pathological process while minimizing the dose to nearby, uninvolved, normal brain. This process involves accurately tailoring a dose of radiation to match the shape of a target volume in three dimensions. Linear accelerator-based SRS and SRT is conventionally carried out with circular collimators using single or multiple isocentres, non-coplanar arcing techniques. As an alternative, conformal SRS and SRT (CSRS/T) using an adjustable collimator to conform the beam profile by non-coplanar, individually shaped static beams to a target cross-section in the 'beam's eye view' can be employed [2, 16, 17, 22, 25, 26, 31, 32]. CSRS/T offers a number of advantages over conventional, arcing techniques, in instances such as larger nonspherical irregularly shaped targets within 5 mm of a critical structure, and holds the potential to improve the dose delivery in the vast majority of the SRS and SRT caseload. These advantages include improved normal tissue sparing, more homogeneous dose distributions throughout the target volume and reduced treatment times [2, 17, 23–25, 29].

The design and use of multileaf collimators (MLCs) is now well established, and MLCs are currently regarded as the state-of-the-art device for producing arbitrary, irregularly shaped radiation fields [3, 6, 10, 11, 15, 18, 20, 27]. The advantage of automatic field-shaping devices over conventional lead alloy shielding blocks has also been documented [7, 8, 14, 21]. More recently, MLCs have been shown to have the additional potential for modulating the intensity of radiation across a field [1, 4, 5, 13, 19, 31, 35]. Conformation of dose to small intracranial targets (up to 5 cm in cross-section) using conventional MLCs is impeded by the relatively large leaf width at isocentre (usually > 0.5 cm). To overcome this problem, linear accelerator-based SRS and SRT of these small targets using static non-coplanar beams have up to now been carried out using lead alloy blocks or manually shaped miniature multileaves [2, 9, 22, 28]. Between four and eight static beams shaped using 3D beams eye view image displays are normally used in clinical routine. The process of treatment delivery can be very time consuming and laboured in terms of block construction or manual field shaping, verification and treatment delivery. There has, therefore, been much interest in developing an automated, miniature MLC to improve dose conformation to small target volumes as well as take advantage of the known labour and time-saving attributes of a computer-controlled field-shaping device.

Materials and Methods

We report the dosimetric measurements, initial acceptance testing and commissioning of the m3 computer-controlled micro-MLC (m3). The measurements were principally used to verify that the features of the m3, such as leaf design, positioning and monitoring, fulfilled the demands for high precision, SRT applications. Beam data was then collected and transferred to a BrainSCAN v3.5 stereotactic planning system and used to calculate conformal, multiple-field, non-coplanar treatment plans. Further measurements were carried out in phantom to compare and verify the calculated and delivered dose distributions.

The m3 micro-MLC (a joint development project between BrainLAB GmbH, Germany, and Varian Inc., USA) is a detachable device mounted to the accessory rails of our departmental Varian 2100C Clinac by a specially designed trolley (fig. 1a, b, table 1). The m3 has 26 pairs of tungsten leaves of variable width, which move perpendicularly to the beam central axis (i.e. unfocused). 14 pairs of 3-mm wide leaves are located in the centre of the field area and 6 pairs each of 4.5- and 5.5-mm wide leaves to the edge. From this a maximum square field size of 10.2×10 cm^2 can be defined at isocentre. Loaded onto the linac the m3 connects to a power supply located within the gantry head. Communication to a computer controller, located outside the treatment room, is made via four fibreoptic cables preinstalled within the linac with external, quick-release sockets on the gantry head. Following connection, a leaf initialization process is performed. This involves a software module systematically moving each leaf to break a fine infrared beam located within the m3 casing. The position of each leaf can then be calibrated to an accuracy of 0.1 mm. The mounting and initialization procedure is straightforward and is usually completed within 5–10 min.

All measurements were carried out using 6-MV x-rays, since there is no significant difference between dose distributions at megavoltage energies ranging from 4 to 24 MV [29]. Diagnostic film (X-OMAT V2, Kodak, Inc., Rochester, NY, USA) was principally used for

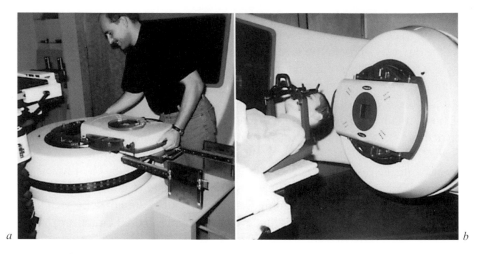

a   b

Fig. 1. a Installation of the m3. *b* The m3 in use.

Table 1. Design specifications of the m3 micro-MLC

Number of leaves	52 (26 pairs)
Leaf width at isocentre	28×3.0, 12×4.5, 12×5.5 mm
Maximum field size	10.2×10 cm
Maximum leaf over-travel	5 cm (across the entire field)
Direction of leaf movement	Parallel to Y jaws
Clearance from isocentre	31 cm
Maximum leaf speed	1.5 cm/s
Weight	30 kg (mounts to gantry using a purpose-built trolley)

dosimetry with films scanned using a computer-controlled digital densitometer (FIPS Plus Laser Scanner, PTW GmBH, Freiburg, Germany). For measurements of leaf transmission, leakage and penumbra, films were positioned perpendicularly to the beam central axis in Solid Water at a depth of 1.5 cm (d_{max}), SSD = 98.5 cm and with the primary jaws of the linac set to 10×10 cm^2. 80–20% beam penumbra was measured as a function of square field size for fields ranging from 2×2 to 10×10 cm^2 in steps of ~ 1 cm. Films were scanned both perpendicular and parallel to leaf motion (i.e. across leaf sides and leaf ends, respectively). The variation in the effective beam penumbra was also investigated as a function of straight but diagonal field edges.

An irregularly shaped phantom was constructed from a hollow aluminium form and Optosil® P dental impression material. The phantom shape was fixed to a BrainLAB stereotactic head frame and CT scanned with slice thickness of 1.5 mm. The data was transferred

Table 2. RTOG Quality Assurance Guidelines and TV/V$_{50\%}$ ratio

	MDPD ratio	PI/TV ratio	TV/V$_{50\%}$ ratio
Per protocol	≤2.0	1–2	≥0.3
Minor deviation (acceptable)	>2 and ≤2.5	>0.9 and <1.0 or >2.0 and <2.5	
Major deviation (unacceptable)	>2.5	<0.9 and ≥2.5	

to the BrainSCAN v3.5 planning system and, using the outer phantom surface as a target volume, conformal m3 fields were shaped using various combinations of collimator, gantry and table angle. The phantom was then irradiated at the defined isocentre position and Portal Vision™ images were collected for each field.

The spatial accuracy of the isodose calculations produced by the planning system was verified using film and a cubic, Solid Water phantom. This was constructed from 14.8×14.8 cm^2 sheets of Solid Water, ranging in thickness from 1 mm to 1 cm. The cubic shape enabled films to be positioned in either the axial, sagittal or coronal planes by simply changing the orientation of the phantom. Various target shapes were defined in various positions within the phantom and six-field, non-coplanar plans were calculated. The treatment isocentre position was marked on each film and was used as the dose normalization point after the film was scanned.

Absolute dose values were measured using an Alderson RANDO® anthropomorphic head phantom and 0.5×6 mm LiF TLDs. The phantom was also fixed inside a stereotactic head frame, immobilized using self-penetrating head pins and CT scanned in the usual way. Six-field, non-coplanar, conformal treatment plans were calculated using arbitrary target volume shapes ranging in size from ~5 to 20 cm^3. Several TLD chips were loaded inside the phantom at the isocentre position. Care was taken so that the planned dose distributions were homogeneous over the length of the TLD chips. TLDs with a reproducibility of ≤3% were selected for the measurements.

Treatment planning differences between non-coplanar arcing techniques around single or multiple isocentres and multiple fixed static conformally shaped beams were assessed by the RTOG Quality Assurance Guidelines [30], and the dose gradient achieved outside the target volume (table 2). The RTOG Guidelines define dose homogeneity within the target volume by the ratio of the maximum dose to the prescription dose (MD/PD ratio). The conformation of the prescription dose to the target is defined by the ratio of the prescription isodose surface volume to the target volume (PIV/TV ratio). The dose gradient achieved outside the target is defined as the ratio of the target volume (TV) to the volume encompassed by the 50% isodose (TV/V50% ratio). Times for treatment set-up and delivery were assessed comparing data from patients treated with non-coplanar arcing techniques and the m3.

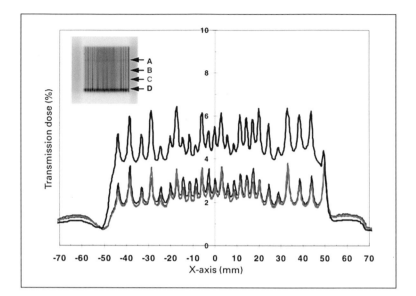

Fig. 2. Transmission through bank A leaves.

Results

Figure 2 illustrates the relative dose distributions obtained from scans across a single bank of leaves (leaves were moved to abut with the opposing leaves 4.5 cm off-axis). Transmission through the leaves had maximum and minimum values of 3.7 and 1.7%, respectively. The mean leakage between leaves was calculated to be $2.8 \pm 0.15\%$, and the mean transmission through the leaves $1.9 \pm 0.1\%$. At the points where opposing leaves abut (scan D), transmission has a maximum value of 6.4% and a mean of $4.5 \pm 0.6\%$. Further scans were made at positions A and C to investigate whether the leaves diverged from each other when extended beyond the central axis. No significant increase in leakage was observed towards the leaf ends. A slight increase in transmission ($\sim 0.3\%$) was observed for scan A, -19.7 mm from the central axis. This coincides with the location of 2-mm diameter holes drilled through the side of each leaf, used to immobilize the leaves during the manufacturing process. The variation of 80–20% beam penumbra as a function of square field size is plotted in figure 3. Penumbra did not vary with field size with any statistical significance, perpendicularly or parallel to leaf motion (i.e. across leaf sides and leaf ends, respectively). Mean 80–20% penumbra values are 2.45 ± 0.1 mm perpendicular to leaf motion and 2.6 ± 0.1 mm parallel with leaf motion. Figure 4 plots a field shape created by defining a number of diagonal, straight

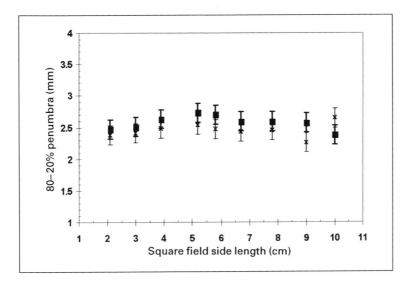

Fig. 3. 80–20% beam penumbra for square fields shapes. × = Perpendicular to leaf motion; ■ = parallel to leaf motion.

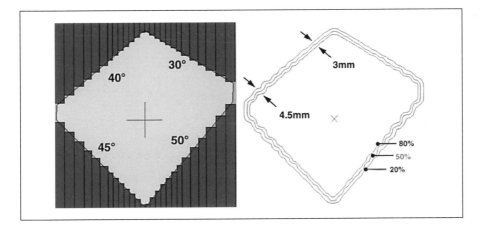

Fig. 4. Two irregular field shapes formed from diagonal, straight field edges. Measured 80, 50 and 20% isodose lines are indicated.

field edges with the indicated angles to the Y-jaws. Beside the field shape are the 20, 50 and 80% isodoses measured with film. The sinusoidal variation in the isodose lines occurs due to the stepping effect between leaf ends. The broadening of the effective 80–20% penumbra resulted as a function of the angle of the diagonal. This broadening is not constant over the whole length of each field edge, due to the variable width of the leaves.

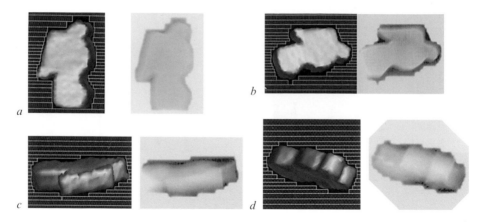

Fig. 5a–d. Four conformal m3 fields shaped to a phantom with corresponding Portal Vision™ images.

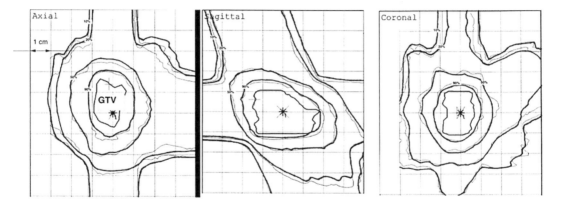

Fig. 6. Isodose distributions for an irregular target volume irradiated with 6 non-coplanar conformal fields. ——— = Film measurements; ——— = BrainSCAN v3.5 calculations.

Four BEV images of the irregularly shaped phantom, as displayed on the BrainSCAN treatment planning system and the respective portal images that were acquired, are shown in figure 5a–d. Measurements using the Portal Vision™ software indicated that the separation between the phantom and m3 field edges was always within 1 mm.

The measured and calculated isodose distributions in the axial, sagittal and coronal orthogonal planes for an irregularly shaped target volume planned and irradiated with six non-coplanar fields are plotted in figure 6. The 6.8-cm³ irregular target volume, transcribed from a patient data set, has dimensions

Table 3. Absolute dose measurements with TLDs in an Alderson phantom

Target volume, cm^3	Planned dose, Gy	Measured dose, Gy
5.8	1.5	1.47 ± 0.07
6.8	1.5	1.53 ± 0.07
19.7	1.5	1.51 ± 0.05

Table 4. Volume of normal tissue contained by the 10–90% isodose lines for an elliptically shaped target with a volume of 7.42 cm^3 treated to the 90% isodose line (20 Gy) with a single and multiple isocentres (5) versus multiple conformally shaped static (6 and 25) beams

Isodose line, %	Normal tissue volume (cm^3) contained by the isodose line			
	single isocentre	multiple (5) isocentre	6 static beams	25 static beams
90	11.31	4.38	1.90	1.36
80	17.99	6.24	4.28	3.90
70	24.46	8.82	7.49	6.44
60	33.14	12.74	11.09	9.46
50	46.65	18.70	17.77	13.73
40	69.36	28.93	31.78	21.21
30	107.91	48.54	57.81	37.52
20	186.44	95.71	165.73	92.70
10	405.83	256.97	269.95	285.99

of approximately $3 \times 2 \times 1.5$ cm. The target was positioned within the cubic phantom so that the treatment isocentre was on the central axial plane but displaced laterally so that it was 30 mm from the left phantom surface.

The measurements of absolute dose obtained with the TLDs for three separate conformal treatment plans using the RANDO head phantom are listed in table 3. The errors represent 1 SD on the mean dose.

Table 4 shows for an ellipsoid shaped target of 7.6 cm^3 in the posterior fossa the volume of normal tissue enclosed by the 10–90% isodose by a single and five isocentre as well as a six and twenty-five static conformally shaped plan prescribed to the 90% isodose. The single isocentre treatment plan offers a MD/PD ratio of 1.25, a PIV/TV ratio of 2.5, and a TV/V$_{50\%}$ ratio of 0.14. For the five isocentre plan the MD/PD ratio is 1.84, the PIV/TV ratio 1.6, and the TV/V$_{50\%}$ ratio 0.28. The volume of normal tissue enclosed by the 10–90% isodose lines is 1.6–2.9 times greater for the single isocentre plan, compared to the five isocentre plan. For the six and twenty-five static beam

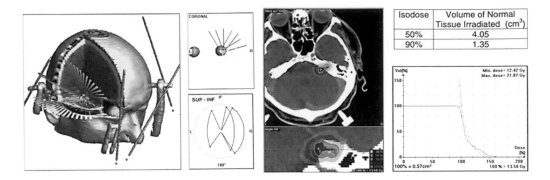

Fig. 7. Vestibular schwannoma treated using two isocentres and eight arced beams.

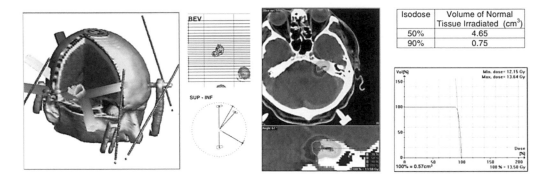

Fig. 8. Vestibular schwannoma treated using a single isocentre and six conformal m3 beams.

plan the MD/PD ratio is 1.25, the PIV/TV ratio 1.3 and 1.2, and the $TV/V_{50\%}$ ratio 0.29 and 0.35, respectively. The volume of normal tissue enclosed by the 10–90% isodose lines for the six static beam is 0.9–1.5 times the volume contained within the same isodose lines by the twenty-five static beam plan. On the contrary, the volume of normal tissue enclosed by the multiple isocentre plan is especially in the high dose area around the 90% isodose line up to 3.2 times greater compared to both static beam plans.

In figures 7 and 8 a small vestibular schwannoma (TV 0.57 cm³; longest dimension 17 mm, shortest 3 mm) is depicted. The vestibular schwannoma's location poses two distinct challenges. First, acoustic schwannomas are often irregular in shape, which can be aggravated by the underlying bony anatomy. Second, the nearby brainstem, and trigeminal nerve as well as the direct involvement of the facial and acoustic nerve need to be considered as structures carrying a considerable risk of serious radiation induced late adverse normal tissue effects. An optimum arc plan required in this case two isocentres (PIV/TV ratio 2.1 and $TV/V_{50\%}$ ratio 0.14) and, therefore, lead to dose inhomogeneity within and around the acoustic schwannoma (MD/PD ratio 1.5). The m3 plan, using six non-coplanar fields, provided a much more homogeneous dose distribution (MD/PD ratio 1.25) while at the same time irradiating a smaller volume of surrounding, normal tissue (PIV/TV ratio 2.1 and $TV/V_{50\%}$ ratio 0.12). However, the volume of normal brain enclosed by the two isocentre plan was in the high dose area around the 90% isodose line by a factor of two greater compared to the single isocentre plan using six static beams.

The m3 micro-MLC is currently being used clinically for CSRS/T. An assessment of the first 40 patients treated shows that one of the main practical advantages of using the m3 is that very irregularly shaped target volumes can now be treated using single isocentres instead of employing multiple isocentre arcing plans. This can considerably reduce the amount of time spent by a physicist planning and also the time spent by a patient being irradiated. A comparison with 87 patients treated with SRS using one or multiple isocentres showed that a single isocentre treatment with arcs or m3 fields can take about 20–30 min in treatment time. Multiple isocentre treatments required a further 15–20 min per isocentre. Based on our departmental quality assurance programme involving light-field checks of each beam both at isocentre and on projected films attached to the patient positioning box, together with the m3 installation and initialization, an extra 20-min treatment preparation time can be necessary compared to a treatment with arcs.

Discussion

SRS and SRT has gained widespread acceptance for the treatment of both benign and malignant intracranial lesions with high cure rates and minimal complications. Necessary requirements for this reputation is the combination of highly precise systems for treatment delivery and a maximum degree of dose conformality achieved in the treatment planning process.

The dosimetric characteristics of the m3 micro-MLC have proved to conform to the manufacturer's specification (leaf leakage <4%). Transmission through and leakage between leaves are slightly higher than those reported elsewhere for the standard Varian MLC. For 6-MV x-rays, mean values of 2.0% for leaf leakage and 1.5% for leaf transmission were measured [11, 15]. However, the values are still lower than for standard lead-alloy shielding blocks of similar thickness. For 6-MV x-rays, transmission values of around 3.5–4% were reported [11, 15].

Values for beam penumbrae were seen be small and did not significantly vary as a function of leaf position. The width of the leaves of the m3 can cause additional broadening of the beam penumbra when fitted to diagonal, straight field edges, due to the stepping between leaf ends. This broadening, however, is significantly smaller than has been reported with an MLC with 1-cm wide leaves at isocentre [27].

From the comparisons between planned fields and portal films (fig. 5a–d) it was clearly seen that the m3 was correctly and accurately shaped to the phantom structure. Image reconstruction of the phantom shape by the planning software agreed well with the portal images. It should be noted that this test is also a verification of the accuracy of CT localization, target positioning and irradiation. The Portal Vision™ software made it possible to measure the separation between the phantom and m3 field edges. In all cases an accuracy of within 1 mm was observed.

Of the irregular target volumes so far investigated, calculations of dose distribution using the BrainSCAN v3.5 planning system have compared well with measured distributions using TLDs and film. In figure 6, comparisons between the calculated dose distributions and the film measurements were most consistent with the higher isodose values ($\geq 50\%$) where curves were spatially correct to ~ 1 mm. Larger deviations (up to 5 mm) were only observed between the lower (10 and 20%) isodose curves.

Most linear accelerator SRS and SRT groups are currently using a certain number of multiple non-coplanar arcs and isocentre techniques focused on a target to achieve the necessary high dose conformity. This treatment essentially relies on a number of circular collimators and spherically symmetric beam placements, and the resultant dose distribution is therefore spherical. The standard arc set used at the Charité takes into account that the volume outside the target treated to more than 50% of the prescribed dose is not further reduced by increasing the number of arcs above four arcs [12, 29]. For irregular-shaped targets dose conformity has been optimized until the clinical commissioning of the m3 by the use of single or multiple isocentres and manipulation of arc weighting, collimator diameter, arc start and stop angle. Since then, we have been able to achieve substantial normal tissue sparing in the region treated to more than 50% of the prescribed dose with m3 plans compared to conventional arc plans. As shown for an ellipsoid target (table 3) in the majority of cases treated so far we did not find any improvement in normal tissue sparing by increasing the number of static beams above six. This result is in agreement with the comparison between static conformal beams and non-coplanar arcs by Laing et al. [17]. It should be noted that the benefit of using multiple isocentre non-coplanar arcs and static conformal beams becomes less pronounced for small targets below 1 cm^3 and the ratio TV/V$_{50\%}$ shows a loss of beam penumbra for both techniques. The advantage of static beams in SRS and SRT is obvious. In SRS and SRT there is an inevitable need to spare sensitive structures, such as the chiasm, other cranial nerves, and eloquent areas, in the direct vicinity of the target volume. Therefore, comparisons of treatment techniques and plans based on the assessment of dose-volume histograms, the RTOG Guidelines and the ratio $TV/V_{50\%}$ alone neglect that the steep dose gradient at the field border is only fully effective for static beams. On the other hand, a disadvantage may be that larger areas of normal tissue might receive a relatively high dose in comparison to non-coplanar arcing techniques. Our own preliminary results indicate that in this situation the dose distribution may be further optimized by dynamic adjustment of shaped fields with the m3 during arcing. However, more work has to be done to investigate and qualify the plans and dose delivery, and to generate on-line warning interrupts if the dynamic field shapes do not match the predicted shapes.

Conclusions

All the tests with the m3 micro-MLC and BrainSCAN v3.5 stereotactic treatment planning system have indicated that a target volume can be accurately irradiated to the precision demanded by radiosurgery applications. Significant normal tissue sparing in the region treated to more than 50% of the prescribed dose can be achieved with m3 plans compared to conventional arc plans. The use of micro-MLC for CSRS/T should therefore have impact on the probability of treatment-related complications, particularly for lesions located close to critical structures. Furthermore, the rigors and times of treatment planning and irradiation can be substantially reduced when using the m3, given that there is a clear universal tendency to use more and more isocentres and smaller collimators to ensure better conformation of the prescription dose to the target. It is likely that the widespread availability of the m3 and other automated micro-MLC yet to come will dramatically modify treatment techniques for SRS and SRT within the next years.

Acknowledgements

This work has been supported by grants from the Bundesministerium für Bildung, Wissenshaft, Forschung und Technologie, Germany (Grant No. AWO256897, R.E. Wurm) and the Deutsche Forschungsgemeinschaft, Germany (Grant Wu 229/1). Initial discussions and advice on film dosimetry from Andreas Scheffler (Universitäts Klinikum Benjamin Franklin, Berlin, Germany) is also acknowledged.

References

1 Bortfeld TR, Kahler DL, Waldron TJ, Boyer AL: X-ray field compensation with multileaf collimators. Int J Radiat Oncol Biol Phys 1994;28:723–30.
2 Bourland JD, McCollough KP: Static field conformal stereotactic radiosurgery: Physical techniques. Int J Radiat Oncol Biol Phys 1994;28:471–479.
3 Brewster L, Mohan R, Mageras G, Burman C, Leibel S, Fuks Z: Three-dimensional conformal treatment planning with multileaf collimators. Int J Radiat Oncol Biol Phys 1995;33:1081–1089.
4 Burman C, Chui CS, Kutcher G, Leibel S, Zelefsky M, LoSasso T, Spirou S, Wu Q, Yang J, Stein J, Mohan R, Fuks Z, Ling CC: Planning, delivery, and quality assurance of intensity modulated radiotherapy using dynamic multileaf collimator: A strategy for large-scale implementation for the treatment of carcinoma of the prostate. Int J Radiat Oncol Biol Phys 1997;39:863–873.
5 Chui CS, LoSasso T, Spirou S: Dose calculation for photon beams with intensity modulation generated by dynamic jaw or multileaf collimations. Med Phys 1994;21:1237–1244.
6 Du MN, Yu CX, Symons M, Yan D, Taylor R, Matter RC, Gustafson G, Martinez A, Wong JW: A multileaf collimator field prescription preparation system for conventional radiotherapy. Int J Radiat Oncol Biol Phys 1995;32:513–520.
7 Fernandez EM, Shentall GS, Mayles WP, Dearnaley DP: The acceptability of a multileaf collimator as a replacement for conventional blocks. Radiother Oncol 1995;36:65–74.
8 Frazier A, Yan D, Du M, Wong J, Vicini F, Matter R, Joyce M, Martinez A: Effects of treatment setup variation on beam's eye view dosimetry for radiation therapy using the multileaf collimator vs the cerrobend block. Int J Radiat Oncol Biol Phys 1995;33:1247–1256.
9 Gademann G, Schlegel G, Debus J, Schad L, Bortfeld T, Hover KH, Lorenz WJ, Wannenmacher M: Fractionated stereotactically guided radiotherapy of head and neck tumours: A report on clinical use of a new system in 195 cases. Radiother Oncol 1993;29:205–213.
10 Galvin JM, Smith AR, Moeller RD, Goodman RL, Powlis WD, Rubenstein J, Solin LJ, Michael B, Needham M, Huntzinger CJ, et al: Evaluation of multileaf collimator design for a photon beam. Int J Radiat Oncol Biol Phys 1992;23:789–801. [Published erratum appears in Int J Radiat Oncol Biol Phys 1992;24:579.]
11 Galvin JM, Smith A, Lally B: Characterization of a multileaf collimator system. Int J Radiat Oncol Biol Phys 1993;25:181–192.
12 Galvin JM, Chen XG, Smith RM: Combining multileaf fields to modulate fluence distributions. Int J Radiat Oncol Biol Phys 1993;27:697–705.
13 Graham JD, Nahum AE, Brada M: A comparison of techniques for stereotactic radiotherapy by linear accelerator based on 3-dimensional dose distributions. Radiother Oncol 1991;22:29–35.
14 Helyer SJ, Heisig S: Multileaf collimation versus conventional shielding blocks: A time and motion study of beam shaping in radiotherapy. Radiother Oncol 1995;37:61–64.
15 Klein EE, Harms WB, Low DA, Willcut V, Purdy JA: Clinical implementation of a commercial multileaf collimator: Dosimetry, networking, simulation and quality assurance. Int J Radiat Oncol Biol Phys 1995;33:1195–1208.
16 Kubo HD, Pappas CTE, Wilder RB: A comparison of arc-based and static mini-multileaf collimator based radiosurgery treatment plans. Radiother. Oncol 1997;45:89–93.
17 Laing RW, Bentley RE, Nahum AE, Warrington AP, Brada M: Stereotactic radiotherapy of irregular targets: A comparison between static conformal beams and non-coplanar arcs. Radiother Oncol 1993;28:241–246.
18 Leibel SA, Kutcher GJ, Zelefsky MJ, Burman CM, Mohan R, Ling CC, Fuks Z: 3-D conformal radiation therapy at the Memorial Sloan Kettering Cancer Centre. Radiat Oncol 1992;2:274–289.
19 Ling CC, Burman C, Chui CS, Kutcher GJ, Leibel SA, LoSasso T, Mohan R, Bortfeld T, Reinstein L, Spirou S, Wang XH, Wu Q, Zelefsky M, Fuks Z: Conformal radiation treatment of prostate cancer using inversely planned intensity modulated photon beams produced with dynamic multileaf collimation. Int J Radiat Oncol Biol Phys 1996;35:721–730.
20 LoSasso T, Chui CC, Kutcher GJ, Leibel SA, Fuks Z, Ling CC: The use of a multileaf collimator for conformal radiotherapy of carcinomas of the prostate and nasopharynx. Int J Radiat Oncol Biol Phys 1993;25:161–170.

21   LoSasso T, Kutcher GJ: Multileaf collimation versus alloy blocks: Analysis of geometric accuracy. Int J Radiat Oncol Biol Phys 1995;32:499–506.
22   Lutz W, Kimball W: A method to produce fixed shaped fields for stereotatic radiosurgery. Med Phys 1994;21:890.
23   Marks LB, Sherouse GW, Das S, Bentel GC, Spencer DP, Turner D: Conformal radiation therapy with fixed shaped coplanar or non-coplanar radiation beam bouquets: A possible alternative to radiosurgery. Int J Radiat Oncol Biol Phys 1995;33:1209–1219.
24   Nedzi LA, Kooy H, Alexander E III, Gelman RS, Loeffler JS: Variables associated with the development of complications from radiosurgery of intracranial tumors. Int J Radiat Oncol Biol Phys 1991;21:591–599.
25   Otto-Oelschläger S, Schlegel W, Lorenz W: Different collimators in convergent beam irradiation of irregularly shaped intracranial target volumes. Radiother Oncol 1994;30:175–179.
26   Perez CA, Brady LW: Principles and Practice of Radiation Oncology, ed 3. New York, Lippincott Raven, 1997.
27   Powlis WD, Smith AR, Cheng E, Galvin JM, Villari F, Boch P, Kligerman MM: Initiation of multileaf collimator conformal radiation therapy. Int J Radiat Oncol Biol Phys 1993;25:171–179.
28   Schlegel W, Pastyr O, Bortfield T, Becker G, Schad L, Gademann G, Lorenz WJ: Computer systems and mechanical tools for stereotactically guided conformation therapy with linear accelerators. Int J Radiat Oncol Biol Phys 1992;24:781–787.
29   Serago CF, Houdek PV, Bauer-Kirpes B, Lewin AA, Abitbol AA, Gonzalez-Arias S, Marcial-Vega VA, Schwade JG: Stereotactic radiosurgery: Dose-volume analysis of linear accelerator techniques. Med Phys 1992;19:181–185.
30   Shaw E, Kline R, Gillin M, Souhami L, Hirschfeld A, Dinapoli R, Martin L: Radiation Therapy Oncology Group; Radiosurgery Quality Assurance Guidelines. Int J Radiat Oncol Biol Phys 1993; 27:1231–1239.
31   Shiu AS, Kooy HM, Ewton JR, Tung SS, Wong J, Antes K, Maor MH: Comparison of miniature multileaf collimation with circular collimation for stereotactic treatment. Int J Radiat Oncol Biol Phys 1997;37:679–88.
32   Webb S: Optimization by simulated annealing of three-dimensional conformal treatment planning for radiation fields defined by a multileaf collimator. Phys Med Biol 1991;36:1201–1226.
33   Webb S: The Physics of Conformal Radiotherapy. Bristol, IOP Publ, 1997.
34   Winston KR, Lutz W: Linear accelerator as a neurosurgical tool for stereotactic radiosurgery. Neurosurgery 1988;22:454–464.
35   Yu CX, Symons MJ, Du MN, Martinez AA, Wong JW: A method for implementing dynamic photon beam intensity modulation using independent jaws and a multileaf collimator. Phys Med Biol 1995;40:769–87.

Dr. med. R. Wurm, Klinik für Strahlentherapie, Charité, Humboldt University,
Schumann Strasse 20–21, D–10117 Berlin (Germany)
Tel. +49 30 2802 2633. Fax +49 30 2802 8306, E-Mail reinhard.wurm@charite.de

Wiegel T, Hinkelbein W, Brock M, Hoell T (eds): Controversies in Neuro-Oncology.
Front Radiat Ther Oncol. Basel, Karger, 1999, vol 33, pp 78–87

....

Neuronavigation and Magnetic Source Imaging in Brain Tumors

K. Ebmeier, N. Haberland, J. Steenbeck, A. Hochstetter, R. Kalff

Department of Neurosurgery, Friedrich-Schiller-University, Jena, Germany

Introduction

Decisionmaking in the treatment of any patient with a brain tumor should always be an individualized process. The neurosurgeon has to take into account the specific biology and geography of the lesions, as well as the functional grade, the age, and the neurological status of the patient. The length of survival for patients suffering with a variety of brain tumors has been statistically associated with the extent of resection. Furthermore, the amount of residual tumor on postoperative images correlates with the length of survival in patients with malignant astrocytoma and glioblastoma multiforme. The neurosurgical management of intracranial lesions involving eloquent cortex is a challenging endeavor with a high risk of significant functional morbidity. Thus, exact localization of eloquent cortex is essential preoperatively and intraoperatively. Since the pioneer work of Roberts et al. [20] in 1986, several frameless stereotactic systems were developed for localization and resection guidance of small superficial or deep-seated lesions [4, 21, 28]. The use of these systems allows a reliable intraoperative orientation and assists the neurosurgeon in the localization of critical structures, in the definition of the lesion border, and in resection control [1]. The next step in minimizing the surgical morbidity of lesions in close proximity to sensitive functional cortex was the integration of functional mapping information with anatomic imaging. Since Penfield and Boldray [17] reported their landmark study of motor and sensory representation in human cerebral cortex, several reports have described the usefulness of cortical surface recording of somatosensory evoked potentials for the functional localization of the human cortex during surgery [11, 14, 30]. Furthermore, several clinical studies have demon-

Table 1. Summary of the 12 cases undergoing MSI-navigated neurosurgical procedures according to histopathology

Histopathology	n
Glioblastoma	4
Benign astrocytoma	3
Metastasis	2
Ganglioglioma	1
Oligoastrocytoma	1
Malignant astrocytoma	1

strated that the noninvasive technique of magnetoencephalography can perform localizations of the somatosensory, motor and auditory cortex with high spatial resolution and validity [9, 13, 16]. The new developed method of magnetic source imaging (MSI) superimposes sources of magnetic fields measured with multichannel biomagnetometers onto magnetic resonance images. The use of this new type of information in the operating room with the help of a neuronavigator, which was first described by Watanabe et al. [27], allows intraoperatively a detailed 3-D real-time visualization of the lesion itself and the surrounding functional cortex. Several clinical studies [6, 10, 12, 13, 18, 19] have recently demonstrated the clinical usefulness of MSI in the presurgical localization of the somotosensory cortex in lesions adjacent to the central sulcus. This report summarizes our own clinical experiences in the surgical treatment of 12 patients with a variety of brain tumors in the region of the somatosensory, the motor and the auditory cortex using the spatial physiological information derived noninvasively with MEG mapping for presurgical planning and stereotactic operative procedures.

Patients and Methods

Patients

From July 1997 to April 1998, 21 patients (11 men and 10 women; mean age 53 years, range 19–78) were examined. The data from 12 patients (7 men, 5 women; 11 right-handed patients; mean age 54 years, range 37–63) with various brain tumors as shown in table 1 were transformed from the 3-D MEG coordinates into the neurosurgical stereotactic database and used for real-time visualization during surgery. Eight patients had lesions located in the central region, 3 patients had lesions in the frontal, in the temporal and in the occipital lobe in close proximity to the central region. One female patient had a ganglioglioma in the left ventricle, where a navigation-guided transcortical approach was chosen after localization of the postcentral gyrus. Informed consent was obtained from all patients before the MEG examination and prior to surgery.

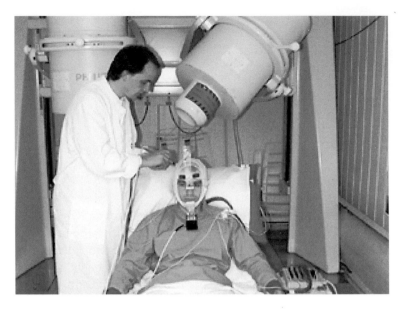

Fig. 1. Physician placing the hemispherical sensor array over the patient's central scalp.

MEG Recording and Data Analysis

MEG recordings were performed by using a dual 31-channel biomagnetometer (Philips) placed in the magnetically shielded room of the Center for Biomagnetism at the Friedrich Schiller University of Jena (fig. 1). The hemispherical sensor array (144 mm in diameter, 25 mm distance between the sensors) was placed contactless over the patient's central or temporal scalp, respectively. Simultaneous ECG and EOG recording were used as a detector of artifacts and involuntary movements. To evoke somatosensory fields (SEFs) we stimulated the median nerve near the retinaculum flexorum carpi or the tibial nerve near the malleolus medialis tibiae, respectively, using square current pulses (repetition rate 2 Hz; duration 200 μms; amplitude = individual + sensory threshold) contralaterally to the measured hemisphere. 512 trials of 500 ms duration were recorded. For the derivation of motor evoked fields (MEF) we used a pneumatic balloon switch. The patient was instructed to carry out self-paced movements of the thumb against index and middle finger of the hand contralaterally to the measured hemisphere 256 times in a constant and fast manner. The switch provided the trigger impulse. The sampling frequency was set to 1,000 Hz, pretrigger to 50 ms, the data was filtered 500 Hz low pass and 0.3 Hz high pass. Auditory evoked fields (AEFs) were recorded after stimulation with tone bursts (1 kHz, 50 ms duration and 70–90 dB SPL). These test tones were led to the contralateral ear through a tested tube system. The evaluation of the measured data was carried out using the Curry® Software (Philips). The data sets were digitally filtered (Hann, 0.3–250 Hz for SEFs, 0.3–40 Hz for MEFs and AEFs) and averaged after rejection of trials contaminated by artifacts.

We localized sources at the maximum of the first cortical response of the evoked field, that means $N_{20}m$ of median nerve SEF, $P_{40}m$ of tibial nerve SEF and/or MEF after self-paced finger movements, respectively, to identify the central sulcus. AEFs were localized

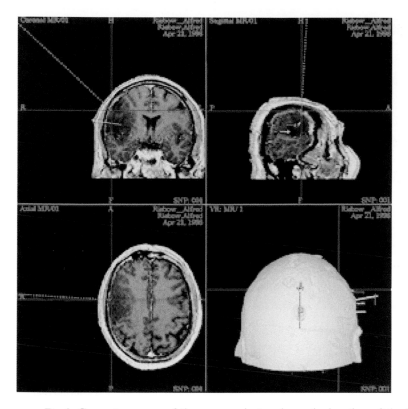

Fig. 2. Computer screen of the neuronavigator shows the location of the focus point of the operating microscope displayed into the MR images every time during surgery.

after about 100 ms after trigger (N_{100}m). For the fitting procedure the single equivalent current dipole model (ECD) in a realistic shaped head model (BEM) segmented from the individual MRI data set was used. All dipole solutions showed a goodness of fit $> 80\%$.

To combine the MRI- and MEG-coordinate system, the position of 10 localization coils fixed on the scalp was recorded in regular intervals during the MEG measurement. The same coils were digitized together with the position of those at least six fiducials, which served as reference points in the frameless stereotactic procedure. The 3-D digitizer system Polhemus® was applied immediately before or after the MEG session for this recording. The fiducials can be recognized and marked in the MRI. Thus all localization results of the MEG were transformed into the MRI and neuronavigation-coordinate system and could be overlaid on MR images (fig. 2).

MRI Data Acquisition and Neuronavigation

After placement of at least six external fiducials (skin markers) on the scalp of the patient, image data were acquired by MR tomography (1.5 Tesla Gyroscan ACR 2; Philips, The Netherlands). We used a standardized protocol for all of our patients (T1-weighted,

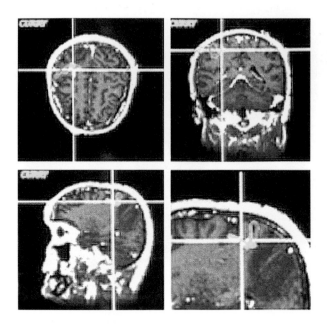

Fig. 3. Multiplanar screen demonstrates the location of motor evoked fields in a patient with a glioblastoma in the central region.

gadolinium-enhanced axial images with a 1-mm slice thickness). The data transfer to the neuronavigation system (Surgical Microscope Navigator; Zeiss, Oberkochen, Germany) was done by magneto-optical disc. This neuronavigational device is a light-emitting, diode-based localization and computer system for frameless stereotactic navigation which consists of six main components: a mobile planning workstation (Digital alpha station 266/4, 250 MHz), a position digitizer (including a camera array), the operating microscope (OPMI-ES, Zeiss), a pointing device, a dynamic reference frame and a universal instrumental tracking tool. During surgery, the neurosurgeon sees superimposed in his binocular the position of the preoperatively defined trajectory in relation to the optical axis of the microscope, the distance of the target from the focal point of the microscope as well as the predefined contours of the lesion and possible risk zones whose size varies as a function of the zoom. The MEG dipole localization results were imported into the neuronavigation system as trajectories. The coordinates of the dipole itself are used to define a target point, whereas the entry point is defined as the result of the radial projection of the dipole on the cortical surface (fig. 3).

Intraoperative Procedures

The patient was positioned on the operating table and the skull was fixed in a Mayfield-Kees clamp. After performing the patient-image registration procedure, the projection of the lesion and the MEG dipole localizations were marked on the patient's head to plan an exactly centered craniotomy. The physical localization of the radial projection of the dipole to the surface of the gyrus was performed using the information of the neuronavigator. The sulcus located in close proximity to the projected dipole in an anterior direction was defined

Table 2. Correlation between MEG dipole localization and anatomical criteria in preoperative MR images

	SEF (median nerve)	SEF (tibial nerve)	MEF (hand movement)	AEF
Patients measured	12	7	9	1
Correlation	12	7	6	1
No correlation	0	0	3	1

to be the central sulcus. In a second step, a single electrode strip containing eight electrodes was positioned on the cortex within the shortest distance between the estimated central sulcus and the projected MEG dipole to record somatosensory evoked potentials using the neurophysiological diagnostic device Nicolet Viking IV. The stimulation paradigm for these measurements is equivalent to that used in MEG recording. The point of maximum amplitude is generally assumed to be situated directly on the surface of the postcentral gyrus. To identify primary motor cortex, we stimulated electrically the region anterior to the once identified postcentral gyrus (500-Hz train stimulus, anodal). By evaluating the simultaneously derived electromyogram of the musculus abductor pollicis brevis, the motor hand area on the precentral gyrus is defined. Postoperatively we evaluated whether MEG localizations corresponded with ECoG results regarding the antero-posterior position to the central sulcus and measured the rectangular distance to it.

Results

In all the patients included in this study, the MSI results (SEFs) correctly identified the postcentral gyrus. The used motor paradigm however turned out to be not accurate enough to localize the precentral gyrus. A number of patients were not able to perform the motor task correctly. Thus a lot of trials are superimposed by sensory responses. This leads to dipole localizations in the postcentral gyrus in 3 cases (table 2).

In 4 patients we performed intraoperative recording of SEPs and direct stimulation of motor cortex. The postoperative evaluation of MEG dipole localization compared with ECoG measurements and radiological criteria showed in the localization of the median nerve SEFs a complete agreement applying MRI criteria and only one disagreement relative to the corresponding ECoG result. Tibial nerve SEF localization agreed with the controls in 1 case while a second case was not assessable because of strong perifocal edema.

The rectangular distances of the SEF dipole sources to the central sulcus ranged from 0 to 6 mm. The values of absolute distances between MEG and ECoG localization results rised up to 33.7 mm for tibial nerve SEFs (table 3).

Table 3. Correlation between MEG dipole localization and corresponding ECoG results

	Patient 1			Patient 2			Patient 3	Patient 4
Stimulation:	m	t	mo	m	t	mo	m	m
Distance 1	31.6	33.7	28.5	24.7	17.9	28.0	20.1	17.2
Distance 2	14.6	17.3	25.1	21.0	4.2	28.3	17.2	12.7
Distance 3	14.0	1.0	25.0	8.0	3.0	17.0	8.8	4.0
Correlation to central sulcus								
MRI criteria	+	+	–	+	–	+	+	+
ECoG criteria	+	+	–	–	–	+	+	+
Rectangular distance to central sulcus	6	0	4	0	–	5	4	0

m = Median nerve; t = tibial nerve; mo = motor cortex. Distance 1 = Calculated MEG-ECoG distance; distance 2 = calculated distance between ECoG and MEG projected on cortical surface; distance 3 = antero-posterior distance; distances measured in mm.

In 1 patient with a left temporal located lesion, we recorded AEFs preoperatively. The results showed that the auditory cortex was not involved into the lesion so that a complete resection of the tumor was possible. The patient had postoperatively no additional neurological deficits. Based on the MSI localization results, complete tumor removal was performed in 10 cases. In 2 cases the neurosurgeon decided intraoperatively as a result of brain mapping and cortical recording to only take an extended biopsy. The neurological status was unchanged in 8 patients and improved in 4 patients. Two patients showed postoperatively an aggravated hemiparesis. The MEG examinations required between 30 min and 2 h to complete depending on the type of examination. The data analysis and the transforming procedure takes up to 8 h of work for a specialized person. Intraoperatively the progression of the procedure was delayed approximately 15 min by the registration procedure, the localization of the dipoles and the performing of electrocorticography. During surgery there is the need of two additional specialized persons to handle the neuronavigator and the electrophysiological diagnostic device.

Discussion

The surgical management of lesions involving eloquent cortex requires an accurate localization of these critcal structures to minimize postoperative functional morbidity. Numerous MEG studies have indicated the accurate and reproducible localization of the sensorimotor cortex [8, 23–25]. The validity of MEG sensorimotor mapping has also been confirmed by intraoperative sensory and motor evoked potentials recorded directly from the cortical surface [5, 6, 13, 18, 25]. The use of functional mapping in stereotactic neurosurgery has been reported previously [6, 10, 12, 18, 19, 27]. Our results showed that a safe and accurate localization of the postcentral gyrus and in the same manner of the central sulcus is possible and reproducible. The localization of MEFs seems to be more complicated because of the task design which combines motor and somatosensory brain activity. A new task design which has been developed at the Center for Biomagnetism in recent months will probably improve the results of MEF recording. The measured distances between the located sources of brain activity with MEG and ECoG are greater than reported in the literature [2, 7, 10] but the methods to measure these distances are different in the reported studies [26]. Thus, a comparison of these results is difficult and questionable. The most important question for the neurosurgeon at this time is the location of the central sulcus. This information in combination with an intraoperative real-time visualization allows an excellent orientation in the central region. Based on this information, the neurosurgeon himself decides intraoperatively about the extent of resection. The recording of AEFs as performed in 1 patient is still under investigation at this time. Preoperative functional brain mapping using PET, fMRI and MEG is becoming increasingly common in neurosurgical practice [3, 6, 8, 10, 12, 15, 16, 18, 29]. Each of these techniques has particular advantages and limitations for neurosurgical application. The method of magnetoencephalography includes several advantages because it is one of few truly noninvasive methods without requirement for application of radionucleotides or X-rays. Other techniques like PET, SPECT and fMRI record brain activity only indirectly by measuring metabolic and hemodynamic changes. Recent regional CBF measurement studies highlighted the usefulness and potential pitfalls of functional mapping [15, 22, 29]. Metabolic techniques have a long integration time which make them useful for complex language and motor mapping in functions distributed over multiple cortical areas. The mapping of circumscribed cortical activity however requires a spatial and temporal resolution within milliseconds. Indeed, only electromagnetic techniques can measure brain electrophysiology directly. In addition, they are the only techniques with the temporal resolution required to capture the millisecond events used by the brain to encode and transmit information. At present, one limitation of MSI is that the source localization model (equivalent current dipole model) can detect only one active region that suits the stimulation task of the sensorimotor cortex. There is a need for further investigations concerning the comparison and correlation of the various brain mapping strategies in an individual patient. In addition to that, the task design has to be developed to create standarized conditions for the mapping of special brain functions and areas. It should be noted that every image-guided resection procedure carries the risk of a shift in intracranial structures secondary to cerebrospinal fluid loss and the progress of the resection. Thus, the identification of functional cortex has to be performed before tumor resection.

Conclusion

Preoperative MEG mapping and the transformation of this information into a neuronavigation system allows intraoperatively a safe localization of the central sulcus and a real-time orientation within this eloquent brain area during surgery. This may contribute to a safer and more radical surgery in lesions adjacent to the motor cortex and reduces the risk of postoperative functional morbidity. Further investigations are necessary to improve the mapping of more complex and spatially distributed cortical activity and to correlate the results of several mapping methods. At present, the availability of MSI is limited to only a few institutions but its use and the use of other functional mapping strategies in clinical and neurosurgical practice will become routine during the next decade.

References

1   Black PM, Moriarty T, Alexander E III, Stieg P, Woodard EJ, Gleason L, Martin CH, Kikinis R, Schwartz RB, Jolesz FA: Development and implementation of intraoperative magnetic resonance imaging and its neurosurgical applications. Neurosurgery 1997;41:831–845.
2   Buchner H, Fuchs M, Wischmann HA, Dossel O, Ludwig I, Knepper A: Source analysis of median nerve and finger-stimulated somatosensory evoked potentials: Multichannel simultaneous recording of electric and magnetic field combined with 3D-MR tomography. Brain Topogr 1994;6:299–310.
3   Fried I, Nenov VI, Ojeman SG, Woods RP: Functional MR and PET imaging of rolandic and visual cortices for neurosurgical planning. J Neurosurg 1995;83:854–861.
4   Friets EM, Strohbehn JW, Hatch JF, Roberts DW: A frameless stereotaxic operating microscope for neurosurgery. IEEE Trans Biomed Eng 1989;36:608–611.
5   Gallen CC, Bucholz R, Sobel DF: Intracranial neurosurgery guided by functional imaging. Surg Neurol 1994;42:523–530.
6   Gallen CC, Schwartz BJ, Bucholz RD, Malik G, Barkley GL, Smith J, Tung H, Copeland B, Bruno L, Assam S, Hirschkopf E, Bloom F: Presurgical localization of functional cortex using magnetic source imaging. J Neurosurg 1995;82:988–994.
7   Gallen CC, Schwartz B, Reike K: Intrasubject reliability and validity of somatosensory source localization using a large array biomagnetometer. Electroencephalogr Clin Neurophysiol 1994;90:145–156.
8   Gallen CC, Sobel DF, Waltz T, Aung M, Copeland B, Schwartz BJ, Hirschkoff EC, Bloom FE: Non-invasive pre-surgical neuromagnetic mapping of the somatosensory cortex. Neurosurgery 1993; 33:260–268.
9   Gallen CC, Schwartz B, Rieke K, Pantev C, Sobel D, Hirschkoff E, Bloom FE: Intrasubject reliability and validity of somatosensory source localization using a large array biomagnetometer. Electroencephalogr Clin Neurophysiol 1994;90:145–156.

10   Ganslandt O, Steinmeier R, Kober H, Vieth J, Kassubek J, Romstöck J, Strauss C, Fahlbusch R: Magnetic source imaging combiend with image-guided frameless stereotaxy: A new method in surgery around the motor strip. Neurosurgery 1997;41:621–628.
11   Gregorie EM, Goldring S: Localization of function in the excision of lesions from the sensorimotor region. J Neurosurg 1984;61:1047–1054.
12   Hund M, Rezai AR, Kronber E, Cappell J, Zonenshayn M, Ribary U, Kelly PJ, Llinás R: Magnetoencephalographic mapping: Basis of a new functional risk profile in the selection of patients with cortical brain lesions. Neurosurgery 1997;40:936–943.
13   Kamada K, Takeuci F, Kuriki S, Oshiro O, Houkin K, Abe H: Functional neurosurgical stimulation with brain surface magnetic resonance images and magnetoencephalography. Neurosurgery 1993; 33:269–273.
14   King RB, Schell GR: Cortical localization and monitoring during cerebral operations. J Neurosurg 1987;67:210–219.
15   Latchaw RE, Hu X, Ugurbil K, Hall WA, Madison MT, Heros RF: Functional magnetic resonance imaging as a management tool for cerebral arteriovenous malformations. Neurosurgery 1995;37:619–626.
16   Orrison WW Jr, Douglas FR, Blaine LH, Edward LM, Sanders JA, Willis BK, Marchand EP, Wood CC, Davis LE: Noninvasive preoperative cortical localization by magnetic source imaging. Am J Neuroradiol 1992;13:1124–1128.
17   Penfield W, Boldrey E: Somatic motor and sensory representation in the cerebral cortex of man as studied by electrical stimulation. Brain 1937;60:389–443.
18   Rezai AR, Hund M, Kronberg E, Deletis V, Zonenshayn M, Cappel J, Ribary U, Llinas R, Kelly PJ: Introduction of magnetoencephalography to stereotactic techniques. Stereotact Funct Neurosurg 1995;65:37–41.
19   Rezai AR, Hund M, Kronberg E, Zonenshayn M, Cappell J, Ribary U, Kall B, Llinas R, Kelly PJ: The interactive use of magnetoencephalography in stereotactic image-guided neurosurgery. Neurosurgery 1996;39:92–102.
20   Roberts DW, Strohbehn JW, Hatch JF, Murray W: A frameless stereotaxic integration of computerized tomographic imaging and the operating microscope. J Neurosurg 1986;65:545–549.
21   Roberts DW, Nakajima T, Brodwater B, Pavlidis J, Fagan E, Hartov A, Strohbehn J: Further development and clinical application of the stereotactic operating microscope. Stereotact Funct Neurosurg 1992;58:114–117.
22   Sergent J: Brain-imaging studies of cognitive functions. Trends Neurosci 1994;17:221–227.
23   Sobel DF, Gallen CC, Schwartz BJ, Waltz TA, Copeland B, Yamada S, Hirschkoff EC, Bloom FE: Central sulcus localization in humans: Comparison of MR anatomic and magnetoencephalographic functional methods. Am J Neuroradiol 1993;14:915–927.
24   Suk J, Ribary U, Cappel J, Yamamoto T, Llinás R: Anatomical localization revealed by MEG recording of the human somatosensory system. Electroencephalogr Clin Neurophysiol 1991;78:185–196.
25   Sutherling WW, Crandall PH, Darcey TM: The magnetic and electrical fields agree with intracranial localization of somatosensory cortex. Neurology 1991;38:1705–1714.
26   Suzuki A, Yasui N: Intraoperative localization of the central sulcus by cortical somatosensory evoked potentials in brain tumor. J Neurosurg 1992;76:867–870.
27   Watanabe E, Mayanagi Y, Kaneko Y: Identification of the central sulcus using magnetoencephalography and neuronavigator. No To Shinkei 1993;45:1027–1032.
28   Watanabe E, Mayanagi Y, Kosugi Y, Manaka S, Takakura K: Open surgery assisted by the neuronavigator, a stereotactic, articulated, sensitive arm. Neurosurgery 1991;28:792–800.
29   Wise R, Hadar U, Howard D, Patterson K: Language activation studies with positron emission tomography; in Symposium CIBA: Exploring Brain Functional Anatomy with Positron Tomography. Chichester, Wiley, 1991, pp 218–234.
30   Wood CC, Spencer DD, Allison T, McCarthy G, Willimason PD, Goff WR: Localization of human sensorimotor cortex during surgery by cortical surface recording of somatosensory evoked potentials. J Neurosurg 1988;68:99–111.

K. Ebmeier, Department of Neurosurgery, Friedrich-Schiller-Universität,
Bachstrasse 18, D–07740 Jena (Germany)

Wiegel T, Hinkelbein W, Brock M, Hoell T (eds): Controversies in Neuro-Oncology.
Front Radiat Ther Oncol. Basel, Karger, 1999, vol 33, pp 88–93

······················

The Value of 3D Magnetic Resonance Imaging in the Planning of Neurosurgery

T. Hoell [a], *F. Oltmanns* [a], *A. Schilling* [b], *A. Schernick* [a], *M. Brock* [a]

Department of [a] Neurosurgery and [b] Radiology,
University Hospital Benjamin Franklin, Berlin, Germany

Introduction

Magnetic resonance imaging (MRI) is a fast, reliable and inexpensive technique to obtain the data set for 3D reconstruction [1–6]. The procedure introduced in this paper is however able to manage CT data as well. Until present the major problem has been to convey adequate automated software for 3D segmentation. Another problem is the uncontrolled movement of the patient during scanning. The latter has been solved by a fiberoptic image transmission system (fig. 1).

The software discussed in this paper allows semiautomatic and rapid processing of the enormous amount of imaging data. During the last 5 years many types of software have been expected to achieve 3D imaging of the brain. Some software provides good images of the brain but much of the segmentation work has ultimately been done by hand. Processing of imaging data by hand however is too time-consuming to be suitable for clinical purposes.

Methods

The 3D software package is based on the scientific visualization software IDL (Research Systems, Inc., Boulder, Colo., USA) and runs on Windows-, Mac- and Unix-based computers. The software allows semiautomatic visualization of the brain in three dimensions without the surrounding structures (segmentation).

MR angiography data can be attached and functional data can be superimposed. The user interface is optimized for neurosurgical purposes. The software was designed and written by H.M. v. Stockhausen and is commercially distributed (Functional Imaging Technologies GmbH, Berlin, Germany).

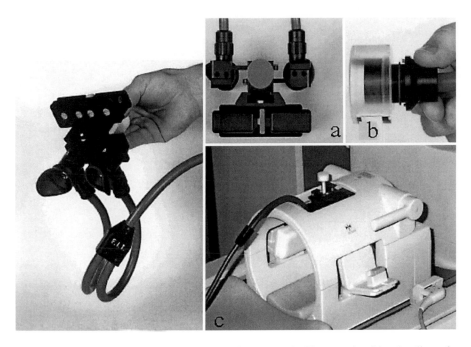

Fig. 1. a Eyepiece (ocular) attached to the receptacle. The round red knob adjusts for individual eye distance. The optical fiber is covered by a multilayer silicon tube for protection against mechanical hazards. *b* Objectives at the tip of both fibers integrated into a plug and ready for placement in front of a monitor. *c* Optical system mounted in the head coil of MRI scanner. Different receptacles allow fitting into all major MR scanner brands.

The fiberoptic system was developed under the auspices of our department in 1993 [5]. The optical device consists of a pair of objective lenses mounted in front of a TV or computer monitor and a pair of ocular lenses mounted in front of the patient's eyes. The 10-meter fiber length allows the monitor to be operated in the MR control room. This is important when working with unshielded scanners. The TV monitor was fixed at the foot of the patient's table. An eyepiece device (fig. 1a) presents the images to the patient. The adjustable lens in the eyepiece device allows vision correction. The virtual angle (opening) is 20°. The eyepiece, made entirely of glass and plastic, is mounted in front of the patient's eyes by means of a special receptacle in the head coil of the MR scanner (fig. 1c). This ensures a comfortable noncontact procedure for the patient.

Procedures

Once the patient had been positioned on the MRI table, the optical system was attached to the head coil of the scanner. During diagnostic MRI, the patient was entertained by cartoon videos which helps to reduce patients head movements. The 3D data set was obtained

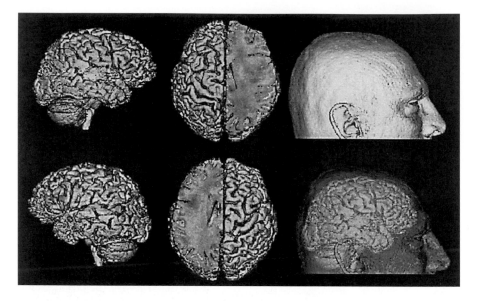

Fig. 2. Morphological reconstruction (segmentation) of the MR data set. The brain surface of left and right hemisphere with functional MR data superimposed. In colored images, speech-activated areas are highlighted in orange on the right hemisphere of a left-handed patient and the blue color indicates areas that are inversely correlated with the cognitive task.

with a Flash 3D sequence in 1 mm resolution in all dimensions, which took about 12 min. Data from the 3D investigation was transferred to an external computer for further statistical analysis via local area network. The software dismisses the header of the single 2D image files and forms a stack of them which is the basic 3D data set. In a next step the user determines a distinct anatomical structure for segmentation via definition of upper and lower thresholds of gray scale values. The segmentation works semi-automatically. Brain segmentation also includes the brain nerves, e.g. the optic nerve. Comparable steps must be performed for the segmentation of the ventricular system, the skin, the vessels and all pathological structures. In case of functional imaging, 3D anatomical data is fused with functional data into one image (fig. 2).

Results

The 'FIT ware' 3D tool provides adequate visualization for neurosurgical purposes. Its main advantage is the essentially semi-automatic segmentation of the brain as well as of brain tumors, AVMs and others. The segmentation quality is high in respect to spatial resolution. No inadequate rendering procedures are processed to soften the brain surface with the aim to reach better design. This prevents the sacrifice of anatomical details.

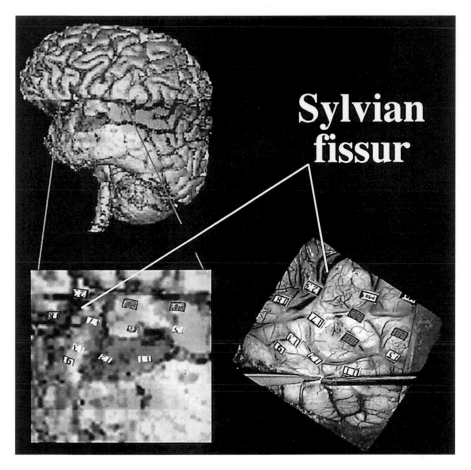

Sylvian fissur

Fig. 3. Top: 3D reconstruction of the left side of a patient's brain. The colored band represents the functional data superimposed on the anatomical site. Bottom right: Photographed brain surface of the same patient. The paper tags are upside down with respect to the intraoperative situation. Bright tags represent speech areas, dark tags show areas with no influence under electrical stimulation. Bottom left: Montage of the 3D reconstruction and picture with paper tags of the brain surface superimposed.

The quality of the imaged brain surface is virtually identical to the intraoperative view, which has been proven with intraoperative photo documentation. The high quality of the 3D data provides its use for neuronavigation. This has been documented in 8 neurosurgical applications of navigation so far.

Disadvantages of the software are that it requires high-priced computers and additional RAM of at least 256 MB. Segmentation near the skull base is not as perfect as at the parietal and temporal brain surface. The user interface needs some hours of adjustment and accommodation to be handled without difficulty.

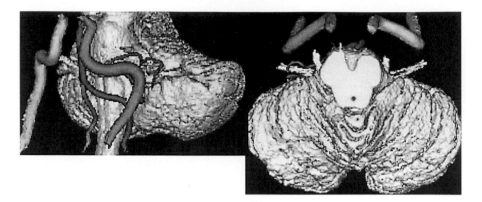

Fig. 4. The image reveals the brain stem and the cerebellum (gray). The vessels are presented darker. Please note the close contact between the trigeminal nerve and a branch of the posterior inferior cerebellar artery in the right image. In this case the contact zone between nerve and vessel was the anatomical correlate of a trigeminal neuralgia.

Technical comments on the optical system: Handling of the optical system was easy and safe. None of the components were accidentally misused. Colors were transmitted true-to-life, and suffered only a slight loss of brilliance. The fiber strands did not suffer any mechanical damage despite their routine application. Another advantage is the improvement of anatomical MR images due to the optimal positioning of the patient's head in the head coil. Patients do not tire, and do not skip, thus movement artifacts are significantly reduced.

Only 2 patients had panic attack during the examination (0.01%) versus the usual 5%. This increases patient compliance and saves time and money. Binocular vision was satisfactory in 116 patients (83%). Sufficient monocular vision was achieved by 137 patients (98%). Some patients had difficulty fusing the left and right image, and several complained about the small opening of the ocular.

The fiberoptic system combined with 3D software is a reliable tool for localizaing speech function. The main advantage is the mechanical robustness of the optical system combined with sophisticated and time-saving software. The 3D image is essential for superimposing functional information. Interpretation of functional information on 2D images is nearly impossible because the interesting cortical functional data is visualized as only a small rim at the border of the brain image. To verify the assessed functional information, intraoperative electrophysiological mapping, e.g. for motor areas and speech areas, was employed.

All speech-eloquent areas identified intraoperatively were likewise identified by functional imaging. However, functional imaging with the introduced equipment identified additional territories not detected by intraoperative mapping. Both methods identify eloquent areas with a spatial resolution of 0.5 cm (fig. 3).

Five cases, in which the MR angiography and the anatomical image were combined, showed acceptable image quality. The contact zones of brain nerves and vessels could be identified on the image as well as in the intraoperative site. The fact that the resolution of MR images is close to the size of the vessels, limits imaging quality and precision. However, this technique is the first that generates images of nerve-vessel junctions that are of clinical value (fig. 4).

Discussion

The high accuracy and the easy handling of soft and hardware components of the system are contributing towards establishing 3D MRI as a useful and safe method in preoperative care. The reliability of the images and the spatial resolution of 1 mm in each dimension well serves neuronavigation purposes and approach planning with the computer. Of disadvantage is still the additional time and work that need to be invested into the preoperative planning. The return on this investment however is the establishment of a high level 3D navigation for surgery as well as for other purposes, e.g. radiation planning. With the reported improvements, it is likely that 3D MRI will soon be widely applied for preoperative detection of eloquent areas. This will improve the general safety of surgery.

References

1   Schmidgen H, Hoell T, Regard M, et al: The Neuropsychological Screening Test (NST): First validation and reliability studies. Zentralbl Neurochir 1994;55:185–192.
2   Herholz K, Petrzyk U, Karbe H, et al: Individual metabolic anatomy of repeating words demonstrated by MRI-guided positron emission tomography. Neurosci Lett 1994;182:47–50.
3   Wada J, Rasmussen T: Intracarotid injection of sodium amytal for the lateralization of cerebral speech dominance. Neurosurgery 1960;17:266–282.
4   Ogawa S, Menon R, Tank D, et al: Functional brain mapping by blood oxygenation level-dependent contrast magnetic resonance imaging. Biophys J 1993;64:803–812.
5   Hoell T, Sander M, Oltmanns F, et al: A new system for image transmission into MRI scanners for functional MRI investigation: MR-EYE. Proc 10th European Congress of Neurosurgery, Berlin 1995, pp 67–68.
6   Ojemann G, Ojemann J, Lettich E, et al: Cortical language localization in left, dominant hemisphere. An electrical stimulation mapping investigation in 117 patients. J Neurosurg 1989;71:316–326.

T. Hoell, Department of Neurosurgery, University Hospital Benjamin Franklin, Hindenburgdamm 30, D–12200 Berlin (Germany)

Wiegel T, Hinkelbein W, Brock M, Hoell T (eds): Controversies in Neuro-Oncology.
Front Radiat Ther Oncol. Basel, Karger, 1999, vol 33, pp 94–99

··········

Intraoperative Radiotherapy in Brain Tumors

Ch. Rübe[a], *P. Schüller* [a], *S. Palkovic*[b], *W. Wagner* [c], *F.J. Prott* [a], *N. Willich*[a]

Departments for [a]Radiotherapy and [b]Neurosurgery, University of Münster, and
[c]Department for Radiotherapy, Paracelsusklinik, Osnabrück, Germany

Introduction

With a median survival time of about 10 months after resection and postoperative radiotherapy [7, 9], the prognosis of patients suffering from malignant brain tumors, especially astrocytomas grade III and glioblastomas, is unsatisfactory. New approaches with combined postoperative radiochemotherapy [2, 6], high-density irradiation (fast neutrons) [5] or the employment of radiosenzitizing substances [11] could not prolong the survival time for brain tumor patients as expected.

A dose escalation from 45 to 60 Gy using external beam fractionated irradiation after surgery could be shown to improve treatment results significantly [14]. Accelerated hyperfractionated radiotherapy or high-dose conformal radiotherapy had no advantage in terms of overall survival [3, 9].

A localized increase of total dose using stereotactic radiosurgery [1] or intraoperative radiotherapy (IORT) with high single doses may lead to an improvement of survival times [8, 12, 13]. Since May 1992, feasibility, perioperative morbidity, early and long-term sequelae as well as survival times following IORT with fast electrons are being examined in a pilot study.

Materials and Methods

Between May 1992 and March 1998, 44 patients with malignant gliomas were treated with IORT at the University of Münster. They formed a heterogeneous collective: 29 patients had primary brain tumors, and 15 patients had recurrent tumors. The male:female ratio was 29:15. The patients' age ranged from 32 to 71 years, with a median of 57 years. The histological tumor types according to WHO grades I–IV were distributed as follows: astrocytoma grade III (n = 16), oligodendroglioma grade III (n = 3), ependymoma grade III (n = 1), glioblastoma (n = 24).

Patients with peripheral and supratentorial tumors of not more than 6 cm in size were included into the treatment study. If they had not received any previous radiotherapy, treatment consisted of surgical resection and 20 Gy intraoperative radiotherapy, followed by 60 Gy external beam radiotherapy after completion of wound healing. Preirradiated patients received an IORT dose of 25 Gy without percutaneous irradiation.

In the neurosurgical operating theater, patients were placed on a movable operating table with their head fixed in a Mayfield clamp. If possible, a radical tumor resection was performed. The craniotomy was carried out in a way that the bone resection surrounded the tumor by about 2 cm on all sides. After complete resection, the operation cavity was measured in all three dimensions by the radiotherapist and then filled up with wet cotton strips for dose homogenization. The intended beam angle was determined by a neuronavigation system and fixed by a device called BDI (beam direction indicator, see below). After covering the wound with sterile plastic foil, the patients were transported to the radiation department lying on the mobile operating table without changing their position.

The gantry angle of the linear accelerator and the table position were chosen according to the position of the patient's head and the resection area. An electron cone was selected according to the diameter of the resection area with a 1–2 cm safety margin. If necessary, the electron field was individually modified with lead absorbers. The electron energy was chosen according to the depth of the tumor bed plus 1 cm safety margin so that the target volume was surrounded by the 80–90% isodose. Electron energy varied from 10 to 18 MeV. Dose prescription usually referred to the 80 or 90% isodose. The irradiation time ranged from 6 to 9 min. After the application, patients were brought back to the operation theater to close the craniotomy wound.

After intraoperative radiotherapy, a reconstruction of the dose distribution was made on the base of thin-sliced CT scans of the patient's head before and after surgery. By using postoperative CT scans for reconstruction, intraoperative mass shifting was not a major problem for exact dose calculation. Fiducial markers visible on CT, MRI, and verification films were fixed on the patient's head at four anatomical landmark points. Before irradiation, a so-called 'beam direction indicator' (BDI) was mounted on the patient's head. This BDI was directed into the incent ray by laser guidance. Verification films of the patient's head with the fixed BDI indicating the direction of the incent ray were then taken in the beam's eye view direction using 10-MV photons. By the use of trigonometric functions, the angle of the incent ray relative to the axes connecting the fiducial markers could be calculated from the length of the projections of these axes on the verification films.

With the use of a radiotherapy planning system (CadPlan), this three-dimensional angle could be translated into a virtual gantry angle and table rotation relative to the CT scans. Knowing the exact angle of the incent ray, the isodose curves for the chosen electron energy and cone diameter could be calculated by the planning system. After radiotherapy, this procedure made it possible to investigate if the tumor volume was completely covered by the target volume dose or not.

Since April 1995, IORT of brain tumors was performed by the help of the neuronavigation system by the Radionics Burlington Company. The base of this system is a 5-joint sensing arm and an HP 9000 workstation (32-bit). The system uses an articulated sensing arm to obtain the three-dimensional coordinates for the operating point. Preoperatively a

Table 1. Postoperative improvement of symptoms after surgery and IORT

Symptom	Improvement	No change	Decline
Brain pressure	20/21	0/21	1/21
Hemiparesis	10/18	4/18	4/18
Aphasia	14/17	3/17	0.17
Convulsions	10/15	5/15	0/15
Psychosyndrome	6/10	3/10	1/10
Hemianopsia	3/5	0/5	2/5

CT scanning is made with 4 markers affixed to the patient's scalp. The fiducial points are intraoperatively touched with the tip of the navigator arm for calibration. This way, the navigator arm can translate the current tip localization into the corresponding CT coordinates. The maximum detection error is 2.5 mm [4, 15]. This neuronavigation device is able to combine various diagnostic images into one database and effectively guides the surgeon during surgery [10].

For the radiotherapist, this neuronavigation system can facilitate the correct choice of electron energy, cone size, and beam angle. When the resection wound has been plaqued for dose homogenization and closed with sterile tapes, by pressing the tip of the sensing arm on the patient's head until the edge of the tumor is reached, the tumor depth can be read on a scale. Furthermore, the localization of the arm tip is projected into the corresponding CT slice with a cursor, and the angle of the incent ray can be determined this way and fixed by the BDI (see above).

In prior unirradiated patients, the IORT dose was 20 Gy followed by percutaneous radiotherapy with doses ranging from 40 to 60 Gy, in single fractions of 1.8–2 Gy/day. The target volume (tumor resp. tumor bed plus 1 cm safety margin) was completely surrounded by the 90% isodose. Preirradiated patients (n = 13) received a single dose of 25 Gy without following external beam therapy.

Follow-up examination in 3-month intervals consists of CT and MRI scans, scintigraphic controls and neurological examination. The median follow-up period was 10 months. Survival probabilities were calculated according to the Kaplan-Meier method.

Results

IORT was well feasible and tolerated by the patients; 2 patients had a wound infection, 1 a hemorrhage and 1 a malignant edema. One of these complications was lethal. No relevant late effects have been observed so far.

After the combined treatment, there was a decrease of neurological symptoms, e.g. intracranial pressure (table 1). Twenty-one of 22 patients who suffered from increased intracranial pressure prior to therapy showed an improvement. Other neurological symptoms, e.g. aphasia, hemiparesis, hemi-

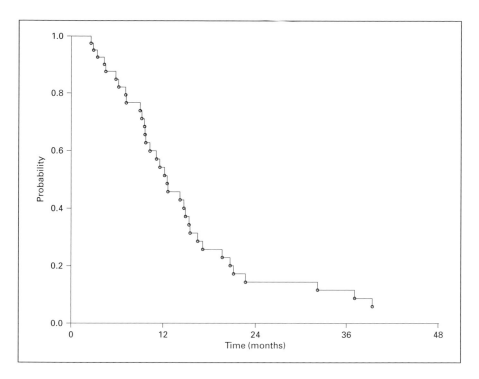

Fig. 1. Survival of patients treated with IORT plus 60 Gy postoperative external beam irradiation (n = 44).

anopsia, psychosyndrome, gyrus angularis syndrome and convulsions, were clearly reduced by the mentioned treatment modality. This improvement also correlates with the development of the Karnofsky performance status before and 6 months after IORT. The Karnofsky status before therapy for all patients was 71% (median 70%) and 6 months after therapy 74.3% (median 80%).

Survival probability for all patients 1 year after IROT was 52%, after 2 years 18% (fig. 1). Median survival was 12.5 months, 1-year survival for astrocytomas III was 64%, for glioblastomas 45% and for recurrent tumors 64%. Median survival time for patients with astrocytomas III was 15 months and therefore significantly better than for glioblastomas (11.8 months, p = 0.04). Recurrent tumors had a median survival of 12.2 months. Recurrence-free survival for all patients after 1 year was 22%.

Karnofsky performance status could be shown to have an influence on survival. Patients with a Karnofsky performance status > 70 showed a 1-year survival of 62%, patients with a Karnofsky performance status < 70 showed a 1-year survival of 36%. Furthermore, the results of surgery influenced survival. If there was a complete tumor resection, the 1-year survival probability was 66%. If because of tumor size and localization only a tumor reduction (R2 resection) was possible, the 1-year survival probability was 18%. Compared to a historical patients' group treated in our clinic with surgery and postoperative external beam irradiation, the patients treated additionally with IORT showed a better survival.

Conclusion

The feasibility of the introduced method was good. Side effects did not increase those known after surgery and postoperative external beam radiotherapy alone. Even though there was a difference comparing the survival probability of the glioblastomas after IORT with a historical patients' group, it has to be taken into account that the comparison is retrospective and the results in the historical group are rather poor. To evaluate a potential advantage of IORT, a randomized trial in comparison to conventional fractionated external beam irradiation alone would be necessary. The efforts which have been made to optimize the intraoperative irradiation technique and postoperative reconstruction of the dose distribution may help to further improve the results.

References

1   Alexander E: Radiosurgery for primary malignant brain tumors. Semin Surg Oncol 1998;14: 43–52.
2   Brandes AA, Rigon A, Zampieri P, Ermani M, Carollo C, Altavilla G, Turazzi S, Chierichetti F, Florentino MV: Carboplatin and teniposide concurrent with radiotherapy in patients with glioblastoma multiforme: A phase II study. Cancer 1998;82:355–361.
3   Buatti JM, Marcus RB, Mendenhall WM, Friedman WA, Bova FJ: Accelerated hyperfractionated radiotherapy for malignant gliomas. Int J Radiat Oncol Biol Phys 1996;34:785–792.
4   Golfinos JG, Fitzpatrick BC, Smith LR, Spetzler RF: Clinical use of a frameless stereotactic arm: Results of 325 cases. J Neurosurg 1995;83:197–205.
5   Griffin TW, Davis RB, Laramore GE, Nelson JS, Hendrickson FR, Rodriguez-Antunez A, Hussey DA: Fast neutron irradiation for glioblastoma multiforme: Results of a RTOG Phase III study. Am J Clin Oncol 1983;6:661–667.
6   Grossmann SA, Wharam M, Sheidler V, Kleinberg L, Zeltzman M, Yue N, Piantadosi S: Phase II study of continuous infusion carmustine and cisplatin followed by cranial irradiation in adults with newly diagnosed high-grade astrocytoma. J Clin Oncol 1997;15:2596–2603.
7   Kristiansen K, Hagen S, Kollevold T, Torvik A, Holme I, Nesbacken R, Hatlevoll R, Lindgren M, Brun A, Lindgren S, Notter G, Anderson AP, Elgen K: Combined modality therapy of operated astrocytomas grade III and IV. Confirmation of the value of postoperative irradiation and lack of potention of bleomycin on survival time: A prospective multicenter trial of the Scandinavian Glioblastoma Study Group. Cancer 1981;47:649–652.
8   Matsutani M, Nakamura O: Intraoperative radiation therapy for cerebral glioblastoma; in Schildberg FW, Willich N, Krämling HJ (eds): Intraoperative Radiation Therapy. Proc 4th Int Symp on IORT, Munich 1992. Essen, Die blaue Eule, 1993, pp 169–171.

9 Nakagawa K, Aoki Y, Fujimaki T, Tago M, Terahara A, Karasawa K, Sakata K, Sasaki Y, Matsutani M, Akanuma A: High-dose conformal radiotherapy influenced the pattern of failure but did not improve survival in glioblastoma multiforme. Int J Radiat Oncol Biol Phys 1998;40:1141–1149.

10 Olivier A, Germano IM, Cukiert A, Peters T: Frameless stereotaxy for surgery of the epilepsies: Preliminary experience. Technical note. J Neurosurg 1994;81:629–633.

11 Prados MD, Scott CB, Rotman M, Rubin P, Murray K, Sause W, Asbell S, Comis R, Curran W, Nelson J, Davis RL, Levin VA, Lamborn K, Phillips TL: Influence of bromodeoxyuridine radiosensitization on malignant glioma patient survival: A retrospective comparison of survival data from the Northern California Oncology Group (NCOG) and Radiation Therapy Oncology Group (RTOG) trials for glioblastoma multiforme and anaplastic astrocytoma. Int J Radiat Oncol Biol Phys 1998;40:653–659.

12 Sakai N, Yamada H, Andoh T, Nishimura Y, Yanagawa S: Clinical results of IORT on malignant glioma and its indications; in Schildberg FW, Willich N, Krämling HJ (eds): Intraoperative Radiation Therapy. Proc 4th Int Symp on IORT, Munich 1992. Essen, Die blaue Eule, 1993, pp 172–177.

13 Wagner W, Schüller P, Willich N, Schober O, Palkovic S, Morgenroth C, Bartenstein P, Prott FJ, Niewöhner U: Intraoperative Strahlentherapie (IORT) maligner Hirntumoren. Strahlenther Onkol 1995;171:154–164.

14 Walker MD, Strike TA, Sheline GE: An analysis of dose-effect relationship in the radiotherapy of malignant gliomas. Int J Radiat Oncol Biol Phys 1979;5:1725–1731.

15 Watanabe E, Mayanagi Y, Kosugi Y, Manaka S, Takakura K: Open surgery assisted by the neuronavigator, a stereotactic, articulated sensitive arm. Neurosurgery 1991;28:792–799.

PD Dr. Christian Rübe, Klinik für Strahlentherapie-Radioonkologie der Universität,
Albert Schweitzer-Strasse 33, D-48129 Münster (Germany)
Tel. +49 251 834 73 89, Fax +49 251 834 73 55, E-Mail ruebech@uni-muenster.de

Wiegel T, Hinkelbein W, Brock M, Hoell T (eds): Controversies in Neuro-Oncology.
Front Radiat Ther Oncol. Basel, Karger, 1999, vol 33, pp 100–113

....

The Role of Radiotherapy in the Treatment of Craniopharyngeoma – Indications, Results, Side Effects

G. Becker [a], *R.D. Kortmann* [a], *M. Skalej* [b], *M. Bamberg* [a]

Abteilungen für [a] Strahlentherapie und [b] Neuroradiologie,
Radiologische Universitätsklinik, Tübingen, Deutschland

Introduction

The treatment of craniopharyngioma is amongst the most controversial issues. Several surgical series recommend the attempt of total excision in order to avoid the potential side effects of radiation [20, 43, 44]. Others have supported the use of limited surgical procedures and radiation therapy because of the frequent inability to carry out a complete excision, the high incidence of recurrence when only a subtotal resection is done and the potential morbidity of aggressive surgery [18]. Similar cautious statements have been made for many years. The lack of knowledge of the natural history of untreated disease and the absence of randomized studies add to the perceived difficulty in defining the best approach of treatment. Over the last 30 years many articles have been published reviewing the results of different treatment strategies. Despite all the problems of retrospective studies, a large amount of information is available to form the basis for settling the long-standing controversy [6].

In the following the different therapeutic strategies are described and compared in terms of local control, survival, side effects and quality of life.

Clinical Considerations

Craniopharyngiomas are benign neoplasms of the suprasellar region occurring in children and adults. They make up 6–9% of the primary intracranial tumors in childhood with a peak age of 8–14 years. Craniopharyngiomas arise from squamous cell rests (Rathke's pouch) in the parasellar area. Typically the tumor consists of a partially calcified, solid nodule and a prominent cystic component. The cystic nature of the tumor is usually evident on computer tomography (CT) and magnetic resonance imaging (MRI) and surrounded by an enhancing cyst wall which is helpful in differential diagnosis. Most of the tumors become symptomatic only after they have reached a diameter of about 3 cm. Intrasellar lesions may compress pituitary and hypothalamic regions, producing hormonal abnormalities, especially antidiuretic and growth hormone insufficiency. Prechiasmatic localization leads to visual field cuts or decreased central visus. Trochiasmal lesions may grow into the third ventricle and lead to hydrocephalus. Symptoms vary and may include obesity, slowing of development, decreased vision, and field defects. The estimated duration of symptoms prior to diagnosis is between 9 and 10 months. Adults typically show visual symptoms, whereas children mostly develop headache, papilledema, endocrinopathies and advanced visual field loss.

Therapeutic Considerations

The best way of managing the treatment of craniopharyngioma remains a controversial issue amongst neurosurgeons and radio-oncologists. Because it is a benign tumor, complete surgical resection can result in long-term local control and should be curative. Because of its localization close to the optic nerves, chiasma, major arteries, and hypothalamus, however, the operability is limited and related to potential morbidity. Published series document excellent and equivalent long-term survival following different approaches of treatment, but reports about the long-term quality of life are still rare.

Surgery
In a survey of the American Society of Pediatric Neurosurgery in which 56 institutions were reviewed, 11 gave detailed information: all surgeons, except 1, reported the attempted gross total resection as the primary approach in all cases [43]. Surgery of craniopharyngioma represents a real challenge in neurosurgery, because of the complexity of neurovascular structures. The tumor is usually adherent to major as well as small perforating arteries at the base of the skull. Tumor adhesion to these vessels is one of the most important reasons for incomplete removal. The natural history of craniopharyngioma following subtotal excision without further therapy shows 71% progressive growth in a relatively short time period requiring further therapy (ranging from 50 to 91%) (table 1). The outcome after microsurgical resection shows a 19.4% recurrence rate, a 5-year survival of 81%, and a 10-year survival of 69% (current results from 15 international groups) (tables 2, 3). Surgical decompression as partial resection or

Table 1. Recurrence after partial tumor removal

Group (first author)	Year	Patients, n	Recurrences	
			n	%
Stalınke [52]	1984	12	6	50
Carmel [9]	1982	14	10	71
Cabezudo [7]	1981	14	12	86
Thomsett [56]	1980	11	10	91
Shapiro [46]	1979	9	7	78
Djordjevic [14]	1979	15	8	53
McMurray [34]	1977	9	9	78
Lichter [32]	1977	9	9	56
Hoffman [21]	1977	15	8	53
Sweet [53]	1976	5	4	80
Hoff [19]	1972	18	16	89
Total	1955–1984	131	93	71

Table 2. Recurrence rate after mircosurgical total resection

Group (first author)	Year	All cases, n	Total resection, n	Recurrences, %
DeVile [13]	1996	59	39	8
Hetelekidis [18]	1993	61	10	50
Pierre-Khan [36]	1994	30	29	0
Tomita [57]	1993	27	23	13
Hoffmann [20]	1992	50	45	29
Fischer [45]	1990	37	7	57
Weiss [60]	1989	31	19	32
Wen [61]	1989	52	20	50
Sorva [50]	1988	22	10	0
Lapras [31]	1987	42	22	14
Shillito [47]	1986	20	7	0
Symon [54]	1985	20	18	6
Total	1980–1996	451	247	19.4

cyst aspiration allows rapid improvement of local symptoms with less morbidity, but lead to tumor progression in 70–100% in less than 3 years. In recent years, the development and refinement of microsurgical techniques and treatment of endocrine disturbances have improved the operative results and patient's postoperative outcome [44]. However, radical resection in this localization is associated with a significant mortality (average 12%; range 0–43%); in contrast, death

Table 3. Survival rate of patients treated with total resection

Group (first author)	Year	Patients, n	Survival, %	
			5 years	10 years
Fischer [15]	1990	8	88	88
Weiss [60]	1989	18	82	
Wen [61]	1989	20	80	
Sorva [50]	1988	10	100	100
Shillito [47]	1986	7	100	
Amendola [1]	1985	12	84	74
Calvo [8]	1983	6	100	
Danoff [12]	1983	3	100	
Cabezudo [7]	1981	16	69	69
Sung [51]	1981	37	79	62
Richmond [42]	1980	8	88	50
Shapiro [46]	1979	22	78	75
Hoffmann [21]	1977	17	73	57
Lichter [32]	1977	7	100	
Katz [24]	1975	34	65	
Total	1970–1990	225	81	69

Table 4. Endocrine disturbances after radical surgery (126 patients analyzed) [data from 11, 43, 48, 49]

Hormone	Deficiency, %	
	pre-operative	post-operative
Growth hormone	5	95
Luteinizing hormone/follicle-stimulating hormone	40	82
Adrenocorticotropic hormone	25	78
Thyroid-stimulating hormone	25	78
Antidiuretic hormone (diabetes insipidus)	10	75–93
Hypothalamic obesity	10	50
Major hormone replacement (2 or more)		95

from limited surgery is < 1%. Severe morbidity occurs in up to 30% of patients, e.g. hemorrhage or infarction in 6–10%, hypothalamic-pituitary dysfunction like diabetes insipidus in 90%, hypothalamic obesity in 50% and visual impairment in 19% (range 3–35%). After radical surgery, major hormone replacement is required in 95% of the patients (table 4).

Table 5. Recurrence rate after partial removal + radiotherapy

Group (first author)	Year	All cases, n	Partial removal + radiotherapy	Recurrences, %
DeVile [13]	1996	75	38	24
Gürkaynak [17]	1994	23	23	26
Hetelekidis [18]	1993	61	37	20
Fischer [15]	1990	37	33	16
Flickinger [16]	1990	21	21	14
Wen [61]	1989	52	8	0
Clayton [10]	1988	23	16	0
Baskin [4]	1986	74	65	9
Shillito [47]	1986	20	10	0
Hoogenhout [22]	1984	29	13	23
Calvo [8]	1983	18	12	0
Danoff [12]	1983	19	14	14
Total	1980–1996	365	204	21

Limited Surgery + Radiotherapy

Tumor control using the combination of limited surgery and radiation therapy was first described by Kramer et al. [28] in 1961. The Royal Marsden Group which has the most experience in this field has published subsequent updates confirming long-term control of disease in 83% of children followed up 20 years after therapy [5, 6, 38, 39]. Numerous series documented reduction of the recurrence rate to 21% (table 5) and excellent survival rates after 5, 10 and 20 years of up to 91, 77 and 66% (table 6), as well as a decline in the morbidity after partial removal followed by radiotherapy (current results from 14 international groups). Radiation-related toxicity includes the gradual onset of endocrine deficits in a large proportion of patients (table 7).

However, the rate of replacement of major hormones is comparable to the rate after total resection surgery (table 4). Around the time of radiotherapy, up to 14% of the patients developed acute complications like visual deterioration or hydrocephalus, assumed to be due to a suprasellar or parasellar mass pressing on the surrounding structures and obstructing CSF flow [39].

Technical Considerations

Radiotherapy
Target Volume. The clinical target volume for craniopharyngioma is closely related to the tumor volume, including the solid component and cysts. In cases

Table 6. Survival rate of patients treated with limited surgery + radiotherapy

Group (first author)	Year	Patients, n	Survival, %	
			10 years	20 years
Rajan [38]	1993	173	77	66
Regine [41]	1993	12	82	78
Hetelekidis [18]	1993	37	86	62
Flickinger [16]	1990	21	82	
Fischer [15]	1990	27	93	
Manaka [33]	1985	45	69	
Hoogenhout [22]	1984	9	86	
Danoff [12]	1983	14	66	
Vyramuthu [59]	1983	15	69	
Cabezudo [7]	1981	13	94	
Sung [51]	1981	32	71	
Richmond [42]	1980	20	62	
Lichter [32]	1977	10	87	
Onoyama [35]	1977	32	60	
Total	1950–1993	10 years: 460	77	
		20 years: 222		66

Table 7. Endocrine disturbances after limited surgery + radiotherapy (103 patients analyzed) [data from 18, 43, 45]

Hormone	Deficiency, %	
	before treatment	after treatment
Growth hormone	30	59
Luteinizing hormone/follicle-stimulating hormone		55
Adrenocorticotropic hormone	15	59
Thyroid-stimulating hormone	20	82
Antidiuretic hormone (diabetes insipidus)	25	5.5–38
Hypothalamic obesity		30
Major hormone replacement (2 or more)		94

where cyst aspiration or limited resection are performed, it is important to cover the cyst wall. It is appropriate to limit the target volume to the postoperative residual tumor if large cystic components are removed surgically [29]. The planning of the target volume depends on the accuracy of the immobilization system and the imaging method used. Using a three-dimensional treatment planning system with MRI correlation, a security distance up to 1 cm would be enough, mainly defined by the inaccuracy of the fixation system. Treatment planning based only on CT scans should have a greater safety margin of 1.5–2 cm [26]. Using a rigid head fixation attached to a stereotactic frame, a safety margin could be minimized of 0.5–1.0 cm [3, 27].

Radiotherapy Technique. High-energy photons, a mixture of non-coplanar and coplanar beams and three-dimensional planned irregular field conformation should be recommended.

Radiation Dose. A dose response is apparent with improved disease control at doses of 50–60 Gy, using a conventional fractionation of 1.8 Gy once daily [5, 16, 29, 38, 39]. Failures are more common with doses < 50 Gy and toxicity is usually associated with doses > 60 Gy.

Time Schedule. The results of primary irradiation are superior to those of delayed therapy or incompletely resected tumors. It is usually preferable to administer postoperative irradiation rather than to await tumor progression [18]. Furthermore, qualitative measures of outcome are less favorable in patients with attempted radical resection and requiring subsequent irradiation than with planned, more limited resection and postoperative radiation therapy [43].

Intracavitary Irradiation

The large cystic nature of craniopharyngiomas has led to trials of intracystic applications of β-emitting radionuclides. In selected settings, the use of ^{90}Y or ^{32}P has resulted in shrinking and fibrosing of the cystic part, improving the symptoms (60%) and long-term tumor control (80% 5-year survival and 64% 10-year rates) with a 13% incidence of side effects [30, 37, 58]. While it may be effective in reducing the need for reaspiration of the cystic component, it is unproven as the only form of primary therapy [6]. Intracavitary irradiation should be considered as a salvage therapy after unsuccessful microsurgical resection and radiotherapy and growing cyst.

Radiosurgery

Radiosurgery in the treatment of small residual or recurrent tumors has only been described in a small number of patients [2, 25], so currently there are no valid results available. However, it can only be considered for selected patients because of the high risk of side effects in this localization by a single-dose application compared to the lower risk by stereotactically guided fractionated conformation radiotherapy [3].

There is considerable enthusiasm for fractionated stereotactic radiotherapy and introduction of three-dimensional conformal therapy, limiting the high-dose volume to the well-circumscribed neoplasm. This technique should provide the same rate of local control but significantly reduce the side effects. However, the results of long-term follow-up will determine if stereotactic conformation radiotherapy causes reduced neuropsychological sequelae compared to conventional radiotherapy.

Discussion

In order to compare the two controversial therapeutic strategies for craniopharyngioma, five aspects have to be discussed: recurrence rate, survival, salvageability if recurrence does occur, side effects and quality of life after the therapy.

Recurrence Rate

The natural history of craniopharyngioma following subtotal excision without further therapy leads in approximately 71% to progressive growth in a relatively short period of time (table 1). Therefore limited surgery alone does not seem to be indicated. In contrast, using modern microsurgery techniques for total resection, the recurrence rate in greater patient series ranges from 8 to 29% [13, 18, 20, 57] with an average of 19.4% (time period 1985–1996; table 2). Comparable to that is the average recurrence rate of 21% after partial removal followed by radiotherapy (table 5). Thus the risk of recurrence is equal for both treatment regimens and cannot be used as base for the treatment strategy.

Survival

Survival rates for patients treated with total resection are 81% for 5 years and 69% for 10 years (table 3). Limited surgery followed by radiotherapy achieves a 10-year rate of 66% up to 77% (table 6, fig. 1). These data from the literature are difficult to compare because they were collected over a period from 1950 to 1993. Treatment techniques in surgery as well as in radiotherapy have dramatically changed and improved. Furthermore, most studies include 10–30 patients, only the Royal Marsden Group followed up 173 patients over 20 years [5, 38, 39]. Considering the absence of randomized studies and the problems of the published retrospective results, the survival rate of both strategies are comparable and cannot be the base for preferring one of the treatment regimens.

Salvageability

Of the 20% of patients who suffer a regrowth of their tumor after micro-surgical gross total resection, approximately 80% can expect salvage by radi-

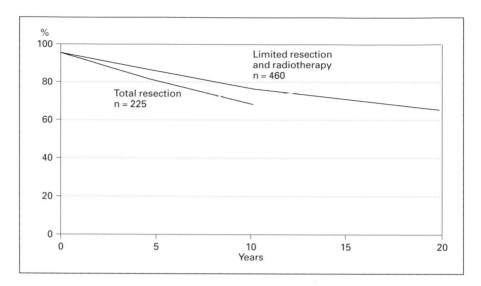

Fig. 1. Comparison of survival between total resection versus limited resection + radiotherapy; review of the literature 1950–1995.

ation as reported in a survey of the American Society of Pediatric Neurosurgery [43]. The greatest single study was reported by Jose et al. [23] with a 77% 10-year survival in 25 patients who showed a recurrence after radical surgery. A more difficult issue are the 21% of patients in whom the tumor recurs after limited surgery followed by radiotherapy. There is controversy among the neurosurgeons about the feasibility of radical surgery in a previously irradiated field. The more radical the initial surgical procedure, the more extensive the postoperative scarring and the greater the difficulties encountered [23, 43]. But up to now, there are no conclusive data about the salvageability after limited surgery plus radiotherapy and resection after the recurrence. A therapeutic alternative could be the intracavitary irradiation if the cystic parts are regrowing, or stereotactic radiotherapy for the solid part.

Side Effects

With the improvement of modern microsurgery techniques, mortality decreased continuously. The range in the literature is from 0 to 43%, with an average of 12%. In highly specialized centers the rate is only 2–4% [20, 55, 62]. In the survey of the American Society of Pediatric Neurosurgery, 7% late complications of irradiation in 57 children (4 children) were reported, 2 resulting in death (radiation vasculitis and a glioblastoma in the field of irradiation). One child suffered an occlusion of the right middle cerebral artery with a severe hemiparesis and 1 child developed a brainstem necrosis (vascular complication 1–2%). Visual

Table 8. Comparison of side effects between total resection versus limited surgery + radiotherapy; review of the literature 1970–1997 (% values)

Side effects	Surgery total resection	Limited surgery + radiotherapy
Mortality	12 (range 0–43)	1–2
Vascular complication	8	1–2
Visual impairment	19 (range 3–35)	1–10
Infections	6	No data
Seizures	14	No data
Cognitive disability	No data	6–15
Necrosis	No data	Rare
Morbidity	30 (range 12–61)	10 (range 2–15)

impairment is reported in 3–35% (average 19%) after radical surgery, in contrast to only in 1.5% after limited surgery plus irradiation. The incidence of endocrine complications is high following both therapies, and major hormone replacement is required in 95% of the cases (tables 4, 7). However, diabetes insipidus occurred in 75–93% of the cases after radical surgery (table 4) and only in 5–38% in children treated with limited surgery and radiotherapy (table 7). Morbid obesity, hypersomnolence and severe endocrine dysfunction only seem to occur as a complication of radical surgery. Comparison of the incidence of all side effects, described in the literature, demonstrates an average morbidity of 30% after radical surgery versus 10% after limited surgery followed by radiotherapy (table 8). This may be a reason for preferring limited surgery plus irradiation. Modern surgery techniques and postoperative care will decrease this rate in future. Also modern conformation radiotherapy will reduce the dose delivery to surrounding healthy tissue and in combination with small single doses will reduce the side effects.

Quality of Life

In a survey of the American Society of Pediatric Neurosurgery the detailed analysis of data from 11 institutions clearly demonstrated that the experience of the surgeon is a major factor in outcome. Centers treating less than 1 child per year reported good results in quality of life in 52%, and poor results in 39%, while centers with more than 2.25 children/year reported 86.6% with a good and only 8.8% with a poor outcome. Regardless of the experience of the surgeon, quality of life after limited surgery followed by radiotherapy was good in 83.3% and poor in 11.1%, which is better than the average outcome of radical surgery. Another important finding was that if radical surgery failed and radiotherapy was required, the result in quality of life was worse (poor

Table 9. Quality of life: a survey of the American Society of Pediatric Neurosurgery, Sanford 1994 [43] (% values)

Outcome (n = 116)	Radical surgery			Radical surgery + radiotherapy			Limited surgery + radiotherapy
	A centers (n = 23)	B centers (n = 45)	total (n = 68)	A centers (n = 7)	B centers (n = 23)	total (n = 30)	total (n = 18)
Good	52.2	86.6	75	42	52	50	83.3
Poor	39.1	8.8	19	57	39	43	11.1
Death	8.7	4.4	6	0	8.6	6.6	5.5

A centers treated <1 child/year; B centers treated 2–3 children/year.

outcome in 43%) because these children suffered the effects of two potentially harmful treatments [43] (table 9).

Conclusion

Most radiation oncologists swear by radiotherapy while a number of neurosurgeons passionately believe in surgery as the best way of treating craniopharyngioma. The lack of knowledge of the natural history of untreated disease and the absence of randomized studies add to the perceived difficulty in defining the best approach of treatment. Despite all the problems of retrospective studies, a large amount of information is available and was analyzed and reviewed with the following results:

Complete surgical resection of craniopharyngiomas can result in long-term local control (80%) and cure (5-year rate 81%, 10-year rate 69%). Although surgical resection rapidly relieves compressive symptoms, some tumors may recur even with complete resection (19.4%). Aggressive resection of these parasellar tumors may also be associated with significant morbidity (30%), including optic nerve and hypothalamic damage with resulting visual (3–35%) and endocrine disturbances (95%). Partial resection or cyst aspiration and biopsy rapidly relieve local compressive symptoms and have a lower operative morbidity but are associated with eventual tumor progression in most cases (71%). Moreover, recurrence is associated with a worse prognosis [29].

Radiation therapy combined with a limited surgical procedure minimizes the potential morbidity (10%) and the recurrence rate to 21%. Just as well, the survival is improved (10-year rate 77%, 20-year rate 66%). About 14% of the patients develop acute complications during radiotherapy, mostly due to cystic enlargement of the tumor. The quality of life after limited surgery and radiotherapy is good in more than 80% and poor in only 11%. The outcome after radical surgery is on average good in 75% and poor in 19%. If radical surgery fails and radiotherapy is required, the quality of life is worse (poor outcome in 43%) because these children suffer the effects of two potentially harmful treatments.

These results led to the recommendation of the preference of radical surgery in young children (e.g. < 5 years of age), small tumors and favorable localization. Limited surgery followed by irradiation is indicated in older children, large tumors and tumors in a critical location.

In the near future in most centers fractionated stereotactic conformation radiotherapy will be available to reduce the dose in the surrounding healthy tissue. This technique should provide the same rate of local control but with the possibility to reduce the side effects so that limited surgery followed by stereotactic radiotherapy may become the treatment of choice.

References

1 Amendola BE, Gebarski SS, Bermudez AG: Analysis of treatment results in craniopharyngioma. J Clin Oncol 1985;3:252–258.
2 Backlund EO: Solid craniopharyngiomas treated by stereotactic radiosurgery; in Szikla G (ed): Stereotactic Cerebral Irradiation. Inserm Symp No 12. New York, Elsevier, 1979, pp 271–280.
3 Becker G, Kortmann RD, Duffner F, Budach W, Buchgeister M, Grote EH, Bamberg M: High-precision external radiotherapy of brain tumors. Onkologie 1998;21:290–297.
4 Baskin DS, Wilson CB: Surgical management of craniopharyngiomas. A review of 74 cases. J Neurosurg 1986;65:22–27.
5 Bloom HJG: Combined modality therapy for intracranial tumors. Cancer 1975;35:111–120.
6 Brada M, Thomas DGT: Craniopharyngioma revisited. Int J Radiat Oncol Biol Phys 1993;27:471–475.
7 Cabezudo JM, Vaquero J, Areitio E, Martinez R, de Sola RG, Bravo G: Craniopharyngiomas: A critical approach to treatment. J Neurosurg 1981;55:371–375.
8 Calvo FA, Hornedo J, Arellano A, Sachetti A, de la Torre A, Aragon G, Otero J: Radiation therapy in craniopharyngiomas. Int J Radiat Oncol Biol Phys 1983;9:493–496.
9 Carmel PW, Antunes JL, Chang CH: Craniopharyngiomas in children. Neurosurgery 1982;11: 382–389.
10 Clayton PE, Price DA, Shalet SM, Gattemaneni HR: Craniopharyngioma recurrence and growth hormone therapy (letter). Lancet 1988;i:642.
11 Curtis J, Daneman D, Hoffman HJ, Ehrlich RM: The endocrine outcome after surgical removal of craniopharyngiomas. Pediatr Neurosurg 1994;21(suppl 1):24–27.
12 Danoff BF, Cowchock FS, Kramer S: Childhood craniopharyngioma: Survival, local control, endocrine and neurologic function following radiotherapy. Int J Radiat Oncol Biol Phys 1983;9:171–175.
13 DeVile CJ, Grant DB, Hayward RD, Stanhope R: Growth and endocrine sequelae of craniopharyngioma. Arch Dis Child 1996;75:108–114.
14 Djordjevic M, Djordjevic Z, Janicijevic M, Nestorovic B, Stefanovic B, Ivkov M: Surgical treatment of craniopharyngiomas in children. Acta Neurochir Suppl Wien 1979;28:344–347.
15 Fischer EG, Welch K, Shillito J Jr, Winston KR, Tarbell NJ: Craniopharyngiomas in children. Long-term effects of conservative surgical procedures combined with radiation therapy. J Neurosurg 1990;73:534–540.

16 Flickinger JC, Lunsford LD, Singer J, Cano ER, Deutsch M: Megavoltage external beam irradiation of craniopharyngiomas: Analysis of tumor control and morbidity. Int J Radiat Oncol Biol Phys 1990;19:117–122.

17 Gürkaynak M, Ozyar E, Zorlu F, Akyol FH, Atahan IL: Results of radiotherapy in craniopharyngiomas analysed by the linear quadratic model. Acta Oncol 1994;33:941–943.

18 Hetelekidis S, Barnes PD, Tao ML, Fischer EG, Schneider L, Scott RM, Tarbell NJ: 20-year experience in childhood craniopharyngioma (see comments). Int J Radiat Oncol Biol Phys 1993;27:189–195.

19 Hoff JT, Patterson RH Jr: Craniopharyngiomas in children and adults. J Neurosurg 1972;36: 299–302.

20 Hoffman HJ, De Silva M, Humphreys RP, Drake JM, Smith ML, Blaser SI: Aggressive surgical management of craniopharyngiomas in children. J Neurosurg 1992;76:47–52.

21 Hoffman HJ, Hendrick EB, Humphreys RP, Buncic JR, Armstrong DL, Jenkin RD: Management of craniopharyngioma in children. J Neurosurg 1977;47:218–227.

22 Hoogenhout J, Otten BJ, Kazem I, Stoelinga GB, Walder AH: Surgery and radiation therapy in the management of craniopharyngiomas. Int J Radiat Oncol Biol Phys 1984;10:2293–2297.

23 Jose CC, Rajah B, Ashley S, Marsh H, Brada M: Radiotherapy for the treatment of recurrent craniopharyngioma. Clin Oncol 1992;4:287–289.

24 Katz EL: Late results of radical excision of craniopharyngiomas in children. J Neurosurg 1975;42: 86–93.

25 Kobayashi T, Tanaka T, Kida Y: Stereotactic gamma radiosurgery of craniopharyngiomas. Pediatr Neurosurg 1994;21(suppl 1):69–74.

26 Kortmann RD, Hess CF, Jany R, Bamberg M: Repeated CT examinations in limited volume irradiation of brain tumors: Quantitative analysis of individualized (CT-based) treatment plans. Radiother Oncol 1994;30:171–174.

27 Kortmann RD, Becker G, Perelmouter J, Buchgeister M, Meisner C, Bamberg M: Geometric accuracy of field alignment in fractionated stereotactic conformal radiotherapy of brain tumors. Int J Radiat Oncol Biol Phys 1999;43:921–926.

28 Kramer S, McKossock W, Concannon JP: Craniopharyngiomas: Treatment by combined surgery and radiation therapy. J Neurosurg 1961;18:217–226.

29 Kun LE: Brain tumors in children; in Perez CA, Brady LW (eds): Principles and Practice of Radiation Oncology, ed 3. Philadelphia, Lippincott-Raven, 1997, pp 2073–2105.

30 Lange M, Kirsch CM, Steude U, Oeckler R: Intracavitary treatment of intrasellar cystic craniopharyngioma with 90-yttrium by trans-sphenoidal approach – A technical note. Acta Neurochir 1995;135:206–209.

31 Lapras C, Patet JD, Mottolese C, Gharbi S, Lapras C Jr: Craniopharyngiomas in childhood: Analysis of 42 cases. Prog Exp Tumor Res 1987;30:350–358.

32 Lichter AS, Wara WM, Sheline GE, Townsend JJ, Wilson CB: The treatment of craniopharyngiomas. Int J Radiat Oncol Biol Phys 1977;2:675–683.

33 Manaka S, Teramoto A, Takakura K: The efficacy of radiotherapy for craniopharyngioma. J Neurosurg 1985;62:648–656.

34 McMurray F, Hardy RW Jr, Dohn DF: Long-term results in the management of craniopharyngioma. Neurosurgery 1977;1:238–241.

35 Onoyama Y, Ono K, Yabumoto E, Takeuchi J: Radiation therapy of craniopharyngioma. Radiology 1977;125:799–803.

36 Pierre-Kahn A, Sainte Rose C, Renier D: Surgical approach to children with craniopharyngiomas and severely impaired vision: Special considerations. Pediatr Neurosurg 1994;21(suppl 1):50–56.

37 Pollock BE, Lunsford LD, Kondziolka D, Levine G, Flickinger JC: Phosphorus-32 intracavitary irradiation of cystic craniopharyngiomas: Current technique and long-term results. Int J Radiat Oncol Biol Phys 1995;33:437–446.

38 Rajan B, Ashley S, Gorman C, Jose CC, Horwich A, Bloom HJ, Marsh H, Brada M: Craniopharyngioma long-term results following limited surgery and radiotherapy. Radiother Oncol 1993;26:1–10.

39 Rajan B, Ashley S, Thomas DGT, Marsh H, Britton J, Brada M: Craniopharyngioma: Improving outcome by early recognition and treatment of acute complications. Int J Radiat Oncol Biol Phys 1997;37:517–521.

40   Regine WF, Kramer S: Pediatric craniopharyngiomas: Long-term results of combined treatment with surgery and radiation. Int J Radiat Oncol Biol Phys 1992;24:611–617.
41   Regine WF, Mohiuddin M, Kramer S: Long-term results of pediatric and adult craniopharyngiomas treated with combined surgery and radiation. Radiother Oncol 1993;27:13–21.
42   Richmond IL, Wara WM, Wilson CB: Role of radiation therapy in the management of craniopharyngiomas in children. Neurosurgery 1980;6:513–517.
43   Sanford RA: Craniopharyngioma, results of survey of the American Society of Pediatric Neurosurgery. Pediatr Neurosurg 1994;21(suppl 1):39–43.
44   Samii M, Tatagiba M: Surgical management of craniopharyngiomas: A review. Neurol Med Chir Tokyo 1997;37:141–149.
45   Scott RM, Hetelekidis S, Barnes PD, Goumnerova L, Tarbell NJ: Surgery, radiation, and combination therapy in the treatment of childhood craniopharyngioma a 20-year experience. Pediatr Neurosurg 1994;21(suppl 1):75–81.
46   Shapiro K, Till K, Grant DN: Craniopharyngiomas in childhood. A rational approach to treatment. J Neurosurg 1979;50:617–623.
47   Shillito J Jr: Treatment of craniopharyngioma. Clin Neurosurg 1986;33:533–546.
48   Sklar CA: Craniopharyngioma: Endocrine abnormalities at presentation. Pediatr Neurosurg 1994; 21(suppl 1):18–20.
49   Sklar CA: Craniopharyngioma: Endocrine sequelae of treatment. Pediatr Neurosurg 1994;21 (suppl 1):120–123.
50   Sorva R, Heiskanen O, Perheentupa J: Craniopharyngioma surgery in children: Endocrine and visual outcome. Childs Nerv Syst 1988;4:97–99.
51   Sung DI, Chang CH, Harisiadis L, Carmel PW: Treatment results of craniopharyngiomas. Cancer 1981;47:847–852.
52   Stahnke N, Grubel G, Lagenstein I, Willig RP: Long-term follow-up of children with craniopharyngioma. Eur J Pediatr 1984;142:179–185.
53   Sweet WH: Radical surgical treatment of craniopharyngioma. Clin Neurosurg 1976;23:52–79.
54   Symon L, Sprich W: Radical excision of craniopharyngioma. Results in 20 patients. J Neurosurg 1985;62:174–181.
55   Symon L, Pell MF, Habib AH: Radical excision of craniopharyngioma by the temporal route: A review of 50 patients. Br J Neurosurg 1991;5:539–549.
56   Thomsett MJ, Conte FA, Kaplan SL, Grumbach MM: Endocrine and neurologic outcome in childhood craniopharyngioma: Review of effect of treatment in 42 patients. J Pediatr 1980;97: 728–735.
57   Tomita T, McLone DG: Radical resections of childhood craniopharyngiomas. Pediatr Neurosurg 1993;19:6 14.
58   Voges J, Sturm V, Lehrke R, Treuar H, Gauss C, Berthold F: Cystic craniopharyngioma: Long-term results after intracavitary irradiation with stereotactically applied colloidal β-emitting radioactive sources. Neurosurgery 1997;40:263–270.
59   Vyramuthu N, Benton TF: The management of craniopharyngioma. Clin Radiol 1983;34:629–632.
60   Weiss M, Sutton L, Marcial V, Fowble B, Packer R, Zimmerman R, Schut L, Bruce D, D'Angio G: The role of radiation therapy in the management of childhood craniopharyngioma. Int J Radiat Oncol Biol Phys 1989;17:1313–1321.
61   Wen BC, Hussey DH, Staples J, Hitchon PW, Jani SK, Vigliotti AP, Doornbos JF: A comparison of the roles of surgery and radiation therapy in the management of craniopharyngiomas. Int J Radiat Oncol Biol Phys 1989;16:17–24.
62   Yasargil MG, Curcic M, Kis M, Siegenthaler G, Teddy PJ, Roth P: Total removal of craniopharyngiomas. Approaches and long-term results in 144 patients. J Neurosurg 1990;73:3–11.

Dr. Becker Gerd, Abteilung für Strahlentherapie, Radiologische Universitätsklinik,
Hoppe-Seyler Strasse 3, D-72076 Tübingen (Germany)
Tel. +49 7071 2986557, Fax +49 7071 295894

Wiegel T, Hinkelbein W, Brock M, Hoell T (eds): Controversies in Neuro-Oncology.
Front Radiat Ther Oncol. Basel, Karger, 1999, vol 33, pp 114–122

....

Craniopharyngeomas, Results in Children and Adolescents Operated through a Transsphenoidal Approach Compared with an Intracranial Approach

Bénédict Rilliet[a], *Vincent de Paul Djientcheu*[a], *Olivier Vernet*[a],
José Montes[b], *Jean-Paul Farmer*[b], *Gilles Bertrand*[c]

[a] Service de Neurochirurgie, Geneva and Lausanne, Switzerland;
[b] Department of Neurosurgery, The Montreal Children's Hospital, Canada, and
[c] Department of Neurosurgery, Montreal Neurological Institute, Canada

Introduction

The ultimate goal of craniopharyngioma surgery is the radical removal of this benign dysembryoplastic tumor. This pretension is nevertheless far from being attained in every case because of sometimes tight adherences between the craniopharyngioma and the noble anatomical structures, mainly the hypothalamus, pituitary stalk, hypophysis and the optic nerves and chiasm and to a lesser extent the arteries of the circle of Willis and their perforating branches to the deep part of the brain and the brainstem. This fact is particularly prominent in children where the surgeon fears to inflict a lifelong hypothalamic syndrome. On the other hand, relapses, mostly occurring before the 5-year limit, are much more often diagnosed in patients who could not benefit from a total removal.

The operative mortality in a collection of pediatric series analyzed by Choux et al. [1] varies from 0–15% (average 3.7%) and is not closely correlated with the extent of removal. Owing to the better topographical and anatomical preoperative evaluation of craniopharyngiomas with MRI, treatment strategies and surgical approaches are at present better defined and achieved.

According to the topographic distribution of craniopharyngiomas in relation to their embryological origin, a significant proportion of tumors enlarge the sella and may have a suprasellar extension and can be suitable for transsphenoidal surgery. The proportion of children operated for a craniopharyngioma by the transsphenoidal approach is small, representing not more than 8% in a collection of 371 cases who benefited from a unique surgical approach [1]. Most of the surgical papers [2–7], comparing the extracranial approach for infradiaphragmatic craniopharyngiomas to the intracranial approach for the other intracranial type of craniopharyngioma, report results on mixed adult and children populations. To our knowledge, such a comparison has not yet been published, considering only pediatric cases.

Patients and Methods

This is a retrospective review of the files of 46 children and adolescents (mean age 9.75, extremes 2–19, sex ratio 1:1) operated for a craniopharyngioma in three institutions (Geneva, Lausanne and Montreal) during a 23-year period (1973–1995). Their medical records were reviewed and endocrine and ophthalmological follow-up were obtained in all the survivors (37 cases). Other data such as level of education and quality of life were obtained through a questionnaire sent to the patient or by a direct phone call to the family doctor.

The outcome of 10 patients that were operated by a primary transsphenoidal approach (TS) and 31 by a primary intracranial approach (IC) are compared. The mean age was 12 years (range 5.5–18) in the TS group, and 9 years (2–19) in the IC group. Five other children who had multiple surgical approaches (TS before or after IC) were not included in this comparison but are also briefly reported in the Results.

Before the introduction of CT scan, the diagnosis was done on skull radiographs, pneumoencephalography and carotid angiography. After 1978, preoperative CT scan, and more recently MRI was obtained in every patient. The TS approach was considered when the anatomical criteria for an infradiaphragmatic craniopharyngioma were met, namely an enlarged sella with a purely intrasellar location or an intrasellar location plus a predominantly cystic suprasellar extension. Completeness of removal was determined by postoperative CT scan or MRI performed during the follow-up period.

To assess the hypothalamic-pituitary-adrenal axis, the basal cortisol and the stimulated secretion to ACTH or insulin-induced hypoglycemia was measured. Basal prolactin level, thyroid and gonadal axis were evaluated by the dosage of the level of TSH, LH, FSH, and the peripheral hormones, T_3, T_4, estradiol or testosterone, according to gender. The growth hormone axis was evaluated by the dosage of GH or IGF-1 after stimulation by insulin-induced hypoglycemia or arginine together with evaluation of osseous age compared with the chronological age. Diabetes insipidus was diagnosed on the measurement of the total fluid intake, the urine volume and the urine-specific gravity. Water deprivation testing was rarely performed.

Results

Preoperative Data

The endocrine symptoms were more common in the TS group: short stature in 24% of cases, 20% of delayed puberty, 8% of diabetes insipidus, 4%

of secondary amenorrhea in adolescent girls compared respectively to 11, 4, 7 and 0% in the IC group. Symptoms and signs of intracranial pressure were more common in the IC group: 36% of headaches, 29% of papilledema, 9% of vomiting, indicating at once a more severe disease as compared respectively to 24, 0 and 4% in the TS group. Obesity was associated to 8% of cases in the TS group and to 11% of cases in the IC group. The diagnosis was fortuitous in 1 case in both groups, a CT being done after a trivial head injury and revealing a craniopharyngioma. Visual field deficit, essentially bitemporal hemianopsia, was the most frequent clinical findings: 70% of cases in the TS group and 35% in the IC group. Visual acuity was decreased in 30% of cases in the TS group and signs of severe visual impairment were present only in the IC group with 25% of optic pallor or atrophy, indicating again a more severe disease. No signs of cranial nerve palsy were seen in the TS group whereas they were found in 19% in the IC group, correlated with lateral extension of the craniopharyngioma.

Preoperative endocrine deficiency was common in the TS group with 40% of ADH deficiency, 30% of TSH deficiency, 40% of GH and 50% of ACTH deficiency, compared respectively to 22, 12, 9 and 12% in the IC group. Only 1 child was hormonally normal in the TS group whereas 54% of children were reported as endocrinologically normal or not specified in the IC group.

Postoperative Data

A total removal was obtained in 7/10 cases (70%) in the TS group against 7/31 (23%) in the IC group. The tumor was cystic in 40% of cases in the TS group and 22% in the IC group; 1 case of solid tumor was found in both groups and the other craniopharyngiomas were of the mixed type.

In 1 case of cystic lesion, the transsphenoidal total removal was not possible by the TS approach and a cystosphenoidal drainage with an H custom-made catheter was inserted. The cyst collapsed as demonstrated on the 4-month postoperative MRI. A small cystic relapse was observed on the 6-month postoperative MRI and the patient was irradiated and there was no sign of relapse after a period of 18 months following radiotherapy. Fourteen patients with total removal (7 TS, 7 IC) were not irradiated, but 2 patients of the IC group who were considered as a total removal were subsequently irradiated for a relapse. All but 1 case (partial TS removal with no subsequent relapse) of incomplete removal or patients who benefited from a palliative cyst aspiration were irradiated. Intracavitary ^{32}P was used in only 1 case.

The postoperative visual function was better in the TS group: 60% of normal vision, 20% of improvement, 20% of patients with a stable deficit and no patient was aggravated compared respectively to 16, 35, 19 and 22% of aggravation in the IC group.

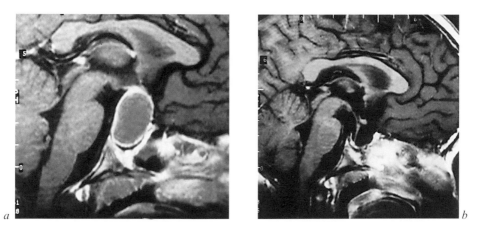

a   *b*

Fig. 1. *a* Preoperative gadolinium-enhanced MRI of an intra- and suprasellar cranio-pharyngioma in a 5-year-old girl who presented with growth retardation. *b* Postoperative MRI shows a total removal of the craniopharyngioma. Although the pituitary stalk is clearly preserved and some remnants of the hypophysis are clearly seen in the sellar floor, this girl is left with a panhypopituitarism.

After the operation, the hormonal status was worsened in both groups: 70% of cases of diabetes insipidus, 60% of panhypopituitarism, and 20% of partial-hypopituitarism in the TS group compared respectively to 74, 74 and 16% in the IC group. 9% of patients had normal endocrine status in the IC group but none in the TS group. Anatomical and radiological integrity of the pituitary stalk and hypophysis was not particularly correlated with preservation of the pituitary function, as demonstrated on the postoperative MRI of a 5-year-old girl who benefited from a total removal by the TS approach and was left with a panhypopituitarism (fig. 1).

There was no neurological complication in patients operated through a TS approach compared to the IC approach where a significant number of complications were encountered, such as hypothalamic syndrome and postoperative obesity in 29%, postoperative seizure in 22%, transient hemiparesis in 13%, transient third nerve palsy in 13%, behavior problems in 9%, transient hemichorea in 3%, subdural hygroma in 3% and as late complication an asymptomatic but radiologically evident fusiform dilatation of the carotid artery in 1 case. There has been no operative mortality in the entire series. The Kaplan-Meier actuarial survival curves clearly show a better prognosis for the TS group compared to the IC group (fig. 2). Three children died from unrelated causes (1 congenital cardiac heart disease in the TS group, 1 subdural hematoma after a fall and 1 drowning in the IC group). On the other hand,

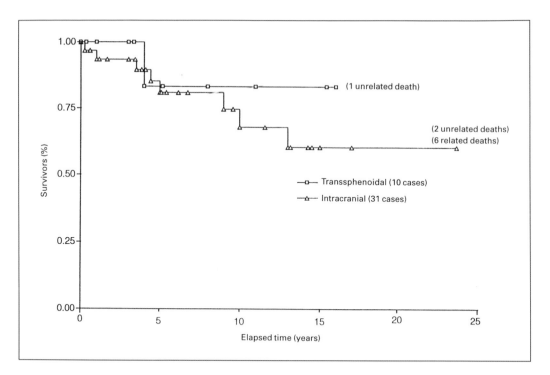

Fig. 2. Kaplan-Meier actuarial survival curves: transsphenoidal versus intracranial approach.

death was related to the disease in 6 children of the IC group (2 cases of endocrine crisis, 2 cases of sudden death, 1 attributed to seizures and the other to a shunt malfunction in a patient who had been treated for hydrocephalus prior to extirpation of the craniopharyngioma and became shunt-dependent, 2 operative deaths after an operation for a relapse).

The local control of the tumor is better in the TS group. 80% of patients are free of relapse in the TS group during the follow-up period against 60% in the IC group (Kaplan-Meier actuarial relapse curves; fig. 3). Nevertheless, these results are biased because 5 patients operated by a combined procedure with transcranial surgery are considered separately. In 3 of the 5 patients, TS surgery was performed as a second procedure and allowed a complete removal, in 1 patient 1 month after an intracranial approach limited to the implantation of an intracystic drain and reservoir, in the second case 1 year after the intracranial approach for an intrasellar relapse and in the third case after several unsuccessful intracranial operations combined with radiotherapy. These 3 patients have no signs of recurrence respectively 10, 8 and 11 years

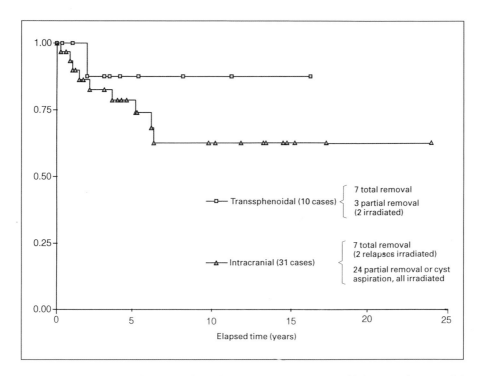

Fig. 3. Kaplan-Meier actuarial relapse curves: transsphenoidal versus intracranial approach.

after the TS operation. In the 2 other cases, a partial removal after a primary TS approach was followed by a transcranial approach. The first patient was definitively cured, the second one was irradiated and reoperated on several occasions 12 years after the first operation for a huge intracranial and intra-sphenoidal relapse. Although this patient had already been irradiated, a persistent solid portion in the sphenoid sinus was successfully treated recently with an injection through the nose of colloidal [186]Re. The outcome in the surviving patients is far better in the TS group. 100% of the patients are alive and well with a normal schooling and no neurological problems. Only 8 out of 23 survivors of the IC group fall in the same good results category, whereas 13 patients, although most of them have been able to attend school and eventually succeeded to complete their education to an apprenticeship level or even to an academic level, suffer from visual impairment, hypothalamic sequelae, mainly obesity, or postoperative seizures needing an antiepileptic medication. Two patients in the IC group are unfortunately considered as dependent with severe disability.

Discussion

Although already performed by Cushing [8] in 14% of his patients, the TS approach is used in only 8% of cases in a multicenter compilation of pediatric series reported by Choux et al. [1]. Laws [6] has certainly the greatest series of TS extirpations of craniopharyngiomas in 76 patients (23 pediatric cases) from a series of 146 patients representing a proportion of 52% of the cases. In other important series [2, 3, 7, 9] the percentage of cases requiring TS surgery varies from 23.6 to 61%. In the present pediatric series, the TS approach was used in 24% of cases.

Intrasellar and suprasellar tumor with an enlarged sella are suitable for this approach providing that the craniopharyngioma does not cross the limit of the diaphragm of the sella. Surgery is easier when the suprasellar extension is predominantly cystic. Some authors [5, 6] consider that an enlarged sella is a prerequisite for the TS approach whereas others do not accept this condition as an absolute finding [4], describing slight or even no enlargement of the pituitary fossa in the cases they have operated through a TS approach. In the present series all the patients operated by the TS approach had an enlarged sella. The absence of the development of the sphenoidal sinus in children is not a contraindication to the TS approach. In 1 of our patients, aged 5, a nonpneumatized sphenoid sinus was drilled.

Neurologic complications of the TS approach are rare compared to the transcranial surgery for craniopharyngioma as observed in the present series and reported cases. Although there is no local or general complication in present series, this approach should not be considered as a completely benign procedure. Laws [6] in his vast experience of 76 patients operated by a TS approach reported 2 deaths presumably due to carotid injuries, 6 cases of meningitis, 12 cases of CSF rhinorrhea, 1 case of visual loss, 1 case of mental changes and 3 cases of nasal perforation. To prevent CSF leak, we have always used a graft of muscle fascia, fat and fibrin glue to pack the sphenoid sinus. As an additional measure, a lumbar catheter has been systematically inserted in all cases during the operation to inflate a small quantity of air to bring down the suprasellar tumor extension in the operative field. The lumbar drainage of CSF is maintained during 3 days should a CSF leak happen during the procedure.

The TS approach allows a rapid decompression of the optic pathways and greatly influences positively the visual outcome. The postoperative visual status in this series compares to other series which reported 94% of normal or visual improvement after TS surgery [5]. No difference was seen between the two groups concerning the endocrinological outcome and the particularly good endocrinological results reported in recent series [2, 7, 10] were not reproduced in this pediatric series.

The debate between the defenders of radical surgery who claim that a total removal provides the best control of craniopharyngioma and those who produce data about excellent results achieved by limited surgery and radiotherapy [11, 12] is not closed. Owing to the rarity of this pathology, much effort and time for collecting more data will be needed to solve this question. Nevertheless, the completeness of removal and the excellent results obtained by the TS approach, confirmed in other reports [2, 6, 7, 10] should prompt the surgeons to identify the patients who may benefit from TS surgery as a unique treatment, mainly by studying the anatomical criteria of the preoperative MRI study.

Conclusion

In this series of pediatric craniopharyngiomas, 24% of children have been operated with a TS approach. Considering the initial symptoms and signs in this subgroup of patients, the infradiaphragmatic localization certainly represents a milder form of a disease that is often not easy to cure. The group of patients that may benefit from TS surgery should be identified and selected because of the possibility of radical surgery as a unique treatment with an excellent visual outcome and a small percentage of complications due to a less aggressive surgery because the intracranial cavity is not virtually entered. Long-term outcome with no mortality and morbidity, excellent quality of life and a low recurrence rate in the TS group compares very favorably with the IC group. The TS approach can also be used as a combined procedure before or after craniotomy during a staged surgery or as a secondary procedure for relapse when the residual cystic tumor has progressively entered and dilated the sella.

References

1   Choux M, Lena G, Genitori L: Le craniopharyngiome de l'enfant. Neurochirurgie 1991;37(supp 1): 1–174.
2   Abe T, Lüdecke D: Recent results of primary transnasal surgery for infradiaphragmatic craniopharyngioma. Neurosurg Focus (an electronic journal published on the Internet by J Neurosurg). 1997;3:article 4:1–11.
3   Fahlbusch R, Honegger J, Paulus W, Huk W, Buchfelder M: Surgical treatment of craniopharyngiomas: Experience with 168 patients. J Neurosurg 1999;90:237–250.
4   Honegger J, Buchfelder M, Fahlbusch R, Däubler B, Dörr H: Transsphenoidal microsurgery for craniopharyngioma. Surg Neurol 1992;37:189–196.
5   König A, Lüdecke D, Herrmann H: Transnasal surgery in the treatment of craniopharyngiomas. Acta Neurochir 1986;83:1–7.
6   Laws EJ: Transsphenoidal removal of craniopharyngioma. Pediatr Neurosurg 1994;21(suppl 1):57–63.

7 Maira G, Anile C, Rossi G, Colosimo C: Surgical treatment of craniopharyngiomas: An evaluation of the transsphenoidal and pterional approaches. Neurosurgery 1995;36:715–725.
8 Cushing H: The craniopharyngiomas; in Intracranial Tumors: Notes Upon a Series of Two Thousand Verified Cases with Surgical Mortality Percentages Pertaining Thereto. Springfield, Thomas, 1932, pp 93–98.
9 Baskin D, Wilson C: Surgical management of craniopharyngioma. A review of 74 cases. J Neurosurg 1986;65:22–27.
10 Honegger J, Buchfelder M, Fahlbush R: Surgical treatment of craniopharyngiomas. Endocrinological results. J Neurosurg 1999;90:251–257.
11 Brada M, Thomas DGT: Craniopharyngioma revisited. Int J Radiat Oncol Biol Phys 1993;27: 471–475.
12 Rajan S, Ashey C, Gorman C, Jose C, Horwich A, Bloom H, Marsh H, Brada M: Craniopharyngioma – Long-term results following limited surgery and radiation therapy. Radiother Oncol 1993; 26:1–10.

Dr. Benedict Rilliet, PD, Hôpitaux Universitaires de Genève,
Rue Micheli-du-Crest 24, CH-1211 Genève 14 (Switzerland)
Tel. +41 22 372 82 08, Fax +41 22 372 82 20, E-Mail Benedict.Rilliet@hcuge.ch

Wiegel T, Hinkelbein W, Brock M, Hoell T (eds): Controversies in Neuro-Oncology.
Front Radiat Ther Oncol. Basel, Karger, 1999, vol 33, pp 123–138

······················

New Developments and Controversies in the Neuropathology of Malignant Gliomas

Otmar D. Wiestler, Matthias C. Schmidt, Andreas von Deimling,
Guido Reifenberger, Martina Deckert-Schlüter, Herbert Radner,
Torsten Pietsch

Institut für Neuropathologie und Hirntumor-Referenzzentrum,
Universitätskliniken Bonn, Deutschland

Significant progress has been made in the neuropathological evaluation of gliomas. The introduction of immunohistochemical reactions for many cell-type-specific and tumor-related antigens was particularly instrumental. Several novel tumor entities have been identified, the histogenesis and classification of others have been redefined and new standards have been introduced for the grading of gliomas. However, several issues remain controversial. In this contribution we will summarize the current diagnostic concept for the analysis of malignant gliomas, highlight topics of continuous debate and introduce novel approaches.

Immunohistochemical Tools and the Revised WHO Classification of Brain Tumors

Immunohistochemical studies are based on the principal that cellular antigens can be reliably identified following incubation of microscopic sections with specific antibodies. With the exception of oligodendrogliomas, specific antibodies are now available for all major normal and neoplastic cell types in the brain. As many of these reagents can be applied to routinely processed paraffin sections, they have gained wide distribution in surgical neuropathology. Data obtained with immunohistochemical analyses have played a major role in the revision of the WHO classification for brain tumors [1].

For the assessment of malignant gliomas, antibodies to the glial fibrillary acidic protein (GFAP) have evolved as particularly valuable tools. Even highly anaplastic and poorly differentiated astrocytic gliomas continue to express GFAP. This protein is only rarely detectable in tumors of nonglial origin. It has to be kept in mind, however, that the presence of GFAP or other cell-type-specific antigens does not distinguish per se between neoplastic and non-neoplastic glial cells.

Major New Developments in Brain Tumor Classification

In 1993, an international panel of experts presented a revision of the WHO classification of brain tumors [1]. This updated classification has not only incorporated major new findings in brain tumor pathology; it has also gained the widest international distribution. We, therefore, strongly advocate to use these WHO guidelines for both daily diagnostic work and for reference neuropathology purposes.

The WHO panel has reconsidered the *cellular origin* of some tumor entities. In the field of gliomas, the consistent detection of GFAP led to a reclassification of glioblastomas as astrocytic rather than embryonic neoplasms. Immunoreactivity for GFAP has also allowed to redefine the monstrocellular sarcoma which was originally described by Zülch, as a variant of glioblastoma, the giant cell glioblastoma.

Several *new tumor entities* have been introduced. Novel clinicopathological entities now recognized by the WHO classification include the pleomorphic xanthoastrocytoma (PXA), the desmoplastic infantile ganglioglioma (DIG) and the central neurocytoma (NC) [2–4]. Of particular relevance for this contribution is the pleomorphic xanthoastrocytoma, a polymorphic, superficially localized astrocytic tumor in children and young adults [2]. Its properties will be specifically discussed in the paragraph on pediatric gliomas.

For some CNS neoplasms, *distinct histopathological variants* have been defined including morphological subtypes of meningiomas and schwannomas. Anaplastic astrocytoma, anaplastic oligoastrocytoma, anaplastic oligodendroglioma, glioblastoma multiforme, pediatric gliomas and pleomorphic xanthoastrocytoma are the major subjects of our contribution (table 1).

Anaplastic Oligodendroglioma and Oligodendroglial Components in Malignant Gliomas

Another matter of debate relates to the classification and grading of oligodendrogliomas or gliomas with an oligodendroglial component (fig. 1). Without available specific immunohistochemical markers for oligodendrogli-

Table 1. Selected glioma entities included in this review: Individual entities are listed according to the WHO classification of brain tumors

Astrocytic tumors	
Pilocytic astrocytoma	WHO grade I
Pleomorphic xanthoastrocytoma	WHO grades II or III
Anaplastic astrocytoma	WHO grade III
Glioblastoma multiforme	WHO grade IV
Oligodendroglioma and oligoastrocytoma	
Anaplastic oligodendroglioma	WHO grade III
Anaplastic oligoastrocytoma	WHO grade III

oma cells, the diagnosis of these entities relies on classical histopathological properties such as clear cell morphology, uniform round nuclei, chicken-wire capillary pattern, and microcalcification. The histogenesis of oligodendrogliomas and of oligoastrocytomas is unresolved. Surprisingly, antigens characteristically encountered in oligodendrocytes including myelin basic protein, galactocerebroside, proteolipid protein, myelin oligodendrocyte glycoprotein and other myelin components are usually not expressed in these neoplasms. This led some investigators to question an origin from the oligodendroglial lineage. The frequent detection of GFAP-positive elements in oligodendrogliomas and oligoastrocytomas would be compatible with a development from the O-2A progenitor, a bipotential precursor for both oligodendroglia and type 2 astroglia. Further experiments will be required to address this hypothetical model.

Several studies have demonstrated that anaplastic oligodendroglioma (WHO grade III) and anaplastic oligoastrocytoma (WHO grade III) exhibit a considerably better prognosis compared to anaplastic astrocytomas (WHO grade III). Clinical data indicate that both entities frequently respond to chemotherapy. A reliable histopathological identification of anaplastic oligodendrogliomas and of oligodendroglia components in malignant gliomas is, therefore, of critical importance. We propose the following diagnostic criteria:

(1) Significant mitotic and proliferative activity constitutes the key diagnostic feature for the grading of an anaplastic oligodendroglioma or anaplastic oligoastrocytoma (WHO grade III). The Ki-67 labeling index should exceed 10% of the tumor cell population. Other morphological parameters such as high cellularity, vascular endothelial proliferation and necrosis are also helpful indicators of anaplasia (fig. 1).

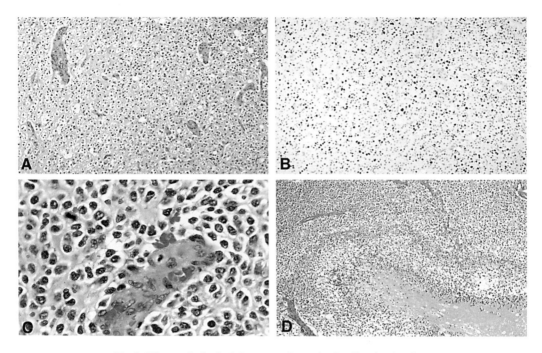

Fig. 1. Histopathological features of anaplastic oligodendroglioma (WHO grade III). An increased Ki-67 labeling index (*B*) and mitotic activity (*C*) represent the decisive criteria for the diagnosis of anaplastic oligodendroglioma. Marked vascular endothelial proliferation (*A, C*) and tumor necrosis (*D*) occur frequently but are of undetermined significance.

(2) The diagnosis of oligoastrocytoma (mixed glioma) requires a minimum of 20% for the smaller of the two components. In the diffuse variant of oligoastrocytoma, the two elements are intermingled (fig. 2). In other cases, they appear well separated.

(3) Tumor necrosis may not be sufficient as criterion to classify an anaplastic oligodendroglioma as glioblastoma of oligodendroglial origin. The diagnosis of this glioblastoma variant should only be made in cases with an unequivocally detectable malignant astrocytic component.

Glioblastomas with focal oligodendroglioma elements have recently received considerable attention. Preliminary reports suggest that they may exhibit sensitivity to PCV chemotherapy [5]. In order to identify this potentially relevant subgroup of glioblastoma patients, stringent histopathological criteria need to be defined. Prospective clinico-neuropathological studies will be required to resolve this important question.

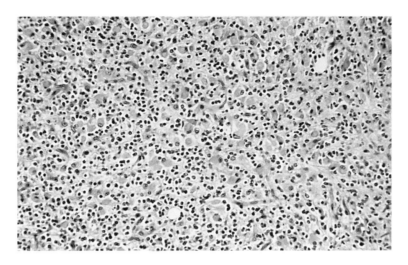

Fig. 2. Oligoastrocytoma (mixed glioma, WHO grade II). In this case, the two cellular elements are diffusely intermingled; in others, the astrocytoma and oligodendroglioma components appear separated.

Malignant Pediatric Astrocytomas

The histopathological diagnosis of astrocytic gliomas in children poses a major challenge to the neuropathologist. Brainstem gliomas constitute a prominent example. In cases with poorly differentiated phenotype, marked cellularity and high mitotic or proliferation index, malignant astrocytic gliomas can be readily identified (fig. 3B). Some investigators have proposed to classify all anaplastic gliomas in the posterior fossa of children as malignant brainstem gliomas, irrespective of their individual microscopic properties. We prefer to apply the WHO classification in these cases as well and differentiate between anaplastic astrocytoma (WHO grade III) and glioblastoma multiforme (WHO grade IV) based on the absence or presence of tumor necrosis. It has, however, not yet been demonstrated that such a distinction is clinically relevant for this group of patients. The frequent use of stereotactic biopsies for the diagnostic assessment of brainstem astrocytomas raises the problem of representative tissue sampling. A reliable classification and grading can be obscured in samples from peripheral tumor regions. Serial biopsies and neuroradiological documentation of the biopsy tract may increase diagnostic accuracy in these patients. There is some indication that proliferation markers can be helpful in this situation.

Cerebral glioblastomas in children frequently exhibit a prominent small cell morphology. This pattern can render their distinction from primitive neu-

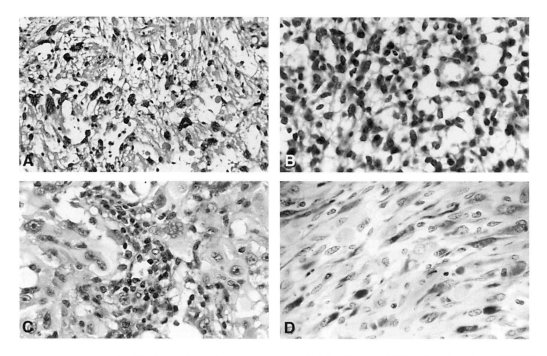

Fig. 3. Morphological appearance of pediatric gliomas. *A* Pilocytic astrocytoma (WHO grade I). Marked cellular and nuclear pleomorphism are not uncommon in these tumors. In contrast to adult astrocytomas, these properties are not associated with anaplasia. *B* Anaplastic astrocytoma (WHO grade III) of the pons (malignant brainstem glioma). Malignant features include high cellularity, poorly differentiated phenotype and increased mitotic rate. *C, D* Pleomorphic xanthoastrocytoma (WHO grade II). The photomicrographs illustrate the polymorphic nature and foamy appearance of the tumor cell population (*C*) and immunoreactivity for astrocytic GFAP (*D*).

roectodermal tumors difficult. Transitional forms between the two entities, both of which originate from a neural precursor cell, may indeed exist. Immunohistochemical detection of glial (GFAP) or early neuronal antigens (neuron-specific enolase, neuronal β-III tubulin, and synaptophysin) can be helpful to establish this differential diagnosis.

PXA have been added to the family of pediatric gliomas [2]. Clinical properties include a presentation in children or young adults, frequent manifestation with focal epilepsy and superficial location with subarachnoid involvement. Histopathological hallmarks are polymorphic neoplastic astrocytes with foamy cytoplasm and spindle cell morphology, reticulin fiber production, frequent lymphocytic infiltrates and a fairly sharp demarcation towards the adjacent brain (fig. 3C, D). These lesions were previously viewed as histiocytic tumors.

With the consistent immunohistochemical detection of GFAP, they are now unequivocally established as an astrocytoma variant. The grading of PXA remains controversial. Despite the regular presence of pleomorphism and high cellularity, the original reports indicated a benign course in many cases. However, an increasing number of patients with malignant forms of PXA as well as with malignant progression of PXA into anaplastic variants or into glioblastoma multiforme have been observed [6]. In our experience, a significant mitotic activity and/or high Ki-67 proliferation index are associated with anaplastic forms. All patients with PXA require a close clinical follow-up.

Pilocytic astrocytomas represent another pediatric glioma entity with unusual histopathological properties. They may display microscopic features, i.e. pleomorphism, extensive neovascularization and, in some instances, necrobiotic change which would indicate malignancy in adult astrocytomas (fig. 3A). The distinction of rare anaplastic pilocytic astrocytoma variants requires the presence of high proliferative activity (Ki-67 index higher than 10%) and/or a poorly differentiated aggressive tumor cell component [7]. It remains to be established whether all pilocytic astrocytomas (WHO grade I) are associated with benign biological behavior. This issue deserves more attention in the future.

Grading of Gliomas

An area clearly in need for further improvement is the histopathological grading of astrocytic and oligodendroglial gliomas. So far, it mainly relies on classical morphological parameters such as cell density, cellular morphology and differentiation, mitotic activity, vascular endothelial proliferation, thrombosis of tumor vasculature and necrosis. Increased nuclear and cellular pleomorphism, mitotic and/or proliferative activity, increased cellularity and an early stage of vascular endothelial proliferation are decisive properties for the distinction of astrocytoma (WHO grade II) and anaplastic astrocytoma (WHO grade III) (fig. 4). The diagnosis of GBM relies on the detection of marked vascular endothelial proliferation and tumor necrosis (fig. 5). Necrosis constitutes the most important among these criteria. Several clinicopathological studies have demonstrated the prognostic significance of necrosis in malignant astrocytic gliomas [8]. However, necrotic change should only be used as a key diagnostic factor in untreated gliomas. Following surgery, radiotherapy and/or chemotherapy its diagnostic significance is uncertain.

Histopathological grading of gliomas has gained critical importance for the clinical management of patients. At many neuro-oncology centers, the treatment for tumors of WHO grades I and II is neurosurgical. Patients with malignant gliomas WHO grade III or IV usually receive postoperative radio-

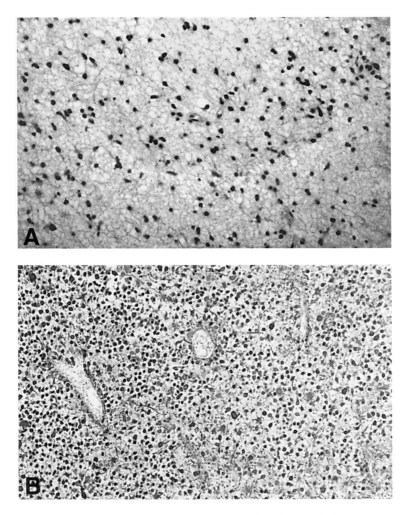

Fig. 4. Grading of astrocytomas. *A* A fibrillary, low-grade diffuse astrocytoma (WHO grade II). *B* An anaplastic astrocytoma (WHO grade III) of gemistocytic morphology.

and/or chemotherapy. A significantly different clinical course for distinct glioma entities should be kept in mind, however. It has been demonstrated that anaplastic oligodendrogliomas and anaplastic astrocytomas show significant differences in their prognosis although both tumors are classified into the WHO grade III category [9].

Antibodies to proliferation-associated antigens have received considerable attention as novel tool in the grading of brain tumors. A monoclonal antibody to the Ki-67 antigen (MiB-1) is now widely used in surgical neuropathology

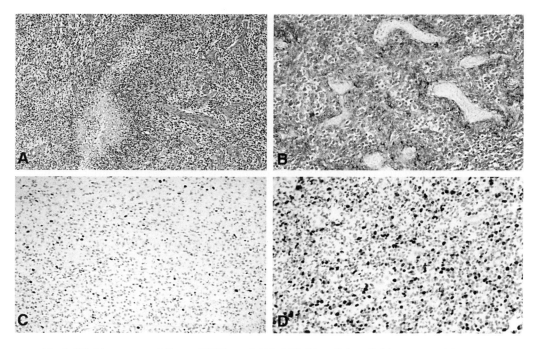

Fig. 5. Glioblastoma multiforme WHO grade IV. *A* Highly cellular glioblastoma multiforme with focal necrosis, pseudopalisading and vascular endothelial proliferation. This glioma exhibits strong immunoreactivity for the angiogenic peptide VEGF. *B* A striking regional variation of tumor cell proliferation is not uncommon in glioblastomas. *C, D* An example of regional heterogeneity in tumor cell proliferation. Significantly different Ki-67-positive fractions can be observed in two different fields of the same tumor.

[10]. The Ki-67 antigen was identified as a nuclear protein associated with the G1, S, G2 and M phases of the cell cycle. Significant levels cannot be detected in quiescent cells of the G0 phase. The percentage of Ki-67 immunoreactive nuclei can be used to determine the proliferating tumor cell fraction. Many investigators have been able to demonstrate that different histopathological grades of astrocytic and other gliomas exhibit significant differences in their average Ki-67 index. However, there is considerable overlap between WHO grades and significant interindividual variation. In addition, striking regional heterogeneity can be observed in different areas of the same tumor (fig. 5C, D). In astrocytic gliomas, Ki-67 scores above 5% appear to be helpful as an additional tool for the recognition of anaplastic forms [11]. Low proliferation values per se are of uncertain relevance as even malignant gliomas may contain components with a majority of resting tumor cells. A representative example for this phenomenon is given in figure 5C. It illustrates that classical histopatho-

logical grading parameters are of critical importance for the clinical neuro-pathologist.

Gliomas with histopathological features intermediate between WHO grade II and III represent a particularly challenging group. Recent data indicate that Ki-67-staining may be helpful in establishing the diagnosis of anaplastic astrocytoma in such cases [11]. The significance of vascular endothelial prolif-eration has also stirred some debate. In our experience, a moderate extent of proliferated endothelia can be applied as an additional parameter to distinguish anaplastic astrocytomas (WHO grade III) from diffuse low-grade astrocytomas (WHO grade II). Only marked or glomeruloid vascular aggregates should prompt the diagnosis of glioblastoma multiforme. Astrocytomas with border-line morphology often display gemistocytic properties. This observation has led to the hypothesis that gemistocytic astrocytomas carry a significantly higher risk for malignant progression [12]. Although frequently proposed, this notion remains to be confirmed in a controlled setting.

Molecular Neuropathology of Malignant Gliomas

Molecular genetic studies in many laboratories have identified an increas-ing number of glioma-associated tumor genes and genetic loci [13]. Some of these genes appear to be involved at defined stages of glioma development and many have been specifically associated with malignant gliomas, in particular glioblastoma multiforme. Preliminary observations indicate that the detection of specific molecular alterations in individual tumors may evolve as an adjunct tool for the diagnostic evaluation of gliomas. Prominent examples of glioma-associated genes include:

TP53
TP53 encodes a protein of 53 kD (p53) involved in important cellular functions including transcriptional control, cell cycle regulation, genome integ-rity and apoptosis [14]. The TP53 tumor suppressor gene carries mutations in 30–50% of astrocytomas WHO grade II and III and glioblastomas WHO grade IV. This suggests that TP53 plays an important role in the formation of astrocytic gliomas. Mutations cluster in exons 4–8 of TP53. They can be detected with molecular genetic approaches such as SSCP screening and DNA sequence analysis. In some cases, mutant p53 protein accumulates in the nucleus of affected glioma cells and can be visualized immunohistochemically. Some investigators have proposed a potential involvement of TP53 in the malignant progression of astrocytomas. However, subsequent studies have provided evi-dence that mutant TP53 may act at an early stage of glioma development.

A Putative Tumor Suppressor Gene on Chromosome Arm 19q

A putative tumor suppressor gene on chromosome 19q13.3-4 has evolved as an interesting candidate for a genetic locus associated with malignant progression of low-grade astrocytomas to anaplastic forms [15]. This chromosomal region shows allelic deletions in approximately 50% of anaplastic astrocytomas WHO grade III but only a low 10–15% incidence of changes in diffuse low-grade astrocytomas WHO grade II. Despite intense research efforts, the responsible gene has not yet been cloned. Once identified, this gene may be useful as a molecular tool to identify those low-grade astrocytomas with a high risk for malignant progression.

Cyclin-Dependent Kinase Inhibitors 2A and 2B (CDKN2A and CDKN2B)

Cyclin-dependent kinases are members of an increasing family of molecules involved in cell cycle regulation. Structural changes in such regulatory molecules have been detected in many cancers. In brain tumors, alterations of cell cycle control elements can be encountered predominantly in glioblastomas. This property of glioblastomas may well account for their high proliferative potential. The genes for cyclin-dependent kinase inhibitors 2A and 2B (CDKN2A and CDKN2B) on chromosome 9p21 represent examples of cell cycle-associated tumor suppressors which show a high incidence of homozygous deletions of both alleles in glioblastomas [16–18]. Their inactivation is likely to contribute to the malignant transformation of anaplastic astrocytic gliomas into glioblastoma multiforme. In addition to deletion, these genes may be inactivated by hypermethylation.

Glioblastoma-Associated Tumor Suppressors on Chromosome 10

Almost 90% of glioblastomas show structural changes on the long arm of chromosome 10. This finding strongly suggests the presence of a gene or genes on chromosome 10 whose inactivation contributes to the formation of glioblastomas. Recently, the PTEN gene was identified as a candidate. It encodes a novel class of tumor suppressor with domains homologous to protein tyrosine phosphatases and to the cytoskeleton-related protein tensin. PTEN mutations have been found in various human cancers and in several hereditary tumor conditions including Cowden's disease [19]. Several studies reported that the PTEN gene carries mutations in approximately 20% of glioblastomas [20]. Additional tumor suppressors on chromosome 10q need to be identified.

Oncogene Activation in Malignant Gliomas

Oncogene activation constitutes another mechanism of neoplastic transformation. In human tumors, gene amplification appears to represent the most common mode of oncogene activation. Activated oncogenes have only rarely been identified in low grade or anaplastic human gliomas of WHO grades II and III. However, this genetic alteration occurs in a significant fraction of glioblastomas, which carry an amplified epidermal growth factor receptor oncogene (EGFR) in 30–40% [21]. This results in overexpression of the receptor protein and in growth stimulation. Attempts to use antibodies to EGFR for diagnostic and therapeutic purposes are currently under investigation. Amplification of the cyclin-dependent kinase 4 gene (CDK4) whose product functions as a cell cycle regulator, has been reported in 10–20% of glioblastomas [22]. The MDM-2 gene encodes a product interacting with p53. It represents a third example of a gene with genomic amplification in a subfraction of glioblastomas. The overexpressed mdm-2 protein inactivates p53 through complex formation.

Neoangiogenesis in Malignant Gliomas

Vascular endothelial proliferation has been established as a morphological parameter associated with malignancy in adult supratentorial astrocytomas. Molecules, which regulate neoangiogenesis, would, therefore, be expected to contribute to malignant progression of gliomas. Recent molecular studies have unraveled some of the factors responsible for neoangiogenesis and vascular endothelial proliferation in malignant gliomas. Vascular endothelial growth factor, a 167 (VEGF167) or 189 (VEGF189) amino acid polypeptide, produced and secreted by glioma cells is one of the key players [23]. VEGF binds to the flk-1 and flt-1 receptor molecules on vascular endothelial cells and this ligand binding triggers angiogenesis. Experimental strategies interfering with this signaling event are beginning to emerge. However, several studies suggest that other angiogenic molecules including FGF-2 and PDGFs may also be required for endothelial growth in gliomas [24].

The Concept of Molecular Glioblastoma Variants

A hallmark of glioblastomas is the accumulation of several molecular genetic changes in the tumor genome. This property prompted us to examine if such alterations combine in a random fashion or if they occur in distinct patterns. Surprisingly, it turned out that two molecular subtypes of glioblastoma multiforme could be distinguished at a molecular genetic level [25]. The glioblastoma type 1 is characterized by a high incidence of allelic losses on chromosome arm 17p and TP53 mutations and an activated PDGF/PDGFR pathway (fig. 6). Characteristic features of the more common glioblastoma type 2 include an amplified EGFR oncogene, amplification of the cyclin-dependent kinase 4 and MDM-2 genes and an unaffected TP53 gene. Alterations of chromosome arm 10q and VEGF overexpression occur in both variants. The two molecular entities exhibit remarkable clinical differences.

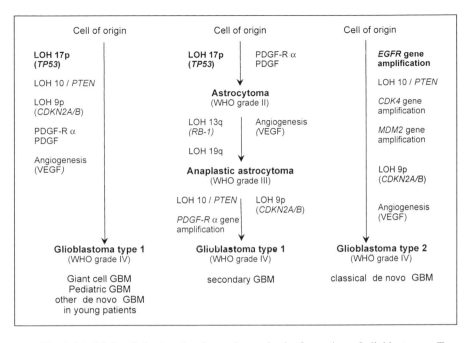

Fig. 6. Model for distinct molecular pathways in the formation of glioblastomas. Two molecular variants can be clearly distinguished: glioblastoma type 1 and 2 are not only characterized by mutually exclusive patterns of molecular genetic alterations, they also display significant clinical/age and histopathological differences. Glioblastoma type 2, the more common variant, arises de novo in patients beyond the age of 45 years. An amplified EGFR oncogene and unaffected TP53/chromosome 17p constitute the key molecular properties. Glioblastomas type 1 occur in young patients and may evolve from pre-existing astrocytomas (secondary glioblastoma). However, the majority of the type 1 tumors also manifest without evidence for a symptomatic precursor lesion. Molecular genetic features include mutant TP53 and/or allelic losses on the short arm of chromosome 17 (LOH 17p), an intact EGFR oncogene, and an activated PDGF/PDGFR pathway.

Glioblastoma type 2 comprises the classical de novo glioblastoma in patients beyond the age of 50 years. In contrast, the type 1 form develops in young patients, evolves from a lower grade lesion in approximately 30% of the cases and includes specific clinical and morphological variants of glioblastoma such as pediatric glioblastomas and giant cell glioblastoma. As many studies have identified young age as one of the few prognostically significant parameters in glioblastoma patients, we propose that the prognostic impact of age at diagnosis may be related to the fact that glioblastomas in young patients are molecularly and biologically distinct. This intriguing hypothesis requires verification in controlled trials. Key features of the two molecular glioblastoma variants are summarized in table 2.

Table 2. Key features of the molecular type 1 and type 2 variants of glioblastoma multiforme

Glioblastoma type 1	Glioblastoma type 2
LOH 17p/TP53 mutation	TP53 wild type
EGFR single copy	EGFR amplification
PDGF-R α activated	CDK4 amplification
	MDM2 amplification
Secondary GBM in 30%	De novo glioblastoma
Young patients	Higher age

LOH = Loss of heterozygosity.

Molecular Neuropathology of Oligodendrogliomas and Mixed Oligoastrocytomas

The molecular pathogenesis of oligodendrogliomas and oligoastrocytomas is clearly distinct from astrocytic gliomas. Most of the genetic lesions encountered in astrocytomas can not usually be observed in these gliomas. LOH studies have identified high rates of allelic defects on the short arm of chromosome 1 and on the long arm of chromosome 19 in these tumors [26]. Putative tumor suppressor genes at the two loci appear to be important players in the development of oligodendroglioma and oligoastrocytoma. It remains to be seen if the gene affected on chromosome 19q will be identical to the astrocytoma progression-associated tumor suppressor discussed above. In a detailed molecular genetic analysis of oligoastrocytomas, we have been able to distinguish two molecular variants with patterns related either to oligodendrogliomas or astrocytomas [27]. A recent clinical study reports a significant association of these two loci with chemotherapy response in oligodendroglioma patients. This finding points to yet another clinical application of molecular neuro-oncology.

A Diagnostic Potential for Molecular Neuropathology?

Some of the pitfalls and deficits in the surgical neuropathology of gliomas have been outlined above. Major areas of debate include the issue of grading and assessment of the risk for malignant progression in individual patients, significant interindividual variations in the clinical course of histopathological entities and the reliable identification of chemotherapy-responsive gliomas. The application of molecular tools promises advances in all three areas.

In a recently completed study on astrocytomas WHO grade II and III, we have evaluated molecular genetic parameters for the diagnostic assessment of stereotactic glioma biopsies [28]. Biopsy specimens obtained during stereotactic procedures and during open neurosurgery were compared in this analysis. The results show that a significant fraction of stereotactic biopsies with a histopathological diagnosis of astrocytoma WHO grade II exhibit molecular alterations characteristically encountered in higher grade gliomas. These findings will have to be confirmed in a larger series of patients. They do, however, indicate that molecular neuropathology can be applied as a valuable additional tool for the classification and grading of gliomas. The further development and evaluation of molecular techniques poses an important interdisciplinary challenge for both molecular and clinical neuro-oncologists.

References

1   Kleihues P, Burger PC, Scheithauer BW: Histological typing of tumours of the central nervous system. World Health Organization International Classification of Tumours. Berlin, Springer, 1993.
2   Kepes JJ: Pleomorphic xanthoastrocytoma: The birth of a diagnosis and a concept. Brain Pathol 1993;3:269–274.
3   Van den Berg SR: Desmoplastic infantile ganglioglioma and desmoplastic cerebral astrocytoma of infancy. Brain Pathol 1993;3:275–281.
4   Hassoun J, Soylemezoglu F, Gambarelli D, Figarella-Branger D, von Ammon K, Kleihues P: Central neurocytoma: A synopsis of clinical and histological features. Brain Pathol 1993;3:297–306.
5   Cairncross G, Macdonald D, Ludwin S, Lee D, Cascino T, Buckner J, Fulton D, Dropcho E, Stewart D, Schold C Jr: Chemotherapy for anaplastic oligodendroglioma. National Cancer Institute of Canada Clinical Trials Group. J Clin Oncol 1994;12:2013–2021.
6   Pahapill PA, Ramsay DA, Del Maestro RF: Pleomorphic xanthoastrocytoma: Case report and analysis of the literature concerning the efficacy of resection and the significance of necrosis. Neurosurgery 1996;38:822–829.
7   Dirks PB, Jay V, Becker LE, Drake JM, Humphreys RP, Hoffman HJ, Rutka JT: Development of anaplastic changes in low-grade astrocytomas of childhood. Neurosurgery 1994;34:68–78.
8   Burger PC, Vollmer RT: Histologic factors of prognostic significance in the glioblastoma multiforme. Cancer 1980;46:1179–1186.
9   Shaw EG, Scheithauer BW, O'Fallon JR, Tazelaar HD, Davis DH: Oligodendrogliomas: The Mayo Clinic experience. J Neurosurg 1992;76:428–434.
10 Gerdes J, Dallenbach F, Lennert K, Lemke H, Stein H: Growth fractions in malignant non-Hodgkin's lymphomas as determined in situ with the monoclonal antibody Ki-67. Hematol Oncol 1984;2: 365–371.
11 Hsu DW, Louis DN, Efird JT, Hedley-Whyte ET: Use of MIB-1 (Ki-67) immunoreactivity in differentiating grade II and grade III gliomas. J Neuropathol Exp Neurol 1997;56:857–865.
12 Krouwer HG, Davis RL, Silver P, Prados M: Gemistocytic astrocytomas: A reappraisal. J Neurosurg 1991;74:399–406.
13 Kleihues P, Cavenee WK: Pathology and Genetics of Tumors of the Nervous System. Lyon, IARC, 1997.
14 Fulci G, Ishii N, Van Meir EG: p53 and brain tumors: From gene mutations to gene therapy. Brain Pathol 1998;8:599–613.
15 Von Deimling A, Bender B, Jahnke R, Waha A, Kraus J, Albrecht S, Wellenreuther R, Fassbender F, Nagel J, Menon AG: Loci associated with malignant progression in astrocytomas: A candidate on chromosome 19q. Cancer Res 1994;54:1397–1401.

16   Jen J, Harper W, Bigner SH, Bigner DD, Papadopoulos N, Markowitz S, Willson JKV, Kinzler KW, Vogelstein B: Deletion of p16 and p15 genes in brain tumors. Cancer Res 1994;54:6353–6358.

17   Nishikawa R, Furnari FB, Lin H, Arap W, Berger MS, Cavenee WK, Su Huang HJ: Loss of P16INK4 expression is frequent in high grade gliomas. Cancer Res 1995;55:1941–1945.

18   Schmidt EE, Ichimura K, Reifenberger G, Collins VP: CDKN2 (p16/MTS1) gene deletion or CDK4 amplification occurs in the majority of glioblastomas. Cancer Res 1994;54:6321–6324.

19   Liaw D, Marsh DJ, Li J, Dahia PL, Wang SI, Zheng Z, Bose S, Call KM, Tsou HC, Peacocke M: Germline mutations of the PTEN gene in Cowden disease, an inherited breast and thyroid cancer syndrome. Nat Genet 1997;16:64–67.

20   Duerr EM, Rollbrocker B, Hayashi Y, Peters N, Meyer-Puttlitz B, Louis DN, Schramm J, Wiestler OD, Parsons R, Eng C: PTEN mutations in gliomas and glioneuronal tumors. Oncogene 1998;16: 2259–2264.

21   Von Deimling A, Louis DN, von Ammon K, Petersen I, Hoell T, Chung RY, Martuza R, Schoenfeld D, Yasargil MG, Wiestler OD: Association of epidermal growth factor receptor gene amplification with loss of chromosome 10 in human glioblastoma multiforme. J Neurosurg 1992;77:295–301.

22   Reifenberger G, Reifenberger J, Ichimura K, Meltzer PS, Collins VP: Amplification of multiple genes from chromosomal region 12q13-14 in human malignant gliomas: Preliminary mapping of the amplicons shows preferential involvement of CDK4, SAS, and MDM2. Cancer Res 1994;54: 4299–4303.

23   Plate KH, Risau W: Angiogenesis in malignant gliomas. Glia 1995;15:339–347.

24   Pietsch T, Valter MM, Wolf HK, von Deimling A, Huang HJ, Cavenee WK, Wiestler OD: Expression and distribution of vascular endothelial growth factor protein in human brain tumors. Acta Neuropathol (Berl) 1997;93:109–117.

25   Von Deimling A, Louis DN, Wiestler OD: Molecular pathways in the formation of gliomas. Glia 1995;15:328–338.

26   Reifenberger J, Reifenberger G, Liu L, James CD, Wechsler W, Collins VP: Molecular genetic analysis of oligodendroglial tumors shows preferential allelic deletions on 19q and 1p. Am J Pathol 1994;145:1175–1190.

27   Maintz D, Fiedler K, Koopmann J, Rollbrocker B, Nechev S, Lenartz D, Stangl AP, Louis DN, Schramm J, Wiestler OD: Molecular genetic evidence for subtypes of oligoastrocytomas. J Neuropathol Exp Neurol 1997;56:1098–1104.

28   Müller MB, Schmidt MC, Schmidt O, Hayashi Y, Rollbrocker B, Waha A, Fimmers R, Volk B, Warnke P, Ostertag CB: Molecular genetic analysis as a tool for evaluating stereotactic biopsies of glioma specimens. J Neuropathol Exp Neurol 1999;58:40–45.

Dr. Otmar D. Wiestler, Institut für Neuropathologie und Hirntumor-Referenzzentrum, Universitätskliniken Bonn, Sigmund-Freud-Strasse 25, D–53105 Bonn (Germany)
Tel. +49 228 287 6602, Fax +49 228 287 4331, E-Mail neuropath@uni-bonn.de

Wiegel T, Hinkelbein W, Brock M, Hoell T (eds): Controversies in Neuro-Oncology.
Front Radiat Ther Oncol. Basel, Karger, 1999, vol 33, pp 139–149

....

Current Approaches to Radiation Therapy for Malignant Gliomas

Michael Brada

Neuro-Oncology Unit and Academic Unit of Radiotherapy and Oncology,
The Institute of Cancer Research and The Royal Marsden NHS Trust, Sutton,
Surrey, UK

Conventional External Beam Radiotherapy

Effectiveness of Radiotherapy

The role of conventional external beam radiotherapy (RT) in patients with high-grade glioma has been tested in two randomized studies [1, 2]. Both demonstrated unequivocal survival benefit in patients receiving whole-brain irradiation with an approximate 6-month gain in median survival, even though the overall median survival of 9–12 months remains poor with no apparent long-term cure. The results are supported by a Scandinavian study comparing chemotherapy with radiation with a clear survival benefit for RT in younger patients [3]. A 6-month prolongation of survival may only be of value if it is of good quality but an objective quality of life benefit has not been fully documented. However, performance status measured by Karnofsky Performance Status Scale (KPS) improved after treatment and patients who received RT maintained the improvement for longer [1].

Radiotherapy Dose

The optimum dose to large volume using conventional RT technique is 55–60 Gy at 1.8–2 Gy per fraction. Initial nonrandomized studies suggested a dose-response relationship with prolongation of median survival with doses increasing from 45–50 to 60 Gy [4]. This has been confirmed in a randomized MRC study comparing 45 Gy in 20 fractions with 60 Gy in 30 fractions [5] with a prolongation in median survival in patients receiving 60 Gy. A randomized study comparing 60 Gy whole-brain irradiation with 60 Gy followed by a 10 Gy boost failed to show a survival benefit for a higher radiation dose to large volume [6].

Volume of Irradiation

The policy of whole-brain irradiation used in initial RT trials was based on historical information of the spread of tumour beyond the suspected margin visualized surgically or by radioisotope scan. With CT and MR imaging, most centres have adopted localized treatment techniques with margins of 2–5 cm beyond the region of enhancement or low density on CT/high signal intensity on T2W MRI. The policy of such localized irradiation is supported by histological evidence of tumour spread beyond the enhancing CT margin [7, 8] and the local nature of recurrence in the majority of tumours [9]. One randomized study which suggests equal efficacy of localized irradiation demonstrated equivalent survival following whole-brain irradiation with a localized boost in comparison to whole-brain irradiation alone [10]. Despite incomplete information on the equivalence of whole-brain and localized irradiation, the potential toxicity of irradiating large volumes of normal brain and the lack of clear benefit of whole-brain radiotherapy has led to the policy of local RT alone.

Tailoring Therapy to Prognosis

Age, performance status and histology are the principal determinants of survival in patients with malignant glioma [11, 12]. Using a method of recursive partitioning it is possible to separate patients into prognostic subgroups with predicted median survival ranging from 5 months in elderly disabled patients with glioblastoma multiforme to 59 months in young, fit patients with anaplastic astrocytoma [13]. An intensive course of RT as daily treatment over 6 weeks may be inappropriate for patients destined to survive less than 6 months with no prospect of long-term cure. Conversely, radical intensive treatment schedules may be offered to patients with longer life expectancy. However, caution should be exercised in patients with best prognostic features to avoid potential long-term toxicity of intensive treatment strategies.

Palliative Treatment

For severely disabled and elderly patients with high-grade glioma who have a poor prognosis, an aggressive 6-week course of intensive RT may be too onerous. The options are either a shortened hypofractionated palliative course of irradiation as used in the treatment of brain metastases or palliative care alone. A number of palliative RT regimens have been examined in Phase II studies [14–16] with doses ranging from 30 to 45 Gy given in 6–20 fractions over 2–4 weeks. One hundred patients treated at the Royal Marsden Hospital to a dose of 30 Gy in 6 fractions over 2 weeks had a median survival of 6 months [update of 14]. While the results are comparable to radical RT given to a similar group of patients, formal randomized studies comparing radical and short palliative regimens are not available. Hypofractionated RT has some palliative efficacy with a third of surviving patients showing improvement and a third stabilization of functional status 1–3 months after treatment [14]. The overall efficacy of palliative RT in comparison to other approaches needs to be evaluated in future randomized studies. The control group should include either supportive care alone, radical RT alone or both and the choice depends on the prevailing national treatment strategies and expectations for the group of patients with poor life expectancy.

Increasing Intensity of Radiotherapy

RT can be intensified simply by increasing the dose of radiation. However, this is unlikely to achieve the desired aim of improving the therapeutic ratio. This can be theoretically achieved by the use of altered fractionation [17], radiosensitizers and by giving highly localized irradiation through interstitial or external beam stereotactic delivery techniques.

Altered Fractionation

Hyperfractionation, the use of two or three small dose fractions per day in the same overall treatment time, exploits the differences in repair capacity between tumour and late responding normal tissue. In CNS RT it may allow for a higher total dose and may result in increased tumour cell kill without increasing normal tissue toxicity. Small randomized studies of hyperfractionation usually given also in a shorter time (accelerated) have yielded conflicting results [17]. The largest dose searching Phase I/II study tested doses from 64.8 to 81.6 Gy over 5.5–6.5 weeks together with BCNU [18]. There was no survival benefit with higher radiation doses; even a suggestion of worse results with doses ≥ 74.5 Gy, ascribed to neurotoxicity.

Accelerated RT, which shortens the overall treatment time by multiple conventional dose fractions per day, may reduce the repopulation of tumour cells between fractions. It may potentially improve tumour control for a given dose level providing there is no increase in late normal tissue injury. The kinetics of repair of radiation injury in the nervous system is slow and within the time interval between fractions may not be complete. Accelerated

RT may therefore carry a potential risk of increased late normal tissue damage.

Studies of accelerated RT usually combined with hyperfractionation have so far not demonstrated a survival advantage [17]. At the Royal Marsden Hospital, patients are offered conventional or accelerated RT. The median survival of patients treated with accelerated regimen is 10 months [19] which is similar to a matched control cohort treated with conventional daily fractionation to 60 Gy [20]. Despite the lack of survival benefit, the treatment can be completed in shorter overall time with no excess acute toxicity and this may avoid a protracted 6-week course of therapy. Accelerated RT requires the patient to come to the hospital twice a day (with potential financial consequences), is inconvenient for the normal functioning of a busy department and is manpower-intensive. While the approach is reasonable, the short overall survival of patients with high-grade glioma also precludes any definite conclusion about the long-term safety of high-dose accelerated RT in terms of late CNS injury.

Radiosensitizers

Based on the knowledge of the mechanisms likely to contribute to radioresistance, a number of experimental strategies aiming to biochemically enhance the cellular response to irradiation have been evaluated in clinical studies. These have included the use of hypoxic cell sensitizers, hyperbaric oxygen, chemical sensitization with halogenated pyrimidines, and neutron therapy.

The use of radiosensitizers [21], hyperbaric oxygen [22] and neutron beam therapy [23, 24], to overcome the presumed problem of hypoxia have not shown a significant survival advantage. Despite suggestion from a number of Phase II studies of efficacy of BUdR as a radiation sensitizer in the treatment of high-grade glioma, a randomized RTOG study 94-04 has demonstrated inferior survival in patients receiving BUdR [Curran, unpubl. data]. The use of etanidazole as a sensitizer has also been disappointing [25].

Localized Irradiation

Based on the presumed localized nature of glial tumours and the apparent dose-response relationship of gliomas, attempts have been made to increase the dose to the tumour using the technique of interstitial RT (IRT) or stereotactic external beam RT/radiosurgery (SRT).

Interstitial Radiotherapy (Brachytherapy)

The results of IRT boost show a wide variation in median survival ranging from 7–36 months [26, 27]. It is likely that patient selection is the major determinant of survival [28]. Two randomized studies have been carried out to assess the role of implant boost in primary treatment of malignant gliomas. In Brain Tumor Cooperative Group (BTCG) Protocol 87-01 and the University of Toronto trial, all patients underwent conventional surgery, high-dose external beam radiotherapy and BCNU, and were randomized to an implant boost. The results of the University of Toronto trial show no improvement in survival in patients receiving IRT [29]. The treatment is not without toxicity as a large proportion of patients were steroid-dependent and required reoperation for presumed necrosis. The results of the BTCG trial completed some years ago have not been published.

Currently there is no evidence that interstitial irradiation prolongs survival. It is a highly interventionist policy with a need for a number of operative procedures. In patients with high-grade glioma where the treatment is not curative, it is questionable whether such a policy has any role particularly as there is no information of benefit in terms of quality of life.

Stereotactic Radiotherapy

Single fraction radiosurgery can be considered as a noninvasive alternative to brachytherapy. It has been used as a boost after conventional external beam irradiation in patients with newly diagnosed gliomas. This technique is limited to fit patients with small lesions. Following radiosurgery a large proportion of patients require reoperation for necrosis. Survival benefit has been claimed for radiosurgery boost but the data presented are not convincing [30, 31], and the apparently favourable results may be due to patient selection [32].

Despite the almost complete lack of evidence of benefit of localized stereotactic radiotherapy boost in the management of primary malignant glioma, the easy availability of what is a noninvasive treatment technique means that it is frequently offered to patients with appropriate size lesions. However, to obtain objective information about the potential benefit and toxicity of this approach we have to await the result of randomized studies of single fraction radiosurgery boost (RTOG) and fractionated stereotactic radiotherapy boost (EORTC and MRC) in patients with small primary malignant glioma.

Intralesional Radiotherapy

Intralesional radioimmunotherapy offers a biological means of delivering localized RT to malignant glioma. It combines the use of short-lived radioisotopes conjugated to monoclonal antibodies directed against tumour-specific antigenic targets, with the precision of stereotactic localization and catheterization. Clinical studies have predominantly focused on the delivery of ^{131}I to glioma overexpressing either the extracellular protein tenascin, or epidermal growth factor receptor [33, 34]. The toxicity of the approach is acceptable, although it requires invasive intralesional delivery of antibody. Nevertheless, it is possible to achieve clinically relevant intratumoral radiation doses with acceptable systemic irradiation. The homogeneity of dose delivery depends on both the microdosimetry profile of the chosen radioisotope, and the intratumoral distribution of both target and antibody. Early clinical studies of adjuvant intralesional antibody, while claiming survival benefit [34], are difficult to evaluate because of patient selection. On the basis of the available data there is no evidence of significant prolongation in survival.

Particle Radiation and BNCT

Heavy charged particles achieve localized delivery of radiation which is suitable for conformal RT. Particles are also considered beneficial due to higher biological effectiveness although this does not differentiate between tumour and normal tissue and there is no clear potential for improved therapeutic ratio. Randomized study of pion (pi-meson) radiation had not demonstrated survival advantage in comparison to conventional RT [35]. Other particle radiation (protons, neons, helium ions) have not been studied in randomized trials.

Boron neutron capture therapy (BNCT) [36–38] is currently undergoing Phase I/II evaluation using BSH and BPA and there is not yet sufficient published data available to assess its potential efficacy and toxicity.

Recurrent Malignant Glioma

The aim of therapy in patients with recurrent malignant glioma is palliation, yet prolongation of survival continues to be the major endpoint of treatment efficacy in the majority of published studies. Patients offered further active treatment are highly selected in terms of age, performance status, general medical fitness and size of recurrent tumour. Patients suitable for salvage therapy also have relatively slow progression of disease at the time of recurrence. The results of single-arm studies of patients with recurrent disease therefore suffer from lead time, length and selection bias. The prognosis of such patients with recurrent disease is measured in months and prognostic factors at the time of recurrence are the same as those at presentation with initial histology, performance status and age the most important determinants [39].

Interstitial Radiotherapy

Median survival of patients with glioblastoma multiforme treated with IRT at the time of recurrence ranges from 5 to 13 months [27]. With the exception of one study [40], there is no appreciable difference in survival between patients with recurrent anaplastic astrocytoma and gliblastoma multiforme. Late side effects in terms of symptomatic radiation necrosis requiring reoperation have been reported in 50% of patients, but measured in actuarial terms the 2- to 3-year risk of symptomatic necrosis can be up to 100%. Even high doses of radiation are unable to eradicate the tumour as there are often viable tumour cells noted within the necrotic material. The palliative efficacy of IRT is not fully documented. There is a small decrease in mean KPS during follow-up and a large proportion of patients remain steroid-dependent.

Stereotactic Radiotherapy

Single fraction radiosurgery [41] or fractionated SRT [42] have been used in a manner equivalent to brachytherapy in patients with recurrent malignant glioma. Using fractionated SRT at 5 Gy per fraction (to 30–35 Gy) the median survival is 9–10 months, which is similar to that achieved with IRT. The majority of patients remain functionally stable during follow-up, with few showing significant functional improvement. Only 2 patients required reoperation for necrosis, although the incidence of transient steroid-responsive deterioration, which is considered to represent radiation damage, increases with time. Fractionated SRT is a palliative treatment similar in efficacy to single fraction radiosurgery, but assumed to carry lesser toxicity. It is a noninvasive and a relatively well-tolerated outpatient therapy.

Summary

RT remains the mainstay of treatment of malignant glioma. The standard policy is to treat a planning target volume (PTV) confined to the enhancing tumour and a 2- to 5-cm margin. Conventional treatment is given to a dose of 55–60 Gy at <2 Gy per fraction. Such regimens have not been superseded although similar doses may be given using accelerated RT largely with the aim of shortening treatment time.

The standard policy results in a median survival of 9–12 months in patients with glioblastoma multiforme and 12–24 months in patients with anaplastic astrocytoma. There is currently no evidence that high-dose focal irradiation in the form of IRT or as noninvasive SRT prolong survival or improve quality of life. While IRT has been shown not to be of value, we have to await the results of randomized studies of SRT before introducing it into routine practice. All techniques which lead to an increase in the effective radiation dose are potentially toxic and should be introduced into primary therapy with great caution.

In patients with poor prognosis disease, which includes older (usually >65 years) and severely disabled patients (KPS ≤50), the role of RT has not been fully proven. A protracted course of intensive RT is probably too onerous and palliative short regimens may be appropriate. Formal comparison with conventional approaches is required.

While RT continues to be advocated as the most effective primary therapy, a 6-week course of intensive therapy is not without toxicity, particularly in the form of lethargy, and some patients and carers may feel that side effects may outweigh the limited survival benefit. The effects of treatment on health-related quality of life need to be fully evaluated in prospective studies, to enable appropriate advice and treatment selection for each individual patient.

Conclusions

RT is an effective treatment modality in the management of malignant glioma. However, despite many promising results from early Phase II trials, there has been no real progress in offering more effective means of delivering RT either in terms of reduction in treatment toxicity or improvement in survival. Serious examination of the last 20 years of research effort suggests serious problems with the methodology employed in Phase II trials. Anyone reading the glioma clinical literature will be aware of the plethora of positive and encouraging Phase II trials which have all to date failed to yield positive Phase III trials, which must remain the gold standard in assessing new forms of therapy. The lesson for the future must be a serious re-examination of the validity of the Phase II trial methodology. Before embarking on any further costly and time-consuming randomized studies, we should have more certainty that such trials are likely to result in positive results. Dilution of research by a plethora of 'promising' but largely ineffective treatment strategies is not only unhelpful, but positively destructive. Misdirecting research effort into blind alleys prevents the development and evaluation of truly effective new therapies.

The poor prognosis of malignant glioma means that there are desperate patients and equally eager clinicians looking for new and promising treatments. The last decade has seen fast progress in the development of new technology of RT. Apparent innovations such as radiosurgery claim their role early in the development phase as part of the marketing strategy of research organizations, manufacturers and institutions or individuals delivering treatment. The pressing need and the demand to come up with successful new treatments has led to early introduction of apparently novel approaches usually based on limited and often flawed evidence. All clinicians have a responsibility to find truly effective new treatments, which will be of help to future patients with malignant glioma. To achieve this will require more robust and flawless methods of assessment combined with scientific rigour and intellectual honesty beyond that seen in the past.

Advances in the treatment of brain tumours are usually measured in terms of survival benefit. While there is clear need for new treatments, which prolong survival, the management of patients with high-grade glioma is essentially that of care of patients with incurable malignancy. New care strategies therefore constitute an important and often forgotten part of management which should also be subject to research.

References

1   Kristiansen K, Hagen S, Kollevold T, Torvik A, Holme I, Nesbakken R, et al: Combined modality therapy of operated astrocytomas grade III and IV. Confirmation of the value of postoperative irradiation and lack of potentiation of bleomycin on survival time: A Prospective Multicenter Trial of the Scandinavian Glioblastoma Study Group. Cancer 1981;47:649–652.
2   Walker MD, Alexander E, Hunt WE, MacCarty CS, Mahaley MS, Mealey J, et al: Evaluation of BCNU and/or radiotherapy in the treatment of anaplastic gliomas. J Neurosurg 1978;49:333–343.
3   Sandberg WM, Malmström P, Strömblad LG, Anderson H, Borgström S, Brun A, et al: A randomized study of chemotherapy with procarbazine, vincristine, and lomustine with and without radiation therapy for astrocytoma grades 3 and/or 4. Cancer 1991;68:22–29.
4   Walker MD, Strike TA, Sheline GE: An analysis of dose-effect relationship in the radiotherapy of malignant gliomas. Int J Radiat Oncol Biol Phys 1979;5:1725.
5   Bleehen NM, Stenning SP, on behalf of the Medical Research Council Brain Tumour Working Party: A Medical Research Council trial of two radiotherapy doses in the treatment of grades 3 and 4 astrocytoma. The Medical Research Council Brain Tumour Working Party. Br J Cancer 1991;64:769–774.
6   Chang CH, Horton J, Schoenfeld D, Salazar O, Perez Tamayo R, Kramer S, et al: Comparison of postoperative radiotherapy and combined postoperative radiotherapy and chemotherapy in the multidisciplinary management of malignant gliomas. A joint Radiation Therapy Oncology Group and Eastern Cooperative Oncology Group study. Cancer 1983;52:997–1007.
7   Burger P, Heinz E, Shibata T, Kleihues P: Topographic anatomy and CT correlations in the untreated glioblastoma multiforme. J Neurosurg 1988;68:698.
8   Halperin EC, Bentel G, Heinz ER, Burger PC: Radiation therapy treatment planning in supratentorial glioblastoma multiforme: An analysis based on post-mortem topographic anatomy with CT correlations. Int J Radiat Oncol Biol Phys 1989;17:1347–1350.
9   Wallner KE, Galicich JH, Krol G, Arbit E, Malkin MG: Patterns of failure following treatment for glioblastoma multiforme and anaplastic astrocytoma. Int J Radiat Oncol Biol Phys 1989;16:1405–1409.
10   Shapiro WR, Green SB, Burger PC, Mahaley MSJ, Selker RG, VanGilder JC, et al: Randomised trial of three chemotherapy regimens and two radiotherapy regimens in postoperative treatment of malignant glioma. J Neurosurg 1989;71:1–9.
11   Stenning S, Freedman LS, Bleehen NM, Medical Research Council Brain Tumour Working Party: Prognostic factors for high grade glioma: Development of a prognostic index. J Neurooncol 1990;9:47–55.
12   Curran WJ, Scott CB, Horton J, Nelson JS, Weinstein AS, Fischbach J, et al: Recursive partitioning analysis of prognostic factors in three Radiation Therapy Oncology Group Malignant Glioma Trials. J Natl Cancer Inst 1993;85:704–710.
13   Scott CB, Scarantino C, Urtasun R, Movsas B, Jones CU, Simpson JR, et al: Validation and predictive power of Radiation Therapy Oncology Group (RTOG) recursive partitioning analysis classes for malignant glioma patients: A report using RTOG 90-06. Int J Radiat Oncol Biol Phys 1998;40:51–55.

14 Thomas R, James N, Guerrero D, Ashley S, Gregor A, Brada M: Hypofractionated radiotherapy as palliative treatment in poor prognosis patients with high grade glioma. Radiother Oncol 1994; 33:113–116.

15 Bauman GS, Gaspar LE, Fisher BJ, Halperin EC, Macdonald DR, Cairncross JG: A prospective study of short course radiotherapy in poor prognosis glioblastoma multiforme. Int J Radiat Oncol Biol Phys 1994;29:835–839.

16 Kleinberg L, Slick T, Enger C, Grossman S, Brem H, Wharam MD Jr: Short course radiotherapy is an appropriate option for most malignant glioma patients. Int J Radiat Oncol Biol Phys 1997; 38:31–36.

17 Fallai C, Olmi P: Hyperfractionated and accelerated radiation therapy in central nervous system tumors (malignant gliomas, pediatric tumors, and brain metastases). Radiother Oncol 1997;43: 235–246.

18 Nelson DF, Curran WJ, Scott C, Nelson JS, Weinstein AS, Ahmad K, et al: Hyperfractionated radiation therapy and bis-chlorethyl-nitrosourea in the treatment of malignant glioma – Possible advantage observed at 72.0 Gy in 1.2 Gy BID fractions: Report of the Radiation Therapy Oncology Group Protocol 83 02. Int J Radiat Oncol Biol Phys 1993;25:193–207.

19 Brada M, Sharpe G, Rajan B, Britten J, Wilkins P, Guererro D, et al: Modifying radical radiotherapy in high grade gliomas; shortening the treatment time through acceleration. Int J Radiol Oncol Biol Phys 1999;43:287–292.

20 Brada M, Thomas G, Elyan S, James N, Hines F, Ashley S, et al: Improving the acceptability of high dose radiotherapy by reducing the duration of treatment: Accelerated radiotherapy in high grade glioma. Br J Cancer 1995;71:1330–1334.

21 Bleehen NM: Studies of high grade cerebral gliomas. Int J Radiat Oncol Biol Phys 1990;18:811–813.

22 Chang CH: Hyperbaric oxygen and radiation therapy in the management of glioblastoma; in Modern Concepts in Brain Tumour Therapy: Laboratory and Clinical Investigations. Natl Cancer Inst Monogr No 46. Washington, US Government Printing Office, 1977, p 163.

23 Catterall M, Bloom HJG, Ash DV, Walsh L, Richardson A, Uttley D, et al: Fast neutrons compared with megavoltage X-rays in the treatment of patients with supratentorial glioblastoma: A controlled pilot study. Int J Radiat Oncol Biol Phys 1980;6:261–266.

24 Duncan W, McLelland J, Jack WJL: Report of a randomised pilot study of the treatment of patients with supratentorial gliomas using neutron irradiation. Br J Radiol 1986;59:373.

25 Chang EL, Loeffler JS, Riese NE, Wen PY, Alexander ER, Black PM, et al: Survival results from a phase I study of etanidazole (SR2508) and radiotherapy in patients with malignant glioma. Int J Radiat Oncol Biol Phys 1998;40:65–70.

26 Liang B, Weil M: Locoregional approaches to therapy with gliomas as the paradigm. Curr Opin Oncol 1998;10:201–206.

27 McDermott MW, Sneed PK, Gutin PH: Interstitial brachytherapy for malignant brain tumors. Semin Surg Oncol 1998;14:79–87.

28 Florell R, MacDonald D, Irish W, Bernstein M, Leibel S, Gutin P, et al: Selection bias, survival, and brachytherapy for glioma. J Neurosurg 1992;76:179–183.

29 Laperriere NJ, Leung PM, McKenzie S, Milosevic M, Wong S, Glen J, et al: Randomized study of brachytherapy in the initial management of patients with malignant astrocytoma. Int J Radiat Oncol Biol Phys 1998;41:1005–1011.

30 Loeffler JS, Alexander E, Kooy HM, Wen PY: Results of radiosurgery used in the initial management of patients with malignant gliomas. Int J Radiat Oncol Biol Phys 1991;21(suppl 1):171.

31 Mehta MP, Masciopinto J, Rozental J, Levin A, Chappell R, Bastin K, et al: Stereotactic radiosurgery for glioblastoma multiforme: Report of a prospective study evaluating prognostic factors and analyzing long-term survival advantage. Int J Radiat Oncol Biol Phys 1994;30:541–549.

32 Curran WJ, Scott CB, Weinstein AS, Martin LA, Nelson JS, Phillips TL, et al: Survival comparison of radiosurgery eligible and ineligible malignant glioma patients treated with hyperfractionated radiation therapy and carmustine: A report of Radiation Therapy Oncology Group 83 02. J Clin Oncol 1993;11:857–862.

33 Colapinto EV, Zalutsky MR, Archer GE: RIT of intercranial human glioma xenografts with ^{131}I-labelled F(ab)$_2$ fragments of Mab Mel 14. Cancer Res 1990;50:1822–1827.

34 Riva P, Arista A, Tison V, Sturiale C, Francheshi G, Spinelli A, et al: Intralesional radioimmunother-apy of malignant gliomas. Cancer 1994;73:1076–1082.
35 Pickles T, Goodman GB, Rheaume DE, Duncan GG, Fryer CJ, Bhimji S, et al: Pion radiation for high grade astrocytoma: Results of a randomized study. Int J Radiat Oncol Biol Phys 1997;37: 491–497.
36 Soloway AH, Barth RF, Gahbauer RA, Blue TE, Goodman JH: The rationale and requirements for the development of boron neutron capture therapy of brain tumors. J Neurooncol 1997;33: 9–18.
37 Feinendegen LE: Strategic planning workshop on research needs for neutron capture therapy. J Neurooncol 1997;33:179–185.
38 Barth RF, Soloway AH: Boron neutron capture therapy of brain tumors – Current status and future prospects. J Neurooncol 1997;33:3–7.
39 Rajan B, Ross G, Lim CC, Ashley S, Goode D, Traish D, et al: Survival in patients with recurrent glioma as a measure of treatment efficacy: Prognostic factors following nitrosourea chemotherapy. Eur J Cancer 1994;12:1809–1815.
40 Leibel SA, Gutin PH, Wara WM, Silver PA, Larson DA, Edwards MSB, et al: Survival and quality of life after interstitial implantation of removable high activity iodine-125 sources for the treatment of patients with recurrent malignant gliomas. Int J Radiat Oncol Biol Phys 1989;17:1129–1139.
41 Shrieve DC, Alexander EI, Wen PY, Fine HA, Kooy HM, Black PM, et al: Comparison of stereotactic radiosurgery and brachytherapy in the treatment of recurrent glioblastoma multiforme. Neurosurgery 1995;36:275–282.
42 Shepherd SF, Laing RW, Cosgrove VP, Warrington AP, Hines F, Ashley SE, et al: Hypofractionated stereotactic radiotherapy in the management of recurrent glioma. Int J Radiat Oncol Biol Phys 1997;37:393–398.

Dr. M. Brada, The Royal Marsden NHS Trust, Downs Road, Sutton, Surrey SM2 5PT (UK)
Tel. +44 181 661 3272, Fax +44 181 643 5468, E-Mail mbrada@icr.ac.uk

Wiegel T, Hinkelbein W, Brock M, Hoell T (eds): Controversies in Neuro-Oncology.
Front Radiat Ther Oncol. Basel, Karger, 1999, vol 33, pp 150–157

....

Hyperfractionated Reirradiation for Malignant Glioma

C. Nieder, U. Nestle, M. Niewald, K. Walter, K. Schnabel

Department of Radiotherapy, University Hospital Homburg/Saar, Germany

Introduction

Surgery and radiotherapy are the mainstay of treatment of patients with malignant glioma. Additional adjuvant chemotherapy showed at best a moderate improvement of survival for patients with glioblastoma multiforme (gbm), whereas the results for patients with anaplastic astrocytoma (aa) or oligodendroglioma (ao) are more encouraging [1]. However, ultimately most patients develop a tumor relapse and die from uncontrolled local disease.

Treatment options for recurrent glioma are limited. They depend on type of pretreatment, time to recurrence, side of the lesion, performance status and other patient- and tumor-related factors. Therefore it is rather difficult to perform prospective studies, in which a uniform treatment protocol is applied to these patients with very individual history. As a consequence, many reported series were retrospective and included highly selected patients with different glial and other brain neoplasms.

Some groups analyzed the effects of reirradiation (re-rt) [2, 3], which might delay tumor progression, but the risk of acute and late brain injury must be taken into account. In order to reduce toxicity, we started a prospective study of hyperfractionated radiotherapy (hf-rt).

Material and Methods

Between September 1989 and June 1997, a prospective single-arm study of hf-rt for recurrent supratentorial malignant glioma was performed. We included patients younger than 70 years, who were not eligible for radiosurgery or fractionated stereotactic radiotherapy because of tumor size and side, and who gave their informed consent (n = 32). Table 1 shows their pretreatment characteristics. All had a relapse within the previously treated volume.

Table 1. Patients' characteristics

Histology (original – at recurrence)	n
Primary glioblastoma (gbm)	15
Anaplastic astrocytoma (aa) – gbm	2[a]
Anaplastic oligodendroglioma (ao) – gbm	2[a]
Low-grade astrocytoma – gbm	2[a]
aa – aa	2[a]
ao – ao	2[a]
Low-grade astrocytoma – aa	1[a]
aa – high-grade[b]	4
ao – high-grade[b]	1
Low-grade astrocytoma – high-grade[b]	1
Male:female ratio	17:15
Frontal:other side ratio	19:13
<5 cm: ≥ = 5 cm ratio	10:22
Age (median, range), year	44 (26–69)
Karnofsky performance status, %	70 (20–100)
Interval between rt series, months	20 (2–120)

[a] Histologically diagnosed before re-rt.
[b] No histological diagnosis before re-rt.

Whenever possible, a surgical resection was performed before re-rt (n = 14). In 3 other patients the diagnosis was verified with a biopsy. Five of the remainder without new histological diagnosis had a pretreatment equivalent to 60 Gy in 2-Gy fractions (the dose that leads to a 5% risk of radionecrosis during a 5-year interval). All others were pretreated with lower doses.

Individual 2-D treatment planning based on computed tomography (CT) was carried out using contrast-enhanced CT scans taken in the treatment position. Immobilization of the head of the patients was achieved by using a mask. Target volume included tumor and perifocal edema. Fields were shaped with the aim of sparing previously irradiated brain regions as much as possible. Customized lead-alloy blocks were used (if considered appropriate). Radiotherapy was administered using 4–23 MV photons or a combination of photons and electrons. In the beginning, we applied two daily fractions of 1.3 Gy (total dose 45.5 Gy, n = 19). Later on, the protocol was modified in order to reduce treatment time (total dose 45 Gy, two daily fractions of 1.5 Gy, n = 13). The interval between daily fractions was 6 h. Dose descriptions refer to a reference point at a representative point in the target volume. The latter was surrounded by the 80% isodose. Median total dose of original radiotherapy course was 58.6 Gy (25–78 Gy, mostly hyperfractionated). Median single dose was 1.3 Gy (1–5 Gy). Cumulative doses ranged between 58.5 and 123.5 Gy (median 101.6 Gy, including

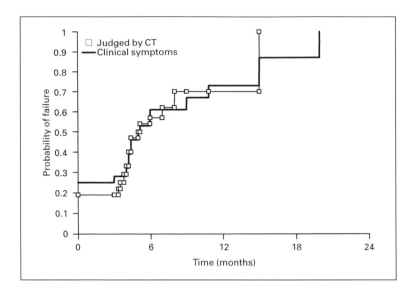

Fig. 1. Actuarial progression-free survival (n = 32, all patients).

patients with incomplete re-rt course). The biologically effective dose (BED) was calculated according to the linear-quadratic model assuming an α/β value of 1 Gy for normal brain tissue without corrections for hyperfractionation (BED = n*d*(1 + d/1). Median BED was 254 Gy_1 (135–296). Normalized to 2-Gy fractions, these values correspond to a median cumulative dose of 84 Gy and a maximum cumulative dose of 98 Gy.

Nearly all patients took dexamethasone in individual doses which were reduced as soon as possible. Chemotherapy was neither part of the first nor the second treatment course.

Follow-up included neurologic examination, assessment of Karnofsky performance status, and brain CT and was done in intervals of 3 months. Late radiation toxicity was defined as a deterioration in the neurological condition more than 3 months after re-rt, and not related to residual or recurrent tumor. Tumor progression was defined as an increase in size of more than 25% or development of new contrast-enhancing lesions. Survival was calculated from first histological diagnosis as well as re-rt according to the method of Kaplan and Meier and compared between the groups using the log-rank test. At the time of evaluation of the study, 7 patients were alive (median follow-up 10 months, range 3–19).

Four patients underwent a third therapy after further tumor progression, 3 of those in form of a further surgical resection, 1 was treated with chemotherapy. In 1 other case a biopsy was performed in order to differentiate between viable tumor and radionecrosis.

Results

Five patients failed to complete their prescribed re-rt. They received doses between 13 and 31.2 Gy. All of them had a Karnofsky performance

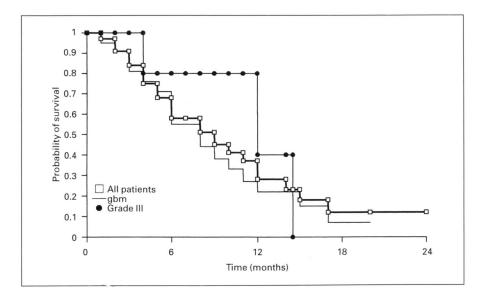

Fig. 2. Actuarial survival (n = 32, 21, 5).

status (Kps) ≤60%. Thus, 50% of the patients with Kps ≤60% (n = 10) failed.

In 19 cases, symptoms improved and corticosteroids could be reduced. Median time to clinical deterioration and local progression (judged by CT) were both 5 months (fig. 1). One-year progression-free survival rate was 30%.

Median survival was 8.5 months. One-year survival rate was 30% (gbm 22%, aa plus ao 40%, $p > 0.1$; fig. 2). Median survival from first histological diagnosis was 18 months for gbm and 4.5 years for aa plus ao. Age, Kps, surgery before re-rt, tumor side, interval between rt series, sex, and histology before re-rt (if available) were tested as prognostic factors in log-rank tests and afterwards in a stepwise Cox proportional-hazards model (table 2). The final model showed 3 independent prognostic factors ($p < 0.05$): Kps >60%, interval >24 months, and frontal side.

Acute neurotoxicity (transient signs of increased intracranial pressure or seizures, which improved after higher steroid doses) was seen in 3 patients.

Altogether, late neurotoxicity was seen in 5 patients (fig. 3). According to the RTOG/EORTC scale, grade I or II symptoms occurred in 3 cases. In 2 patients a radionecrosis was histologically verified. In all other reoperated cases pathological analysis of the surgical specimens showed abundant vital tumor cells. However, most patients who developed contrast-enhancing lesions in a reirradiated area underwent no further surgical treatment, so that in reality some cases of radionecrosis might not have been detected.

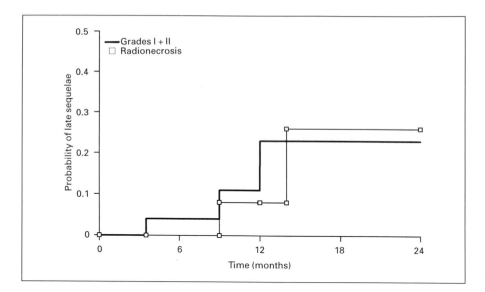

Fig. 3. Actuarial late toxicity-free survival (n = 32, all patients).

Table 2. Prognostic factors

Parameter	p value derived from log-rank test	p value derived from Cox proportional-hazards model
Kps > 60% vs. ≤ 60%	< 0.01	< 0.05
Interval between rt series > 24 vs. ≤ 24 months	< 0.01	< 0.05
Frontal vs. other sides	< 0.05	< 0.05
Surgery before re-rt	< 0.05	> 0.1
Histology before re-rt (gbm vs. sa/ao)	> 0.1	> 0.1
Age > 44 vs. ≤ 44 yeras	> 0.1	Not included
Sex	> 0.1	No included

Discussion

Repeat irradiation within the CNS is rarely performed, largely due to concerns regarding cumulative CNS toxicity. Only a few prospective studies of re-rt for malignant glioma have been published so far [4–6]. Recently, attention was paid to focal radiotherapy, which is one possibility to reduce normal brain toxicity by reducing the irradiated volume. However, only selected patients with rather small tumors are eligible for focal treatment. From the radiobiological point of view, hyperfractionation might also help to avoid late toxicity, although the theoretical advantage could not be demonstrated in the first-line treatment of malignant glioma [7, 8]. This is the first study that evaluates its efficacy as salvage therapy.

When interpreting the results, the following should be taken into account. Reirradiation is usually offered to highly selected patients only. This holds true for previous studies as for the present one, which included 32 patients over a period of 8 years. Histology at the time of recurrence was confirmed in 17 out of 32 and corresponded to the initial histology in 10 out of 17. Seven patients recurred with more aggressive histology. When considering dose of original radiotherapy, time course, and imaging pattern of recurrent lesions, it seems very unlikely that patients without histological diagnosis in fact did not have tumor recurrence. When judging time to progression and risk of radionecrosis, one should be aware that similar CT changes might occur in either case and that further examinations, e.g. [^{18}F]2-fluoro-2-deoxy-D-glucose (FDG) PET imaging, ^{201}Tl SPECT imaging, or re-biopsy, can lead to improved accuracy of diagnosis. However, due to limited availability, cost, and risks associated with invasive procedures, the routine follow-up of the present study did not include such examinations. Open surgery or biopsy were used in selected cases of suspected radionecrosis only, depending on patient's general condition and possible consequence.

Median time to progression was 5 months, median survival 8.5 months. Treatment was feasible without severe acute toxicity. However, mild or moderate late sequelae occurred in 23% after 1 year. Additionally, a substantial risk of radionecrosis (26% after 18 months) was found. In fact, the rate might even be higher, as most patients at risk did not undergo surgical procedures to establish a diagnosis. However, this is a general problem of re-rt trials.

The evaluation of prognostic factors showed that patients with Kps ≤60% have little chance to profit from reirradiation. Kps seems to be the most important selection parameter. A long relapse-free interval also seems to influence prognosis. However, the latter might correlate with tumor histology, which showed no significant influence on prognosis in this trial. Yet, histology at the time of recurrence was not known in each single case, and therefore only a small number of verified grade III tumours could be included. Age also failed to influence survival, but most patients were younger than 45 years. Tumor size was not analyzed, as the majority was rather large (> 5 cm). Frontal tumors were associated with a better prognosis.

A recent report from Heidelberg [6] included 27 recurrent gbm patients treated with radiosurgery (median dose 16 Gy; inclusion criteria: tumor size ≤ 5 cm, Kps ≥ 70%). They had the same median survival from original diagnosis (18 months) as our gbm patients, but 9 months from re-rt. This could be explained by different follow-up intervals or other factors, leading to an earlier diagnosis of relapse, and by the different inclusion criteria. After 4.5 months about 50% of their patients had a deterioration of symptoms, compared to 5 months in our study. Other radiosurgery series reported similar results with median survival times of 6.5 and 10.2 months [9, 10].

Shepherd et al. [5] reported the results of a dose escalation study of hypofractionated stereotactic radiotherapy at 5 Gy/fraction in 29 patients with high-grade astrocytoma. Median survival was 11 months versus 7 months for a matched cohort who received nitrosurea-based chemotherapy ($p < 0.05$). Their patients had a better median Kps, younger median age, and longer median interval to recurrence compared to ours.

Bauman et al. [2] reported 34 patients with primary brain tumors who were retreated with fractionated external beam radiotherapy. This retrospective analysis included 10 patients with high-grade glioma, whose median survival was only 2.8 months. Actuarial incidence of necrosis was 22% at 1 year, and thus comparable to ours. Most complications noted in their patients were seen at or above a cumulative dose of 80–90 Gy (normalized to 2-Gy fractions). In the present study, patients who developed a radionecrosis were treated to 84 and 88 Gy, respectively. However, some uncertainties with regard to BED calculation of hyperfractionated radiotherapy should be considered when comparing our results to others.

Other salvage modalities include repeat surgery, chemotherapy, and gene therapy. Repeat surgery has been associated with median survivals of about 9 months [11, 12]. Salvage chemotherapy is associated with survivals of 2–4 months for gbm and up to 12 months for aa [1]. A phase II study of BCNU plus alpha-interferon ($n = 21$) reported a median time to progression of 4.5 months and survival of 7 months [13]. An RTOG trial achieved 3.8 months to progression and a median survival of 5.7 months in 30 patients treated with all-trans-retinois acid [14].

Comparing the results of the studies mentioned above, progression-free survival seems very similar irrespective of kind of treatment. However, using common follow-up strategies without routine PET and surgical procedures, tumor progression in fact can be mixed up with radionecrosis. Differences in survival might be explained by patient selection. In conclusion, salvage options depend very much upon the primary treatment and will become more and more limited after aggressive first-line treatment, e.g. with high-dose radiation and chemotherapy. In most cases an individual decision will become necessary, taking the patients' preference into account and weighing the risk/benefit ratio carefully considering that, at present, malignant gliomas are not curable.

Compared to our concept, brachytherapy, radiosurgery, and multiple, non-coplanar, 3D conformal beam arrangements might be preferable for eligible patients with smaller tumors in order to avoid toxicity. Other patients with favorable Kps and extended relapse-free interval can be treated with hyperfractionated re-rt, which is able to delay tumor progression in the same amount as other options, and thus might help to improve quality of life for a limited time span. More effective treatments have to be developed in order to improve the prognosis of recurrent malignant glioma.

References

1   Fine HA, Dear KB, Loeffler JS, Black PM, Canellos GP: Meta-analysis of radiation therapy with and without adjuvant chemotherapy for malignant gliomas in adults. Cancer 1993;71:2585–2597.
2   Bauman GS, Sneed PK, Wara WM, Stalpers LJ, Chang SM, Mc Dermott MW, Gutin PH, Larson DA: Reirradiation of primary CNS tumors. Int J Radiat Oncol Biol Phys 1996;36:433–441.
3   Silbergeld DL, Griffin BR, Ojemann GA: Reirradiation for recurrent cerebral astrocytoma. J Neurooncol 1992;12:145–151.
4   Shaw E, Scott C, Souhami L: Radiosurgery for the treatment of previously irradiated recurrent primary brain tumors and brain metastases. Int J Radiat Oncol Biol Phys 1996;34:647–654.
5   Shepherd SF, Laing RW, Cosgrove VP, Warrington AP, Hines F, Ashley SE, Brada M: Hypofractionated stereotactic radiotherapy in the management of recurrent glioma. Int J Radiat Oncol Biol Phys 1997;37:393–398.
6   Van Kampen M, Engenhart-Cabillic R, Debus J, Fuss M, Rhein B, Wannenmacher M: The value of radiosurgery for recurrent glioblastoma multiforme. Strahlenther Onkol 1998;174:19–24.
7   Beck-Bornholdt HP, Dubben HH, Liertz-Petersen C, Willers H: Hyperfractionation: Where do we stand? Radiother Oncol 1997;43:1–21.
8   Fallai C, Olmi P: Hyperfractionated and accelerated radiation therapy in central nervous system tumours (malignant gliomas, pediatric tumours, and brain metastases). Radiother Oncol 1997;43: 235–246.
9   Hall WA, Djalilian HR, Sperduto PW: Stereotactic radiosurgery for recurrent malignant glioma. J Clin Oncol 1995;13:1642–1648.
10 Shrieve DC, Alexander E, Wen PY: Comparison of stereotactic radiosurgery and brachytherapy in the treatment of recurrent glioblastoma multiforme. Neurosurgery 1995;36:275–284.
11 Ammirati M, Galicich JH, Arbit E: Reoperation in the treatment of recurrent intracranial malignant gliomas. Neurosurgery 1987;21:607–614.
12 Harsh GR, Levin VA, Gutin PH: Reoperation for recurrent glioblastoma and anaplastic astrocytoma. Neurosurgery 1987;21:615–621.
13 Brandes AA, Scelzi E, Zampieri P, Rigon A, Rotilio A, Amista P, Berti F, Fiorentino MV: Phase II trial with BCNU plus alpha-interferon in patients with recurrent high-grade gliomas. Am J Clin Oncol 1997;20:364–367.
14 Phuphanich S, Scott C, Fischbach AJ, Langer C, Yung WK: All-trans-retinoic acid: A phase II RTOG study in patients with recurrent malignant astrocytoma. J Neurooncol 1997;34:193–200.

C. Nieder, Department of Radiotherapy, University Hospital,
D–66421 Homburg/Saar (Germany)
Tel. +41 6841 164626, Fax +41 6841 164618

Wiegel T, Hinkelbein W, Brock M, Hoell T (eds): Controversies in Neuro-Oncology.
Front Radiat Ther Oncol. Basel, Karger, 1999, vol 33, pp 158–165

....

Outcome and Side Effects in Radiotherapy of Glioblastoma – Conventional Fractionation versus Accelerated Hyperfractionation

Kirsten Papsdorf, Ulrich Wolf, Guido Hildebrandt, Friedrich Kamprad

Department of Radiotherapy and Radiooncology, University of Leipzig, Germany

Purpose

The prognosis of malignant gliomas, i.e. glioblastomas, remains unsatisfactory. In general, there is a high relapse rate and therefore the survival time is limited. Postoperative radiotherapy continues to be an important treatment modality in high-grade glioma patients. It prolongs survival and usually maintains quality of life by retaining or improving neurological function for the duration of tumor control. We analyzed whether the shortening in overall treatment time (OTT) by accelerated hyperfractionation influences the treatment outcome in such patients without increasing the frequency and intensity of adverse side effects on the central nervous system (CNS).

Material and Methods

Between 1980 and 1995, 416 patients with primary brain tumors were treated at the Department of Radiotherapy of the University of Leipzig. Among the brain tumor group there were 152 glioblastoma patients (WHO grade IV). Whole-brain irradiation with palliative intention was performed in 54 of those patients due to the reduced performance status of the patients or the extended tumor growth. Within the time allocated for this analysis, different irradiation techniques and fractionation schedules have been used for the remaining 98 glioma patients.

Before 1991, irradiation of glioblastoma was performed by conventional fractionation. Among the conventionally treated group with 47 patients the tumor could be resected totally in 23 patients (49%), partially in 16 patients (34%) prior to irradiation, and in 8 patients (17%) tumor removal was not feasible. The median age of the irradiated patients was 47.8 years, and the Karnofsky performance score was in 34 cases (72.3%) higher than 70%.

Irradiation was performed once a day using single doses between 1.8 and 2.0 Gy. The patients were irradiated 5 or 6 times a week with an interfraction interval of 24 h. The applied total dose was between 50 and 57.6 Gy and the OTT ranged between 35 and 42 days.

In general, whole-brain irradiation was performed up to a total dose of 36 Gy, and afterwards a boost of 20 Gy for the tumor region or the tumor burden hemisphere was given (n = 30). In 9 patients only, the tumor and the surrounding tissue was irradiated. The remaining 8 patients were treated with whole-brain irradiation or with hemisphere irradiation.

Since 1992, 51 glioblastoma patients were treated by accelerated hyperfractionated radiotherapy of the tumor burden hemisphere. In this group the tumor could be resected totally in 25 patients (47%), partially in 24 patients (47%) prior to irradiation, and in 2 cases (4%) the tumour remained unresectable. The median age of the irradiated patients was 53.9 years, and the Karnofsky performance score was in 34 cases (66.7%) greater than 70%.

Irradiation was performed twice a day using single doses between 1.2 and 1.7 Gy, with interfraction intervals of more than 6 h, and 10–12 fractions were given per week. The applied daily dose ranged between 2.8 and 3.0 Gy, the total dose was between 57 and 60 Gy and the OTT was between 25 and 28 days.

Results

In the conventionally fractionated group the follow-up ranged between 11 and 50 months, and in the group treated by accelerated hyperfractionation between 7.5 and 35 months. The survival rate was calculated by the Kaplan-Meier method.

In the conventional group the mean survival rate was 15 months, and in the accelerated hyperfractionated group 20 months (fig. 1, table 1). Taking into consideration the surgical radicality prior to irradiation, the comparison of the subgroups revealed a slight but nonsignificant improvement in treatment outcome for the patients who had received accelerated hyperfractionation following surgery. Among the glioblastoma patients who were totally resected prior to radiotherapy, the mean survival rate was 17 months in the conventional group versus 22 months in the hyperfractionated group, and among the glioblastoma patients who were partially resected prior to radiotherapy, the mean survival rate was in the conventional group 13 months versus 16 months in the hyperfractionated group. Due to the small number of patients within the subgroups, significant differences could not be detected.

However, the mean survival rate of glioblastoma patients even after multimodal treatment is still limited. Therefore, the improvement of the quality of the remaining lifetime plays an important role for those patients (table 2). In our analysis we defined 'Improvement of quality of life' as: (1) improvement of the neurological status; (2) improvement of the clinical performance status, and (3) improvement of the subjective general state of health.

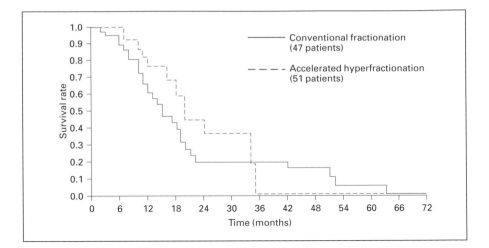

Fig. 1. Overall survival rate of glioblastoma patients following conventional radiotherapy or accelerated hyperfractionation as estimated by Kaplan-Meier method (for details see text).

Table 1. Median survival (MS) of glioblastoma patients following conventional radiotherapy or accelerated hyperfractionation dependent on surgical radicality prior to radiotherapy (for details see text)

Surgical radicality prior to RT	Conventional fractionation (n = 47)		Accelerated hyperfractionation (n = 51)		p value (log-rank)
	MS, months	n	MS, months	n	
Totally resected	17	23	22	25	0.113
Partially resected	13	16	16	24	0.300
Stereotactic biopsy	12	8	4, 18[1]	2	–
All patients	15	47	20	51	0.234

[1] Only 2 patients: 1 survived 4 months, the other 18 months.

Independent on the type of fractionation, the performance status ('quality of life') of the patients could be improved in about 60%; in 20% the status remained stable, and in approximately 20% of all patients deterioration was observed (table 2).

In general, conventional fractionation as well as accelerated hyperfractionation was tolerated well by the treated patients.

Slight acute adverse side effects such as headaches and psychosyndrome occurred temporarily in 40% of the conventionally treated group and in 41% of

Table 2. 'Quality of life' in glioblastoma patients following conventional radiotherapy or accelerated hyperfractionation (for details see text)

'Quality of life'	Conventional fractionation (n = 47)		Accelerated hyperfractionation (n = 51)	
	%	n	%	n
Improvement	63.8	30	60.8	31
Stabilization	19.2	9	19.6	10
Deterioration	17.0	8	19.6	10

Table 3. Adverse side effects in glioblastoma patients following conventional radiotherapy or accelerated hyperfractionation during the treatment course

Adverse side effects	Conventional fractionation (n = 47)		Accelerated hyperfractionation (n = 51)	
	%	n	%	n
No side effects	59.6	28	58.8	30
Slight acute side effects	40.4	19	41.2	21
One symptom only	17.0	8	19.6	10
Multiple symptoms	23.4	11	21.6	11

the hyperfractionated treated group during the treatment course. No severe acute side effects were observed and no treatment interruption was necessary (table 3).

At 4–12 weeks following treatment, slight adverse effects such as headaches, signs of intensified fatigue, sudden drop in performance, lack of concentration or reduction of mental capacity were observed in 36% of the conventionally treated group and 43% of the hyperfractionated treated group. Again, no severe treatment-related side effects were observed (table 4).

Thus, in both groups, the frequency and intensity of adverse side effects during the radiation course as well as 4–12 weeks afterwards was comparable. But, due to hyperfractionated accelerated treatment the overall treatment time could be reduced by approximately 10 days (25–28 vs. 35–42 days).

Discussion

Numerous clinical efforts for decades failed to improve significantly the treatment results for glioblastoma patients. The prognosis of these patients

Table 4. Adverse side effects in glioblastoma patients following conventional radiotherapy or accelerated hyperfractionation 4–12 weeks after radiation treatment

Adverse side effects	Conventional fractionation (n = 47)		Accelerated hyperfractionation (n = 51)	
	%	n	%	n
No side effects	63.8	30	56.9	29
Slight side effects	36.2	17	43.1	22
One symptom only	14.9	7	23.5	12
Multiple symptoms	21.3	10	19.6	10

still remains unsatisfactory due to the high rate of local recurrences or local tumor progression. There is no doubt that surgery is the primary treatment modality for glioblastoma patients and that the extent of tumor removal considerably influences the treatment outcome. But, it is generally acknowledged that postoperative radiotherapy provides nearly a doubling in median survival time as compared to surgery alone (9–12 vs. 4–5 months) [1]. However, median survival of patients following combined treatment is still very limited. Thus, in our opinion the improvement and/or preservation of qualitiy of life for the remaining lifespan is essential.

Concerning the biology of rapidly growing tumors like glioblastoma, having a volume doubling time of about 13 days [28], accelerated treatment schedules seem to be advantageous since tumor cells with a volume doubling time of shorter than 35 days show a decreased survival after accelerated radiation [19]. Furthermore, if repopulation during a protracted course of radiotherapy is an important factor determining relapse rate of glioblastoma, then accelerated radiotherapy might be expected to improve survival. In general, the duration of radiotherapy can be reduced by hypofractionation or accelerated hyperfractionation. Several studies have demonstrated that hypofractionated schedules do obtain similar but not higher survival rates in glioblastoma patients as compared to conventional treatment courses without significant increases in treatment-related toxicity [2, 16, 21, 30]. Also, most of the hyperfractionated treatment schedules published so far could not demonstrate significant prolongation of survival [3, 4, 7, 11, 17, 24].

Dose escalations up to 80 Gy have also been tested [9, 24, 27, 33]. As for example, in a dose escalation phase II study total doses between 61.4, 71.2 and 80 Gy were applied 3 times a day with 0.89 Gy per fraction. An increase in median survival time with higher radiation doses could not be demonstrated [9]. In another randomized dose-searching phase I/II study of the RTOG [24, 33], patients received doses of 1.2 Gy per fraction twice daily. The total doses ranged from 64.8 to 81.6 Gy (four dose levels) and treatment was given over a period of 5.5–6.5 weeks together with adjuvant BCNU. There was no survival benefit with higher radiation doses and even a suggestion of worse results with doses ≥ 74.5 Gy. Taken together, accelerated and/or hyperfractionated radiotherapy seem to provide only little additional survival benefit as compared to conventionally fractionated schedules. Moreover, dose escalation failed to improve treatment results.

Other treatment modalities such as stereotactic radiosurgery [10], the use of other radiation qualities, such as neutrons [13, 20], or pions [12] or heavy ions [5], as well as additional chemotherapy [8, 14, 22, 24] also could not provide any therapeutic breakthrough so far [18]. Concerning intraoperative radiotherapy, ambiguous results have been published [25, 32]. Moreover, the clinical benefit of modalities like boron neutron capture therapy [6, 15], or hyperthermia [29], or the application of radiolabeled antibodies [26, 31] remains to be ultimately proven.

Summarizing the present clinical situation, the treatment modality of choice should be a treatment schedule being feasible and convenient for the patient. This schedule should be kept as short as possible without any decrease in treatment efficiency or any increase in adverse side effects. In our study, the mean survival rate in the conventional group was 15 months, and in the accelerated hyperfractionated group, 20 months. Our better mean survival rates as compared to other authors might be partially due to the relatively high performance status (Karnofsky performance score 7/10 patients $\geq 70\%$) and the age distribution (median age approximately 50 years) of the treated patients, as well as possibly some kind of positive selection due to the retrospective character of the study. In both groups, the frequency and intensity of adverse side effects during the radiation course as well as 4–12 weeks afterwards was comparable. But, due to hyperfractionated accelerated treatment, the overall treatment time could be reduced by approximately 10 days (25–28 vs. 35–42 days).

Conclusions

Accelerated hyperfractionated radiation therapy of glioblastoma is a feasible method. It offers the patients a shortening in overall treatment time without any increase in the frequency and intensity of adverse side effects during treatment as well as afterwards. The mean survival time following accelerated hyperfractionated treatment might be slightly improved, but in general, its effect on the treatment outcome is still not satisfactory. The probability to improve the results by further dose intensification is low.

References

1   Bamberg M, Hess CF, Kortmann RD: Zentralnervensystem; in Scherer E, Sack H (eds): Strahlenthe-
    rapie: Radiologische Onkologie. Berlin, 1996, pp 763–808.
2   Bauman GS, Gaspar LE, Fisher BJ, Halperin EC, Macdonald DR, Cairncross JG: A prospective
    study of shortcourse radiotherapy in poor-prognosis glioblastoma multiforme. Int J Radiat Oncol
    Biol Phys 1994;29:835–839.
3   Brada M, Thomas G, Elyan S, James N, Hines F, Ashley S, Marsh H, Bell BA, Stenning S: Improving
    the acceptability of high-dose radiotherapy by reducing the duration of treatment: Accelerated
    radiotherapy in high-grade glioma. Br J Cancer 1995;71:1330–1334.
4   Buatti JM, Marcus RB, Mendenhall WM, Friedman WA, Bova FJ: Accelerated hyperfractionated
    radiotherapy for malignant gliomas. Int Radiat Oncol Biol Phys 1996;34:785–792.
5   Castro JR, Gademann G, Collier JM, Linstad D, Pitluck S, Woodruff K, Gauger G, Char D, Gutin
    P, Phillips TL: Strahlentherapie mit schweren Teilchen am Lawrence Berkeley Laboratory Laboratory
    der Universität Kalifornien. Strahlenther Onkol 1987;163:9–16.
6   Chadha M, Capala J, Coderre JA, Elowitz EH, Iwai JI, Joel DD, Liu HB, Wielopolski L, Chanana
    AD: Boron neutron-capture therapy (BNCT) for glioblastoma multiforme using the epithermal neut-
    ron beam at the Brookhaven National Laboratory. Int J Radiat Oncol Biol Phys 1998;40:829–834.
7   Curran WJ, Scott CB, Weinstein AS: Survival comparison of radiosurgery-eligible and -ineligible
    malignant glioma patients treated with hyperfractionated radiation therapy and carmustine. A report
    of Radiation Therapy Oncology Group 83-02. Clin Oncol 1993;11:857–862.
8   EORTC Brain Tumor Group: Evaluation of CCNU, VM26 plus CCNU, procarbazine in supraten-
    torial gliomas. Final evaluation of a randomized study. J Neurosurg 1981;55:2731–2737.
9   Fulton DS, Urtasun RC, Scott-Brown I: Increasing radiation dose intensity using hyperfractionation
    in patients with malignant glioma. Final report of a prospective phase I-II dose response study.
    J Neurooncol 1992;14:63–72.
10 Gannett D, Stea B, Lulu BB, Adair T, Verdi C, Hamilton A: Stereotactic radiosurgery as an adjunct
    to surgery and external beam radiotherapy in the treatment of patients with malignant gliomas.
    Int J Radiat Oncol Biol Phys 1995;33:461–468.
11 Goffman TE, Dachowski LJ, Bobo H, Oldfield EH, Steinberg SM, Cok J, Mitchell JB, Katz D, Smith
    R, Glatstein E: Long-term follow-up of National Cancer Institute phase I/II study of glioblastoma
    multiforme treated with iododeoxyuridine and hyperfractionated radiation. J Clin Oncol 1992;10:
    264–268.
12 Goodman GB, Skarsgard LD, Thompson GB, Harrison R, Lam GKY, Lugate C: Pion therapy at
    TRIUMF. Treatment results for astrocytoma grades 3 and 4: A pilot study. Radiother Oncol 1990;
    17:21–28.
13 Griffin BR, Berger MS, Laramore GE: Neutron radiotherapy of malignant gliomas. Am J Clin
    Oncol 1989;12:311–315.
14 Halperin EC, Herndon J, Schold SC, Brown M, Vick N, Cairncross JG, Macdonald DR, Gaspar L,
    Fischer B, Dropcho E, Rosenfeld S, Morowitz R, Piepmeier J, Hait W, Byrne T, Salter M, Imperato
    J, Khandekar J, Paleologos N, Burger P, Bentel GC, Friedman A: A phase III randomized prospective
    trial of external beam radiotherapy, mitomycin C, carmustine, and 6-mercaptopurine for the treatment
    of adults with anaplastic glioma of the brain. Int J Radiat Oncol Biol Phys 1996;34:793–802.
15 Haritz D, Gabel D, Huiskamp R: Clinical phase-I study of Na2B12H11SH (BSH) in patients with
    malignant glioma as precondition for boron neutron capture therapy (BNCT). Int J Radiat Oncol
    Biol Phys 1994;28:1175–1181.
16 Hinkelbein W, Bruggmoser G, Schmidt M, Wannenmacher M: Die Kurzzeitbestrahlung des
    Glioblastoms mit hohen Einzelfraktionen. Strahlentherapie 1984;160:301–308.
17 Hinkelbein W, Hempel M, Gilsbach J, Wannenmacher M: Die Kurzzeitbestrahlung des Glioblas-
    toms: Akzelerierte Superfraktionierung versus hohe Einzelfraktionen; in Bamberg M, Sack H (eds):
    Therapie primärer Hirntumoren. München, Zuckschwert, 1988, pp 122–125.
18 Jeremic B, Grujicic D, Antunovic V, Djuric L, Stojanovic M, Shibamoto Y: Accelerated hyperfrac-
    tionated radiation therapy for malignant glioma. A phase-II study. Am J Clin Oncol 1995;18:
    449–453.

19   Kriester A, Kloetzer KH, Kob D: Zur Dosis-Zeit-Optimierung in der fraktionierten Strahlenthera-
     pie. Strahlenther Onkol 1988;164:459–498.
20   Krishnasamy S, Vokes EE, Dohrmann GJ, Mick R, Garcia JC, Kolker JD, Wollmann RL, Hekmat-
     panah J, Weichselbaum RR: Concomitant chemoradiotherapy, neutron boost, and adjuvant chemo-
     therapy for anaplastic astrocytoma and glioblastoma multiforme. Cancer Invest 1995;13:453–459.
21   Lang O, Liebermeister E, Liesegang J, Sautter-Bihl ML: Radiotherapy of glioblastoma multiforme.
     Feasibility of increased fractionation size and shortened overall treatment. Strahlenther Onkol 1998;
     174:629–632.
22   Levin VA, Silver P, Hannigan J, Wara WM, Gutin PH, Davis RL, Wilson CB: Superiority of
     postradiotherapy adjuvant chemotherapy with CCNU, procarbazine, and vincristine (PCV) over
     BCNU for anaplastic gliomas: NCOG 6C61 final report. Int J Radiat Oncol Biol Phys 1990;18:
     321–324.
23   Krishnasamy S, Vokes EE, Dohrmann GJ, Mick R, Garcia JC, Kolker JD, Wollmann RL, Hekmat-
     panah J, Weichselbaum RR: A randomized comparison of misonidazole-sensitized radiotherapy
     plus BCNU for treatment of malignant gliomas after surgery: Final report of an RTOG study. Int
     J Radiat Oncol Biol Phys 1986;12:1793–1800.
24   Nelson DF, Curran WJ, Scott C, Nelson JS, Weinstein AS, Ahmad K, Constine LS, Murray K,
     Powlis WD, Mohiud-Din M, Fischbach J: Hyperfractionated radiation therapy and bis-chloroethylni-
     trosourea in the treatment of malignant glioma – Possible advantage observed at 72.0 Gy in 1.2-
     Gy bid fractions: Report of the Radiation Therapy Oncology Group Protocol 8302. Int J Radiat
     Oncol Biol Phys 1993;25:193–207.
25   Ortiz de Urbina D, Santos M, Garcia-Berrocal I, Bustos JC, Samblas J, Gutierrez-Diaz JA, Delgado
     JM, Donckaster G, Calvo FA: Intraoperative radiation therapy in malignant glioma: Early clinical
     results. Neurol Res 1995;17:289–294.
26   Riva P, Franceschi G, Arista A, Fratterelli M, Riva N, Cremonini AM, Giuliani G, Casi M: Local
     application of radiolabeled monoclonal antibodies in the treatment of high grade gliomas: A six-
     year clinical experience. Cancer 1997;80(suppl 12):2733–2742.
27   Salazar OM, Rubin P, Feldstein ML, Pizzutiello R: High-dose radiation therapy in the treatment
     of malignant gliomas: Final report. Int J Radiat Oncol Biol Phys 1979;5:1733–1740.
28   Schiffer LM: Cell proliferation in tumors and in normal tissue; in Perez CA, Brada LW (eds):
     Principles and Practice of Radiation Oncology. Philadelphia, Lippincott, 1987, pp 57–65.
29   Seegenschmiedt MH, Feldmann HJ, Wust P, Molls M: Hyperthermia – Its actual role in radiation
     oncology. IV. Thermo-radiotherapy for malignant brain tumors. Strahlenther Onkol 1995;171:560–
     572.
30   Slotman BJ, Kralendonk JH, va Alphen HA, Kamphorst W, Karim AB: Hypofractionated radiation
     therapy in patients with glioblastoma multiforme: Results of treatment and impact of prognostic
     factors. Int J Radiat Oncol Biol Phys 1996;34:895–898.
31   Snelling L, Miyamoto CT, Bender H, Brady LW, Steplewski Z, Class R, Emrich J, Rackover MA:
     Epidermal growth factor receptor 425 monoclonal antibodies radiolabeled with iodine-125 in the
     adjuvant treatment of high-grade astrocytomas. Hybridoma 1995;14:111–114.
32   Wagner W, Schuller P, Willich N, Schober O, Palkovic S, Morgenroth S, Bartenstein P, Prott FJ,
     Niewohner U: Intraoperative Strahlentherapie (IORT) maligner Hirntumoren. Strahlenther Onkol
     1995;171:154–164.
33   Werner-Wasik M, Scott CB, Nelson DF, Gaspar LE, Murray KJ, Fischbach JA, Nelson JS, Weinstein
     AS, Curran WJ: Final report of a phase I/II trial of hyperfractionated radiation therapy with
     carmustine for adults with supratentorial malignant gliomas. Cancer 1996;77:1535–1543.

Dr. K. Papsdorf, Universität Leipzig, Zentrum für Radiologie, Klinik und Poliklinik für Strahlentherapie und Radioonkologie, Liebigstrasse Zoa, D–04103 Leipzig (Germany)
Tel. +49 341 971 8400, Fax +49 341 971 8443, E-Mail kpap@medizin.uni-leipzig.de

Wiegel T, Hinkelbein W, Brock M, Hoell T (eds): Controversies in Neuro-Oncology.
Front Radiat Ther Oncol. Basel, Karger, 1999, vol 33, pp 166–173

Conventionally Fractionated Radiotherapy of Glioblastoma multiforme

Results and Analysis of Possible Influencing Factors

Ursula Maria Schleicher [a], *Demetrios Andreopoulos* [a], *Jürgen Ammon* [a],
Joachim Gilsbach [b]

Departments of [a] Radiotherapy and [b] Neurosurgery, Technical University,
Aachen, Germany

Introduction

Prognosis of patients with glioblastoma is poor with a median survival time after surgery and radiotherapy of about 9–12 months [1]. Postoperative irradiation with doses up to 65 Gy in fractions of 1.8 Gy can improve the 1- and 2-year survival rate [2], but also results in practically no survivors after 5 years. Virtually all patients die of local tumor progression, and only rarely of intracranial or intraspinal spread. All changes of therapy concepts performed in radiotherapy have so far not been able to alter this poor prognosis. Thus, present reflections in therapy are directed to maintenance of quality of life as long and as high as posssible. This implies a postoperative therapy schedule inconveniencing the patient only little. Therefore, radiotherapy schedules have been developed with the aim to shorten overall treatment time by using hyperfractionation or hypofractionation for acceleration of therapy [3]. Before changing treatment policy, however, results of conventional therapy should be evaluated as a standard.

Patients and Methods

From 1990 to 1995, we treated 124 patients for glioblastoma multiforme. The patients were aged 20–77 years with a median of 58 years. The male/female ratio was 70/54 patients.

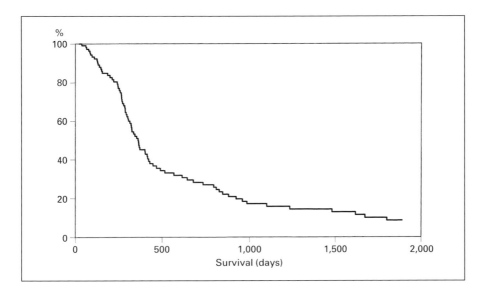

Fig. 1. Survival after surgery (Kaplan-Meier).

Neurologic symptoms at presentation included headache (present in 38% of patients), motor deficit (36%), aphasia (32%), seizure (29%), ataxia or vertigo (23%), loss of consciousness (19%), visual or sensory deficit (14% each) and nausea (12%). 26 patients suffered from only one of these symptoms, 41 of two, 37 of three, 16 of four and only 4 patients suffered from 5 different symptoms. Tumor volume as measured by preoperative diagnostic imaging (CT or MRI) ranged from 0.4 to 216 cm^3 with a median of 34.5 cm^3. Time from onset of symptoms to start of therapy ranged from 4 days to 3 years with a median time of 44 days, whereas time from radiological diagnosis to therapy differed from 1 to 258 days (median 8). Diagnosis of glioma WHO grade IV was histologically proven in 92.7% of patients (tumor resection in 93 patients, open biopsy in 17 and stereotactic biopsy in 5 patients). The others (9 cases) showed unequivocal radiological signs of glioblastoma and were thus included in the analysis. The extent of surgery depended on tumor site and showed no correlation to tumor volume. Radiotherapy was performed as a shrinking field technique, starting with a treatment volume including the preoperative peritumoral edema plus a safety margin, and shrinking the field to the tumor bed after a dose of 30 or 45 Gy. Treatment plans were chosen individually according to tumor size and location. In 7% of the patients, irradiation was terminated before reaching 30 Gy due to neurological deterioration. Of the patients, 11% received a dose between 30 and 40 Gy, 55% a dose of 40–50 Gy and 27% up to 60 Gy at the ICRU reference point. Median dose was 45 Gy. Overall treatment time was up to 110 days with a median treatment time of 45 days.

Follow-up time ranged from 41 days to 3.0 years (median 104 days) for censored data and from 23 days to 5.27 years (median 322 days) for observed data.

Influence of age, tumor size, extent of surgery, radiation dose and overall treatment time on duration of remission and survival was analyzed by Kaplan-Meier estimates and log-rank test. Results were considered significant at a level of p = 0.05.

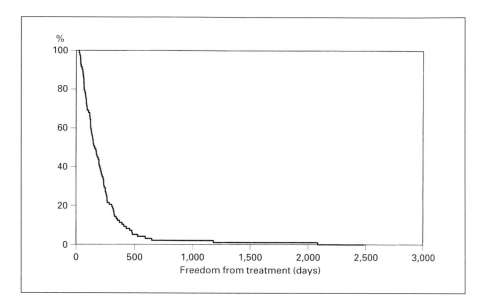

Fig. 2. Freedom from treatment failure (Kaplan-Meier).

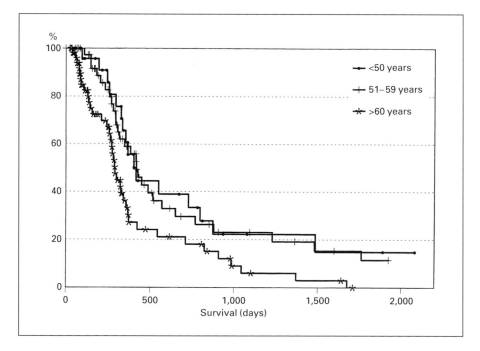

Fig. 3. Correlation of survival and age (Kaplan-Meier, log-rank p = 0.0298).

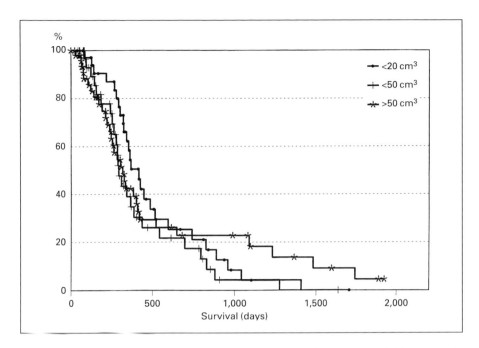

Fig. 4. Correlation of survival and initial tumor volume (Kaplan-Meier, log-rank p=0.4203).

Results

Radiotherapy was well tolerated by all patients. Partial alopecia was seen regularly in all patients treated with >30 Gy and was not completely reversible in patients receiving the full irradiation dose of 60 Gy.

Median survival for all patients (including also those with irradiation dose up to 30 Gy) as estimated by Kaplan-Meier plots was 12 months after therapy onset with a survival rate of 28% after 2 years and 18.5% after 3 years (fig. 1). Freedom from treatment failure lasted 5 months (median) with only 12% of patients being free of tumor progression after 1 year (fig. 2). Survival was closely related to local progression of disease (r=0.62). Two patients developed multiple intraspinal metastases in the further course of disease and 1 of them also intracerebellar metastasis. Patients >60 years of age showed a poorer survival rate than the younger, whereas we did not find a difference between the age group <50 years and 50–60 years (p=0.0298, fig. 3). Neither initial tumor volume (fig. 4), extent of surgery (fig. 5), nor total dose (fig. 6) proved to have a significant effect on survival in our patient group.

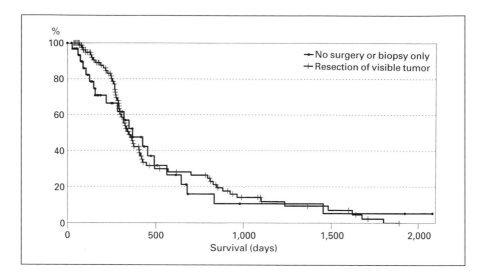

Fig. 5. Correlation of survival and extent of surgery (Kaplan-Meier, log-rank p = 0.958).

Discussion

Patients' age has well been recognized as a prognostic factor for the outcome of patients with glioblastoma in several studies [4–7]. While Peschel et al. [6] distinguish glioma grade III/IV patients older or younger than 70 years, we agree with other authors [5, 7] who consider 60 years as the separation mark for prognosis. In contrast to Simpson et al. [7] in their analysis of several RTOG trials, a difference between the youngest and middle third of patients was not found in our study.

It is a well-known fact from other tumors that tumor burden is an important factor for locoregional control and relapse-free survival [8]. In accordance with Würschmidt et al. [4], we found neither the extent of surgery nor the initial tumor size to be significant, the two parameters not being connected to each other. The significance of irradiation dose was not studied by their group as all their patients received a total dose of approximately 60 Gy. In spite of the fact that most of our patients received a lower dose and also patients discontinuing therapy are included in our Kaplan-Meier plots, our 1-year survival rate is the same (50%), whereas our 3-year survival rate is about twice as high (18.5 vs. 8%). This might also be a hint to the fact that radiotherapy dose of conventional percutaneous irradiation is not of significance in the range from 45 to 60 Gy. As in our study the group receiving 40–50 Gy contained twice as much patients as the group treated with a dose

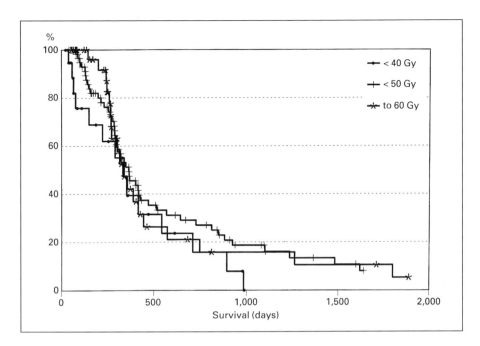

Fig. 6. Correlation of survival and total dose (Kaplan-Meier, log-rank p = 0.1193).

of > 50 Gy, we cannot derive a definite answer on that question from our examination. On the other hand, several studies aim at dose escalation in a small area either by stereotactic radiotherapy boost [9] or brachytherapy to improve local control. This seems necessary because in most cases (86–100%), tumor progression or recurrence is situated in the initial tumor bed and thus in the irradiated area [5, 10]. Liang et al. [10], using the same method of field delineation as we did (tumor plus contrast enhancement plus safety margin and shrinking to a smaller margin around the tumor for a 15-Gy boost at the end of therapy), but based on postoperative imaging, found a median time to recurrence of 8 months. The difference to our data (5 months) might be caused by difference in total dose on the one hand or by the fact that more than 70% of patients received additional radiosensitizing therapy. The role of chemotherapy in the postoperative treatment of glioblastoma, however, is not yet clear. Some data even suggest an adverse effect on survival, such as Fischbach et al. [11] in their analysis of combined RTOG/ECOG studies.

As to the question of hyperfractionation, which was the original motive of our evaluation, most of the clinical studies aim at shortening treatment time not primarily to intensify therapy but to prolong therapy-free interval and thus gain quality of life. Therefore, they are guided by normal tissue tolerance [1, 3, 12] to achieve an acceptable treatment schedule for the patient. Radiobiological studies show a great intra- and intertumor variety of SF_2, α and β values for cell lines derived from surgical specimens [13–16] and a peak of cells in mitosis or G2 phase 20 h after irradiation implying an increased radiosensitivity at this time [2]. On the other hand, no clear correlation was found between clinical and radiobiological tumor parameters [17]. Clinical results of hyperfractionated therapy are comparable to those with conventional fractionation [18, 19]. Practical performance of hyperfractionation, however, requires hospitalization of most patients. With regard to quality of life, this has to be weighted against the reduction of treatment time. This question has to be answered individually in each patient.

References

1   González González D, Menten J, Bosch DA, van der Schueren E, Troost D, Hulshof HCCM, Bernier J: Accelerated radiotherapy in glioblastoma multiforme: A dose-searching prospective study. Radiother Oncol 1994;32:98–105.
2   Marin LA, Smith CE, Langston MY, Quashie D, Dillehay LE: Response of glioblastoma cell lines to low dose rate irradiation. Int J Radiat Oncol Biol Phys 1991;21:397–402.
3   Sautter-Bihl ML, Barcsay E, Liebermeister E, Winheller R, Liesegang J, Heinze HG: Radiotherapy of glioblastoma. Is it justified to reduce the treatment time? (In German) Strahlenther Onkol 1991; 167:7–13.
4   Würschmidt F, Bünemann H, Heilmann, HP: Prognostic factors in high-grade malignant glioma. Strahlenther Onkol 1995;171:315–321.
5   Hess CF, Schaaf JC, Kortmann RD, Schabet M, Bamberg M: Malignant glioma: Patterns of failure following individually tailored limited volume irradiation. Radiother Oncol 1994;30:146–149.
6   Peschel RE, Wilson L, Haffty B, Papadopoulos D, Rosenzweig K, Feltes M: The effect of age on the efficacy of radiation therapy for early breast cancer, local prostate cancer and grade III-IV gliomas. Int J Radiat Oncol Biol Phys 1993;26:539–544.
7   Simpson JR, Horton J, Scott C, Curran WJ, Rubin P, Fischbach J, Isaacson S, Rotman M, Asbell SO, Nelson JS, Weinstein AS, Nelson DF: Influence of location and extent of surgical resection on survival of patients with glioblastoma multiforme: Results of three consecutive Radiation Therapy Oncology Group (RTOG) clinical trials. Int J Radiat Oncol Biol Phys 1993;26:239–244.
8   Dubben HH, Thames HD, Beck-Bornholdt HP: Tumor volume: A basic and specific response predictor in radiotherapy. Radiother Oncol 1998;47:113–124.
9   Loeffler JS, Alexander E III, Shea WM, Wen PY, Fine HA, Kooy HM, Black PMCL: Radiosurgery as part of the initial management of patients with malignant glioma. J Clin Oncol 1992;10:1379–1385.
10 Liang BC, Thornton AF, Sandler HM, Greenberg HS: Malignant astrocytomas: Focal tumor recurrence after focal external beam radiation therapy. J Neurosurg 1991;75:559–563.
11 Fischbach AJ, Martz KL, Nelson JS, Greffin TW, Chang CH, Horton J, Nelson DF: Long-term survival in anaplastic astrocytomas: A report of combined RTOG/ECOG studies. Am J Clin Oncol 1991;14:365–370.
12 Nelson DF, Curran WJ, Scott C, Nelson JS, Weinstein AS, Ahmad K, Costine LS, Murray K, Powlis WD, Mohiuddin M, Fischbach J: Hyperfractionated radiotherapy and bis-chlorethyl nitrosourea in the treatment of malignant glioma – Possible advantage observed at 72.0 Gy in 1.2 BID fractions: Report on the Radiation Therapy Oncology Group Protocol 8302. Int J Radiat Oncol Biol Phys 1993;25:193–207.
13 Allalunis-Turner MJ, Barron GM, Day RS III, Fulton DS, Urtasun RC: Radiosensitivity testing of human primary brain tumor specimens. Int J Radiat Oncol Biol Phys 1992;23:339–343.

14 Allam A, Taghian A, Gioioso D, Duffy M, Suit HD: Intratumoral heterogeneity of malignant gliomas measured in vitro. Int J Radiat Oncol Biol Phys 1993;27:303–308.

15 Malaise EP, Fertil B, Chavaudra N, Guichard M: Distribution of radiation sensitivities for human tumor cells of specific histological types: Comparison of in vitro to in vivo data. Int J Radiat Oncol Biol Phys 1986;12:617–624.

16 Yang X, Darling JL, McMillan TJ, Peacock JH, Steel GG: Heterogeneity of radiosensitivity in a human glioma cell line. Int J Radiat Oncol Biol Phys 1992;22:103–108.

17 Taghian A, Ramsay J, Allalunis-Turner J, Budach W, Gioioso D, Pardo F, Okunieff P, Bleehen N, Urtasun R, Suit H: Intrinsic radiation sensitivity may not be the major determinant of the poor clinical outcome of glioblastoma multiforme. Int J Radiat Oncol Biol Phys 1993;25:243–249.

18 Fallai C, Olmi P: Hyperfractionated and accelerated radiation therapy in central nervous system tumors (malignant gliomas, pediatric tumors, and brain metastases). Radiother Oncol 1997;43: 235–246.

19 Bese NS, Uzel Ö, Turkan S, Okkan S: Continuous hyperfractionated accelerated radiotherapy in the treatment of high-grade astrocytomas. Radiother Oncol 1998;47:113–224.

Dr. med. Ursula M. Schleicher, Department of Radiotherapy of the RWTH,
Pauwelsstrasse 30, D–52057 Aachen (Germany)
Tel. +49 241 80 89 260, Fax +49 241 88 88 425

Wiegel T, Hinkelbein W, Brock M, Hoell T (eds): Controversies in Neuro-Oncology.
Front Radiat Ther Oncol. Basel, Karger, 1999, vol 33, pp 174–191

·······················

Chemotherapy in Adult Malignant Glioma

M.J. van den Bent

Department of Neuro-Oncology, Dr. Daniel den Hoed Cancer Clinic,
Rotterdam, The Netherlands

Introduction

Many years after the first randomized trials on adjuvant chemotherapy for high-grade glioma, the question whether a patient with a high-grade glioma will receive this treatment mainly depends on the country in which he is being treated. This article will review the rationale for adjuvant chemotherapy in anaplastic glioma, and strategies for improvement of efficacy and survival. Next, it will give a short overview of results of recent phase II chemotherapy trials in recurrent glioma, and of recent developments in this field of research. Because of their sensitivity to chemotherapy, oligodendroglial tumors (OD) will be discussed separately. Lastly, attempts to overcome resistance to chemotherapy in glioma by local dose intensification through high-dose chemotherapy, intratumoral chemotherapy, or intracarotid chemotherapy with or without blood-brain barrier modification are reviewed shortly.

Adjuvant Chemotherapy in High-Grade Glioma

Despite a large number of trials on adjuvant chemotherapy after radiation therapy in malignant glioma, there is no consensus of opinion on its value. Even discussions on the design of new phase III chemotherapy trials in newly diagnosed glioma are hampered by a lack of agreement on the kind of treatment in the control arm. Many believers in adjuvant chemotherapy as part of standard treatment in high-grade glioma derive their opinion from large American multicenter randomized studies organized by the Brain Tumor Cooperative Group (BTCG), carried out in the late 60s and 70s (BTSG 69-01, 72-01 and 75-01) [1–3]. In the first two studies, the addition of adjuvant chemotherapy to the postoperative radiation therapy failed to increase the median survival time (MST) in comparison to radiation therapy alone. However, a 10% increase in patients surviving at 18 months in the adjuvant chemotherapy group was observed [1, 2]. A similar increase was observed in the third study (BTSG 75-01) in which adjuvant treatment with BCNU was compared with adjuvant high-dose prednisolone [3]. At the completion of the last trial, a post-hoc analysis without formal statistical testing was done on BTSG 72-01 and 75-01. This showed a 10% increase in 18- and 24-month survival in the adjuvant BCNU group, compared to radiation therapy alone or with prednisolone [3, 4]. Although critics objected that side effects of prednisolone may have had an adverse affect on survival, the BTCG then decided at the start of study 77-02 to consider brain irradiation to 60 Gy plus adjuvant BCNU as the standard treatment for malignant glioma to which all new treatments had to be compared. A similar study started in 1974 by the RTOG/ECOG group also failed to show a significant increase in MST by adjuvant chemotherapy but again 18-month survival was 10% higher in the adjuvant BCNU group [5]. In Europe, some more studies were carried out which included a radiation therapy control arm. As in some of these no benefit of adjuvant chemotherapy was found, many remained unconvinced of the advantage of adjuvant chemotherapy. Table 1 summarizes some of these studies. To resolve this controversy, Fine et al. [6] carried out a meta-analysis of all studies addressing the value of adjuvant chemotherapy. His analysis on 14 studies including more than 3,000 patients confirmed a small benefit of adjuvant chemotherapy. The likelihood of survival at 18 and 24 months was 1.5 times greater if radiation therapy was followed by adjuvant chemotherapy, equivalent with an approximately 10% increase in survival at 12 and 24 months. It was criticized however, for several reasons. Some negative trials had not been identified, and not all trials were from a methodological point of view sound enough for such a comparison [7, 8]. Still, a recent EORTC trial confirmed the analysis of Fine et al: adjuvant BCNU and dibromodulciterol resulted in $\pm 10\%$ – statistical significant – increase in survival at 12–24 months [9].

A constant feature from all survival curves in these reports is the absence of a plateau phase: they show a constant downhill course of the survival curve regardless of treatment (and often the tails of the survival curves meet). The benefit of adjuvant chemotherapy is small: 10 patients must be treated to have two instead of one 2-year survivors, who most likely will relapse within a short time. It should also be noted here that all trials comparing radiation therapy to radiation therapy with adjuvant chemotherapy had survival as endpoint, no trial evaluated cost-effectiveness or quality of life of adjuvant chemotherapy.

Table 1. Overview of median, 1- and 2-year survival of some studies on the value of adjuvant chemotherapy for newly diagnosed glioma

Reference (first author)	Postoperative treatment	Patients n	Survival median (months)	1-year (%)	2-year (%)
Walker [2]	RT	94	8	34.6	9.7
	Me-CCNU	81	6	15.0	7.5
	RT + MeCCNU	91	12	50.0	15.2
	RT + BCNU	92	9.5	36.7	12.2
Chang [5]	RT	148	9.9		19
	RT + boost	105	8.4		22
	RT + BCNU	165	10.0		29
	RT + MeCCNU/DTIC	136	9.8		26
Trojanowski [116]	RT	75	10.2	39.9	25.4
	RT + CCNU	74	12.0	50.4	17.0
Hildebrand [9]	RT	128	10.8		12
	RT + BCNU/DBD	127	13.2		21

RT = Radiotherapy; boost = boost RT on the tumor; Me-CCNU = semustine; CCNU = lomustine; BCNU = carmustine; DTIC = dacarbazine; DBD = dibromodulcitol.

As glioblastoma multiforme (GBM) comprises most of the high-grade gliomas, and phase II studies show these tumors are not very sensitive to chemotherapy, it is clear that with the present available drugs only a minority of patients will really benefit from adjuvant chemotherapy. These meager phase III results warrant a control arm with radiation therapy alone for new phase III trials on adjuvant chemotherapy in combination with a thorough evaluation of quality of life and cost-effectiveness. Even in the USA, the value of adjuvant chemotherapy for all patients with malignant glioma is being questioned, because of the modest survival advantage and the side effects [8, 10].

One possible way of improving the efficacy in the treatment of glioma patients is by recognizing patients with more chemosensitive tumors. In part, this can be done by further refining eligibility criteria for adjuvant chemotherapy. Prognosis of glioma is strongly related to age, which questions the usefulness of treatment in older patients. This holds also for adjuvant chemotherapy; in patients over 60 years of age median time to progression measured from the start of adjuvant chemotherapy was 6 weeks [11]. As serious complications were also more frequent in patients over 60 years of age, the benefit of adjuvant chemotherapy in this age group is highly questionable. In subgroup analysis of the recent EORTC trial, the advantage observed after adjuvant chemotherapy in GBM was statistically significant, but clinically not very relevant: it had disappeared after 18 months. The increase in survival seemed more pronounced in anaplastic astrocytoma (AA), but in this group the difference was not significant from a statistical point of view. This was a post-hoc analysis, and one of the older adjuvant chemotherapy trials did not show a clear difference between AA and GBM [5]. Still, this is an interesting observation; it may well be that the observed differences in the large randomized trials are due to a subset of chemosensitive tumors like oligodendroglioma (OD) or AA [12–14]. An analysis of BTSG studies 72-01 and 75-01 could not confirm however that the benefit of adjuvant chemotherapy could be attributed to the presence of oligodendroglioma [15].

The enzyme O6-methylguanine-DNA methyltransferase (MGMT) in part mediates resistance to the alkylating nitrosoureas. Nitrosoureas alkylate DNA at the O6-guanine position, which damage may be repaired by MGMT. The absence of this enzyme is related to sensitivity to nitrosoureas and temozolomide [16]. In one study on adjuvant BCNU chemotherapy in glioma, it was shown that MGMT correlated with survival [17]. In GBM, survival was more strongly correlated with MGMT levels than with age. If MGMT levels could be measured routinely, this might allow identification of patients with a greater likelihood of response to alkylating chemotherapy. Such an approach will have to prove itself in trials, not in the least because of the many other drug resistance pathways in gliomas. Glioma cells from one tumor show a large heterogeneity in MGMT expression of glioma cells [18, 19]. It may be that the average MGMT level in a tumor is not important but the fraction of cells with high MGMT content which survive treatment and will regrow. Others have attempted to select chemosensitive tumors by testing monoclonal cell populations from patients on their chemosensitivity. This may imply an immunohistochemical assay of MGMT is to be preferred above a quantitated biochemical assay. The same heterogeneity has been observed on chemosensitivity of clonal cell lines. Even clonal cell lines from one parental cell line may show a similar heterogeneity in chemosensitivity and resistant cells may even confer resistance to sensitive cells [20, 21]. It is therefore unlikely clonal cell lines are representative of an entire tumor [20].

Another way of testing new drugs or chemosensitivity in vivo is to treat patients with 1 or 2 cycles of chemotherapy before the start of radiation therapy with new drugs or new combinations [22–25]. This approach necessitates a frequent follow-up to assure delaying radiation therapy does not compromise patient care. Also, postoperative measurable disease – requiring direct postoperative scanning – is mandatory. It is all the same a very interesting approach for two reasons. First, it allows assessment of drug sensitivity in untreated patients. Secondly, it may identify patients responsive to chemotherapy, in whom this can be continued after the radiation therapy.

Phase II Trials in Recurrent Glioma

Until the publication in 1992 of Macdonald's criteria [26] for the measurement of response of recurrent glioma to chemotherapy in phase II trials, a variety of response criteria was used making the interpretation and comparison of trials very difficult. Macdonald's criteria are based on neuroimaging, and are similar to the criteria used for other organ systems in oncology: a partial response means a 50% reduction of tumor size and has to be confirmed with a second scan at least 1 month later. There is still criticism to these criteria, because tumor size is reduced to enhancement, tumors are often difficult to measure and some patients with stable disease remain longer free from progression than patients with a partial response. Clinical experience with OD tumors show however that once a chemotherapy regimen is effective, this translates itself in a better correlation between response and survival [14, 27].

When interpreting the phase II study results, one should not only consider the response criteria, but also the selection of patients. As a result of clinical selection, many phase II trials of recurrent glioma show an overrepresentation of patients in good clinical condition with previous low-grade tumors or AA. In a large study on chemotherapy in recurrent glioma the most important predictive factors for survival and response were a good performance status, young age and low-grade histology [28]. This is the usual phase II population, and this will bias trials to positive results. On the other hand, many of the patients are heavily pretreated (e.g., chemotherapy) which reduces the chance for a response to further treatment [29, 30].

Over the past years, several different approaches for new phase II trials can be distinguished. First, new and promising chemotherapeutic agents have been tested in recurrent glioma like topotecan [31], docetaxel [32], paclitaxel [33, 34], temozolomide [12, 35, 36], amonafide [37], fotemustine [38] and all-trans-retinoic acid [39, 40]. Most of these trials did not report interesting response rates, except for studies on temozolomide and fotemustine. In a first study with temozolomide on 48 patients with recurrent gliomas, a response of 25% was obtained, with a median TTP of 6.1 months, but a later multicenter study including some of these patients observed only 11% objective responses [36, 41]. In AA a 42% response rate was observed with 46% of patients remaining free from progression at 6 months [12]. In 24 patients with high-

Table 2. Response rates of recurrent glioma to some multiagent schedules

Reference (first author)	Drug	n	CR	PR	SD	Objective response %	MTP months
Ameri [113]	Procarbazine, thiotepa, vincristine	20	0	3	1	15	5
Jeremic [44]	Carboplatin, etoposide	38	0	8	12	21	10
Buckner [114]	Cisplatin, etoposide	36	1	5	17	17	3–6
Ameri [115]	Carboplatin, etoposide	31	0	4	10	13	6.5
Van den Bent [45]	Cisplatin, ifosfamide	25	0	5	5	20	6
Sanson [46]	Carboplatin, etoposide, ifosfamide	36	5	5	9	28	5.5

CR = Complete response; PR = partial response; SD = stable disease; Objective response = % of patients with PR or CR; MTP = median time to progression.

grade glioma treated before the initiation of radiation therapy, 3 complete and 12 partial responses were observed [25]. The results of another phase II study in GBM is to be reported soon. Fotemustine, another nitrosourea derivate, induced an objective response in 26% of patients with recurrent glioma, with a median duration of response of 33 weeks [38]. A few studies have tried to modulate MGMT-mediated resistance to nitrosoureas by depleting MGTM prior to the administration of chemotherapy. In one study, MGMT was depleted by procarbazine, after which BCNU was administered [42]. Although the response rate was promising (41% objective responses) a significant increase in toxicity was observed. A similar approach uses O6-benzylguanine to deplete MGMT, a phase II trial is planned [43]. As increased toxicity is to be expected, clinical results will have to be awaited for.

A second approach are phase II trials in which well known combinations of cytostatic agents are tested, like cis- or carboplatin, etoposide, ifosfamide, cyclophosphamide. Single-agent studies with these drugs have reported response rates in the 0–15% range (thus, similar to those of the newer agents!). Although a few of these combinations showed slightly higher response rates (between 20 and 30%; table 2), 65–80% of patients were progressive at 6 months [30, 44–46]. Many of the used schedules were fairly toxic and necessitated frequent hospital admissions. They illustrate that although some patients respond to such schedules, 3–5 patients must be treated to have one responding patient or to have 1 patient free from progression after 6 months. This rarely outweighs the intensity of the administered treatment.

A third approach consists of combinations of known cytostatic drugs and nonclassical cytostatic agents like interleukins, tamoxifen, etc. Interferons have a cytostatic effect on tumor cells. Two studies reported a 30% partial response rate to a combination of BCNU and α-interferon, with a duration of response of 9 months [47, 48]. A study on interferon-α_{2a} and eflornithine appeared inactive [49]. High-dose tamoxifen induced in 8 of 32 patients (25%) a partial response in recurrent glioma, probably by inhibition of protein kinase C [50]. A combination of high-dose tamoxifen and interferon-α_2 was not active [51]. A study on newly diagnosed patients treated with adjuvant carboplatin and tamoxifen after radiation therapy reported a superior survival as compared to a series of matched controls receiving only adjuvant treatment carboplatin; unfortunately details on the matching procedure were not given [52].

There is some evidence AA may be more sensitive to chemotherapy than GBM. In recurrent AA, several phase II studies reported objective response rates of 40–50% [12, 13, 46]. This however has not been a universal finding [36]. Although low-grade astrocytoma, and AA develop from the same astrocytic cells as GBM, they are different with regard to the genetic abnormalities. A distinction can be made between primary (or de novo) and secondary (= developed through progression from low-grade precursors) GBM. Whereas primary GBMs are characterized by EGFR overexpression and loss of heterozygosity on chromosome 10, most secondary GBM show p53 mutations and loss of heterozygosity of chromosome 17p [53–55]. Although the clinical course of these GBMs is similar [56], the differences in abnormalities at the molecular level may have clinical implications in the future. For instance, in many tumors p53 status is related to response to treatment and survival, by either inducing apoptosis or (reversely) protecting the cell by cell cycle arrest to allow DNA repair [57]. In mouse astrocytes, wild-type p53 seemed to make cells resistant to BCNU [57]. Human brain tumors with p53 mutations showed lower MGMT levels and increased growth delay after treatment with procarbazine than those without [58]. In contrast, restoration of wild-type p53 function resulted in sensitization of rat GBM to cisplatin [59]. Thus, response to chemotherapy of astrocytic tumors may be related to p53 status, but at the present time no definite conclusions can be drawn from this basic research. It may even depend on the kind of treatment given. Whether this knowledge can be used to modulate sensitivity to chemotherapy (e.g. with p53 gene transfer into tumor cells) has to prove itself outside the laboratory.

In conclusion, the response rate in glioblastoma is poor. This implies that for nontrial 'compassionate need' chemotherapy in recurrent GBM, easy-to-administer (oral) and nonintensive schedules like the PCV schedule or temozolomide are to be preferred. A somewhat higher response rate may be expected in AA and (previous) low-grade tumors. Phase II trials should explore

Table 3. PCV chemotherapy

Drug	Time	Standard intensity	Intensified
CCNU	Day 1	110 mg/m^2 orally	130 mg/m^2 orally
Vincristine	Days 8, 29	1.4 mg/m^2 i.v.	1.4 mg/m^2 i.v.
Procarbazine	Days 8–21	60 mg/m^2 orally	75 mg/m^2 orally

Cycle to be repeated every 6 weeks, for a maximum of 6 cycles in responding or stabilized patients; patients with progressive disease or unacceptable toxicity go off treatment.

Table 4. Overview of response rates of recurrent OD tumors to PCV chemotherapy

Reference (first author)	n	CR	PR	SD	PD	MTP for CR/PR/SD
Van den Bent [14]	52	17%	46%	19%	17%	25/12/7
Soffietti [62]	26	15%	46%	27%	12%	46/15/9
Cairncross [27]	15	33%[a]	33%	20%	7%	25/16/7[b]
Total	93	18 (19%)	42 (45%)	20 (22%)	13 (14%)	

MTP = Median time to progression; n = number of patients; CR = complete response; PR = partial response; SD = stable disease; PD = progressive disease.

[a] Includes patients with small residual lesions.

[b] MTP in the total study population of 24 patients, of whom 15 had a recurrence after radiation therapy and 9 were radiation-naive.

innovative strategies with new agents, as it is unlikely any of the presently known drugs will add much to the treatment of these tumors.

Chemotherapy in Oligodendroglioma

Several studies have confirmed Cairncross' initial observations of the chemosensitivity of OD tumors, which comprise 5–10% of all gliomas [60, 61]. In recurrent anaplastic OD tumors, a 60–70% response rate with 1–2 year duration to chemotherapy with procarbazine, CCNU and vincristine (PCV; table 3) is the rule (table 4) [14, 27, 62]. Moreover, low-grade oligodendroglioma and mixed oligoastrocytomas may also respond [63–66]. Similar response rates were obtained with other nitrosoureas and with melphalan [65, 66]. The more intensified PCV regimen is more toxic without clearly superior results [14, 27, 63]. It is clear though, that all patients will ultimately relapse.

The explanation for the chemosensitivity of oligodendrogliomas is unclear. OD cells and astrocytic cells probably arise from a common progenitor, but their malignant counterparts have distinct genetic alterations [67]. There is in vitro evidence that cells of OD lineage have a relatively low level of MGMT compared to astrocytic cell lines [68, 69], but studies in human brain tumors have shown conflicting results [70, 71]. Recent studies on second-line chemotherapy in OD tumors reported 40% response rates to cisplatin/etoposide and to paclitaxel, demonstrating that the chemosensitivity of OD is not limited to alkylating agents [72, 73]. Salvage therapy with single-agent carboplatin or oral etoposide was not very effective [62, 74].

With these favorable response rates chemotherapy has become part of standard treatment in oligodendroglioma and mixed oligoastrocytoma. This does not imply that it should be delivered in adjuvant setting after first surgery and radiation therapy, it may be equally effective with regard to survival when administered at recurrence. The question of timing is currently under investigation in both EORTC and North American trials. Future trials must be directed at identifying new active cytostatic agents for oligodendrogliomas, and must identify factors predictive for response to chemotherapy. One study suggested PCV was less effective in patients relapsing within the first year from first treatment, and more effective in patients presenting with seizures and having necrosis at histologic examination [14]. These findings however, need confirmation.

With the favorable response to chemotherapy, the differentiation of OD tumors from astrocytic tumors has important clinical consequences. This differentiation remains and is even troublesome for expert pathologists [75, 76]. A recent study suggested the percentage OD may be much higher (up to 25% of all glioma) [76]. It is hard to imagine an increase in prevalence of OD of this magnitude without an inverse effect on the response rate to chemotherapy. There are no reliable markers to differentiate between astrocytic and OD tumors. The distinction is further impeded by the presence of mixed oligoastrocytomas [75]. Genetic analysis suggests mixed glioma consists of two distinct subsets: one genetically related to OD (allelic losses on chromosome 19q and 1p), and one related to astrocytomas (P53 gene mutations) [77]. Basic research is now focussing on the separation of OD tumors from astrocytic tumors. First reports show they have different phenotypic abnormalities, like EGFR amplification and Trk receptor expression being present in high-grade astrocytic tumors but not in OD, whereas the latter express genes for myelin basic protein and proteolipid protein [78–80]. Perhaps this research results in diagnostic tests and markers improving the differentiation between astrocytomas and OD. From the patient's point of view, the exact histological classification is of course of less importance than a correlation with chemosensitivity.

(Local) Dosis Intensification

One approach that has been used to overcome resistance of cancer cells to chemotherapy is by dosis intensification either by intra-arterial chemotherapy with or without blood-brain barrier modification, by high-dose chemotherapy with autologous bone marrow rescue or by intratumoral administration. Some of these studies are phase II type studies in recurrent glioma, others administered these treatments to newly diagnosed patients and reported on survival. Most of these usually uncontrolled studies are difficult to interpret. All too often, promising outcomes of uncontrolled phase II studies of experimental treatments in glioma are due to selection of patients considered fit and eligible for the experimental treatment (e.g., size of the tumor, Karnofsky) [81–83]. With recursive partitioning, Curran et al. [84] have shown that a group of glioma patients can be identified with an expected median survival >2 years (e.g. <50 years of age, any AA, or GBM with Karnofsky performance status of 90–100). Reports of survival data of new treatments should therefore be compared to a group of controls, matched for the most important prognostic parameters (age, performance status, histology) and the most important eligibility criteria of the trial. If these are not given, a meaningful analysis is very difficult.

Modification or Circumvention of the Blood-Brain Barrier
Even though the penetration of hydrophilic drugs is 10 times higher in the tumor as compared to normal brain and similar to the penetration into extracranial tumors [45, 85–87], the blood-brain barrier (BBB) is still brought up as an explanation for nonresponsiveness of cerebral tumors [88–90]. Although with increasing distance from the tumor drug penetration decreases, most if not all tumor cells receive adequate exposure to the majority of cytostatic agents. Three approaches of BBB modification have been used: first, intracarotid administration of cytostatic agents in combination with BBB modification by intra-arterial (IA) mannitol; secondly, intratumoral administration of chemotherapy, and more recently, by intravenous administration of RPM-7, a bradykinin analogue.

The value of opening the BBB was suggested by an animal study which showed after intracarotid mannitol administration some increase of methotrexate penetration in tumor and brain around the tumor [91]. However, this and subsequent studies also showed that IA BBB modification increased drug delivery to the normal brain far more than it increased drug delivery to the tumor [91–94]. Dexamethasone did not reduce the uptake in the tumor of cytostatic agents, but prevented the increase after BBB modification in normal brain and brain around the tumor [91]. Another study found dexamethasone reduced uptake of cisplatin only in the brain around the tumor area, but not in the tumor itself [87]. These minor changes in drug penetration in the tumor after BBB modification demonstrate the absence of a BBB in brain tumors. The situation is different in brain around the tumor and normal brain, in which area's the barrier is partially or fully intact and can be opened, putting the patient at risk for increased neurotoxicity of the treatment. This again underscores that lack of intrinsic drug sensitivity is the most important factor for the absence of responses, as is nicely demonstrated by the good responses – even of leptomeningeal metastases – in oligodendroglioma [14].

RMP-7 may be a new approach for improving drug delivery to brain tumors. In animal models this bradykinin analogue was found to increase brain tumor and brain around tumor permeability but not of normal brain [95]. The effect was decreased by dexamethasone. Also, animals treated with both carboplatin and RPM-7 lived longer. Studies in humans with PET tracers support the increase of nonlipophilic drugs into brain tumors without increasing transport into normal brain [95]. Such a local dose intensification with drugs that have a steep dose-response curve may greatly enhance antitumor activity. Phase II studies in chemo-naive patients reported a 28% response rate to RPM-7 and carboplatin, which is better than the usual 5–10% response rate to carboplatin alone [96]. A randomized phase II study comparing carboplatin with carboplatin + RPM-7 did not observe significant differences, although a favorable trend in the RPM-7 group was present [Prados, pers. commun.]. Further studies with this drug are planned.

Intra-Arterial Administration

The primary goal of intracarotid chemotherapy for gliomas is to achieve high concentrations of cytostatic drugs in the tumor with only a limited exposure of systemic tissue [97]. The price to be paid is of course the repeated IA procedures to deliver the drug, but also local toxicity (loss of vision, seizures, encephalopathy) perhaps due to the high concentrations of cytostatic drugs in the normal brain [98–100]. Better (supraophthalmic) positioning may prevent some of these complications. In phase II studies in recurrent and newly diagnosed gliomas, promising responses were observed [97, 98, 101, 102], but phase III studies were disappointing. A randomized phase III trial comparing IA versus intravenous BCNU did not show significant differences between both treatments, but in the IA group serious treatment-related side-effects (visual loss, encephalopathy) due to white matter necrosis were observed in up to 15% of IA-treated patients [103]. A comparison between IA cisplatin and intravenous PCNU (a nitrosourea) showed a significant increase in survival in the PCNU group [104]. In the IA group, visual loss occurred in 7% of patients, encephalopathies in 4%. These results are not supportive for further trials in this area, although improvement of the infusion technique may result in decreased toxicity [105]. Even with such techniques, only minor response rates to carboplatin were observed (20% PR). No randomized study has investigated the value of IA administration with BBB modification.

Intratumoral Chemotherapy

One approach to gliomas is to see this as a localized problem, as most gliomas recur within 2 cm of the original tumor site. Localized intratumoral chemotherapy is then an attractive way to treat these tumors, as this circumvents the BBB, allows direct treatment of cancer cells with an increased dosage of cytostatic drugs but at a minimum of systemic exposure to these drugs. A variety of delivery approaches exist, ranging from infusion pomps to biodegradable polymer [88]. The latter approach with BCNU-loaded polymers was tested in a phase III trial in patients with recurrent glioma. A 20% increase in 6-month survival was found, but the effect completely disappeared in the following months [89]. After adjustment for prognostic factors a difference in long-term survival was apparent but this needs confirmation in a prospective study. This study underlines that BNCU is of modest activity in some glioma patients. The advantage of this approach is the delivery during surgery without further care; a major disadvantage is of course that a resection is needed to implant the wafers. Currently a phase III trial with wafers containing a higher dosage of BCNU is underway.

High-Dose Chemotherapy with Autologous Bone Marrow Rescue

Myelotoxicity is the dose-limiting toxicity of most cytostatic drugs, which can in part be circumvented by autologous bone marrow rescue [106]. This allows dose intensification for several drugs like BCNU and etoposide [106]. Phase I and II studies in recurrent glioma have shown relatively good response rates (35%), but with substantial acute toxicity, mortality and delayed neurotoxicity [107–109]. Several phase II studies investigated such regimens as adjuvant chemotherapy, with median survival times of 15–26 months [107, 110–112]. Despite promising reports with long-term survivors, it is quite likely this is at least in part explained by patient selection [84]. Randomized trials have not been carried out.

Conclusions

Until better agents are available, the present increase in survival with adjuvant chemotherapy in newly diagnosed gliomas is of minor clinical significance. This implies a control arm with radiation therapy alone in new phase III trials on adjuvant chemotherapy is fully warranted. Such trials should also assess quality of life, and must separate GBM from AA and OD. One way to improve efficacy of adjuvant is by selecting patients more likely to respond to adjuvant chemotherapy, but this will leave the prognosis for most of the patients unchanged. New research is therefore necessary, but it is doubtful whether any of the presently known agents will substantially improve survival in glioma. Response rates to chemotherapy in recurrent GBM remain poor, but relatively good results have been obtained in OD and – to a lesser extent – in AA. The value of nontrial chemotherapeutic treatment in recurrent primary GBM is doubtful. If treatment is indicated for compassionate need reasons, preferably nonintensive schedules should be used. In OD, chemotherapy must be considered part of standard treatment, but it is yet unclear if this should be administered adjuvantly after radiation therapy or at recurrence. High-grade mixed oligoastrocytomas have a better prognosis than GBM with similar histologic features, and some share the responsiveness of OD. Phase II trials should explore innovative schedules (e.g. modulating resistance, schedules with nonclassical cytotoxic agents), as schedules with the currently used cytostatic agents are unlikely to be effective in GBM, the most important part of gliomas.

References

1 Walker MD, Alexander E, Hunt WE, et al: Evaluation of BCNU and/or radiotherapy in the treatment of anaplastic gliomas. A cooperative clinical trial. J Neurosurg 1978;49:333–343.
2 Walker MD, Green SB, Byar DP, et al: Randomized comparisons of radiotherapy and nitrosoureas for the treatment of malignant glioma after surgery. N Engl J Med 1980;303:1323–1329.
3 Glass J, Gruber ML, Cher L, Hochberg FH: Preirradiation methotrexate chemotherapy of primary central nervous system lymphoma: Long-term outcome. J Neurosurg 1994;81:188–195.
4 Deutsch M, Green SB, Strike TA, et al: Results of a randomized trial comparing BCNU plus radiotherapy, streptozotocin plus radiotherapy, BCNU plus fractionated radiotherapy, and BCNU following misonidazole plus radiotherapy in the postoperative treatment of malignant glioma. Int J Radiat Oncol Biol Phys 1989;16:1389–1396.
5 Chang CH, Horton J, Schoenfeld D, et al: Comparison of postoperative radiotherapy and combined postoperative radiotherapy and chemotherapy in the multidisciplinary management of malignant gliomas. Cancer 1983;52:997–1007.
6 Fine HA, Dear KBG, Loeffler JS, Black PMcL, Canellos GP: Meta-analysis of radiation therapy with and without adjuvant chemotherapy for malignant gliomas in adults. Cancer 1993;71:2585–2597.
7 Graham PH: Meta-analysis of radiation therapy with and without adjuvant chemotherapy for malignant glioma in adults (abstract). Cancer 1993;72:3367.
8 Perry JR, DeAngelis LM, Schold SC, et al: Challenges in the design and conduct of phase III brain tumor therapy trials. Neurology 1997;49:912–917.

9   Hildebrand J, Sahmoud T, Mignolet F, Grucher JM, Afra D, The EORTC Brain Tumor Group: Adjuvant therapy with dibromodulcitol and BCNU increases survival of adults with malignant gliomas. Neurology 1994;44:1479–1483.

10   Mason W, Louis DN, Cairncross JG: Chemosensitive gliomas in adults: Which ones and why? J Clin Oncol 1997;15:3423–3426.

11   Grant R, Lang BC, Page MA, Crane DL, Greenberg HS, Junck L: Age influences chemotherapy response in astrocytomas. Neurology 1995;45:929–933.

12   Levin V, Yung A, Prados M, et al: Phase II study of temodal (temozolamide) at first relapse in anaplastic astrocytoma patients (abstract). Proc ASCO, 1997.

13   Hildebrand J, De Witte O, Sahmoud T: Response of recurrent glioblastoma and anaplastic astrocytoma to dibromodulcitol, BCNU and procarbazine. J Neurooncol 1998;37:155–160.

14   Van den Bent MJ, Kros JM, Heimans JJ, et al: Response rate and prognostic factors of recurrent oligodendroglioma treated with PCV chemotherapy. Neurology 1998;51:1140–1145.

15   DeAngelis LM, Burger PC, Green SB, Cairncross JG: Adjuvant chemotherapy for malignant glioma: Who benefits? (abstract) Ann Neurol 1996;40:491–492.

16   Brent TP, Houghton PJ, Houghton JA: O6-alkylguanine-DNA alkyltransferase activity correlates with the therapeutic response of human rhabdomyosarcoma xenografts to 1-(2-chloroethyl)-3-(trans-4-methylcyclohexyl)-1-nitrosurea. Proc Natl Acad Sci USA 1985;82:2985–2989.

17   Belanich M, Pastor M, Randall T, et al: Retrospective study of the correlation between DNA repair protein alkyltransferase and survival of brain tumor patients treated with carmustine. Cancer Res 1996;56:783–788.

18   Lee SM, Reid H, Elder RH, Thatcher N, Margison GP: Inter- and intracellular heterogeneity of O6-alkylguanine-DNA alkyltransferase expression in human brain tumours: Possible significance in nitrosourea therapy. Carcinogenesis 1996;17:637–641.

19   Belanich M, Randall T, Pastor MA, et al: Intracellular localization and intracellular heterogeneity of the human DNA repair protein O6-methylguanine-DNA methyltransferase. Cancer Chemother Pharmacol 1996;37:547–555.

20   Bradford R, Koppel H, Pilkington GJ, Thomas DGT, Darling JL: Heterogeneity of chemosensitivity in six clonal lines derived from a spontaneous murine astrocytoma and its relationship to genotypic and phenotypic characteristics (abstract). J Neurooncol 1997;34:247–261.

21   Yung WKA, Shapiro JR, Shapiro WR: Heterogenous chemosensitivities of subpopulations of human glioma cells in culture. Cancer Res 1982;42:992–998.

22   Grossman SA, Wharam M, Scheidler V, et al: BCNU/cisplatin followed by radiation in poor prognosis patients with high-grade astrocytomas (abstract). Proc ASCO 1992;11:149.

23   Fetell MR, Grossman SA, Fisher JD, et al: Preirradiation paclitaxel in glioblastoma multiforme: Efficacy, pharmacology, and drug interactions. J Clin Oncol 1997;15:3121–3128.

24   Kirby SH, Macdonald D, Fisher B, Gaspar L, Cairncross G: Pre-radiation chemotherapy for malignant glioma in adults. Can J Neurol Sci 1996;23:123–127.

25   Friedman HS, Dugan M, Kerby T, et al: Temodal therapy of newly diagnosed high grade glioma (abstract). J Neurooncol 1997;35:S51.

26   Macdonald DR, Cascino TL, Schold SC, Cairncross JG: Response criteria for phase II studies of supratentorial malignant glioma. J Clin Oncol 1990;8:1277–1280.

27   Cairncross G, Macdonald D, Ludwin S, et al: Chemotherapy for anaplastic oligodendroglioma. J Clin Oncol 1994;12:2013–2021.

28   Rajan B, Ross G, Lim CC, et al: Survival inpatients with recurrent glioma as a measure of treatment efficacy: Prognostic factors following nitrosourea chemotherapy. Eur J Cancer 1994;30A:1809–1815.

29   Levin VA, Edwards MS, Wright DC, et al: Modified procarbazine, CCNU and vincristine (PCV-3) combination chemotherapy in treatment of malignant brain tumors. Cancer Treat Rep 1980;64:237–241.

30   Kyritsis AP, Yung WKA, Jaeckle KA, et al: Combination of 6-thioguanine, procarbazine, lomustine, and hydroxyurea for patient with recurrent malignant gliomas. Neurosurgery 1996;39:921–926.

31   Macdonald D, Cairncross G, Stewart D, et al: Phase II study of topotecan in patients with recurrent malignant glioma. Ann Oncol 1996;7:205–207.

32   Forsyth P, Cairncross G, Stewart D, Goodyear M, Wainman N, Eisenhauer E: Phase II trial of docetaxel in patients with recurrent malignant glioma: A study of the National Cancer Institute of Canada Clinical Trials Group. Invest New Drugs 1996;14:203–206.

33   Chamberlain MC, Kormanik P: Salvage chemotherapy with paclitaxel for recurrent primary brain tumors. J Clin Oncol 1995;13:2066–2071.

34   Prados MD, Schold SC, Spence AM, et al: Phase II study of paclitaxel in patients with recurrent malignant glioma. J Clin Oncol 1996;14:2316–2321.

35   O'Reilly SM, Newlands ES, Glaser MG, et al: Temozolamide: A new oral cytotoxic chemotherapeutic agent with promising activity against primary brain tumours. Eur J Cancer 1993;29A:940–942.

36   Bower M, Newlands ES, Bleehen NM, et al: Multicentre CRC phase II trial of temozolomide in recurrent or progressive high-grade glioma. Cancer Chemother Pharmacol 1997;40:484–488.

37   Levitt R, Buckner JC, Cascino TL, et al: Phase II study of amonafide in patients with recurrent glioma. J Neurooncol 1995;23:87–93.

38   Khayat D, Giroux B, Berille J, et al: Fotemustine in the treatment of brain primary tumors and metastases. Cancer Invest 1994;12:414–420.

39   Phuphanich S, Scott C, Fischbach AJ, Langer C, Yung WKA: *All-trans*-retinoic acid: A phase II radiation oncology group study (RTOG 91-13) in patients with recurrent malignant glioma. J Neurooncol 1997;34:193–200.

40   Kaba SE, Kyritisis AP, Conrad C, et al: The treatment of recurrent cerebral gliomas with *all-trans*-retinoic acid (tretinoin). J Neurooncol 1997;34:145–151.

41   Newlands ES, O'Reilly SM, Glaser MG, et al: The Charing Cross Hospital experience with temozolamide in patients with gliomas. Eur J Cancer 1996;32A:2236–2241.

42   Beith J, Cook R, Robinson B, Levi J, Bell D, Wheeler H: Modulation of resistance to BCNU by depleting MGMT activity with procarbazine in patients with relapsed gliomas (abstract). J Neurooncol 1997;35:S9.

43   Wedge SR, Porteous JK, Newlands ES: Effect of single and multiple administration of an O6-benzylguanine/temozolomide combination: An evaluation in a human melanoma xenograft model. Cancer Chemother Pharmacol 1997;40:266–272.

44   Jeremic B, Grujicic D, Jevremovic S, et al: Carboplatin and etoposide chemotherapy regimen for recurrent malignant glioma: A phase II study. J Clin Oncol 1992;10:1074–1077.

45   Van den Bent MJ, Schellens JHM, Vecht ChJ, et al: Phase II study on cisplatin and ifosfamide in recurrent high grade gliomas. Eur J Cancer 1998;34:1570–1574.

46   Sanson M, Ameri A, Monjour A, et al: Treatment of recurrent malignant supratentorial gliomas with ifosfamide, carboplatin and etoposide: A phase II study. Eur J Cancer 1996;32A:2229–2235.

47   Buckner JC, Brown LD, Kugler JW, et al: Phase II evaluation of recombinant interferon alpha and BCNU in recurrent glioma. J Neurosurg 1995;82:430–435.

48   Brandes AA, Scelzi E, Zampieri P, et al: Phase II trial with BCNU plus α-interferon in patients with recurrent high-grade gliomas. Am J Clin Oncol 1997;20:364–367.

49   Buckner JC, Burch PA, Cascino TL, O'Fallon JR, Scheithauer BW: Phase II trials of recombinant interferon-alpha-2a and eflornithine in patients with recurrent glioma. J Neurooncol 1998;36:65–70.

50   Couldwell WT, Hinton DR, Surnock AA, et al: Treatment of recurrent malignant gliomas with chronic oral high-dose tamoxifen. Clin Cancer Res 1996;2:619–622.

51   Chang SM, Barker FG, Huhn SL, et al: High dose oral tamoxifen and subcutaneous interferon-alpha-2a for recurrent glioma. J Neurooncol 1998;37:169–176.

52   Mastronardi L, Puzzilli F, Couldwell WT, Farah JO, Lunardi P: Tamoxifen and carboplatin combinational treatment of high grade gliomas. J Neurooncol 1998;38:59–68.

53   Leenstra S, Bijlsma EK, Troost D, et al: Allele loss on chromosomes 10 and 17p and epidermal growth factor gene receptor amplification in human astrocytoma related to prognosis. Br J Cancer 1994;70:684–689.

54   Kleihues P, Ohgaki H: Genetics of glioma progression and the definition of primary and secondary glioblastoma. Brain Pathol 1997;7:1131–1136.

55   Von Deimling A, Louis DN, Wiestler OD: Molecular pathways in the formation of gliomas. Glia 1995;15:328–338.

56   Dropcho EJ, Soong S: The prognostic impact of prior low grade histology in patients with anaplastic gliomas. Neurology 1996;47:684–690.
57   Nutt CL, Chambers AF, Cairncross JG: Wild-type p53 renders mouse astrocytes resistant to 1,3-bis(2-chloroethyl)-1-nitrosourea despite the absence of a p53-dependent cell cycle arrest. Cancer Res 1996;56:2748–2751.
58   Russel SJ, Ye YW, Waber PG, Shuford M, Schold SC, Nisen PD: p53 mutations, O6-alkylguanine-DNA alkyltransferase activity, and sensitivity to procarbazine in human brain tumors. Cancer 1995; 75:1339–1342.
59   Dorigo O, Turla ST, Lebedeva S, Gjerset RA: Sensitization of rat glioblastoma multiforme to cisplatin in vivo following restoration of wild-type p53. J Neurosurg 1998;88:535–540.
60   Cairncross JG, Macdonald DR, Ramsay DA: Aggressive oligodendroglioma: A chemosensitive tumor. Neurosurgery 1992;31:78–82.
61   Cairncross JG, Macdonald DR: Chemotherapy for oligodendroglioma. Arch Neurol 1991;48:225–227.
62   Soffietti R, Borgogne M, Bradac GB, Schiffer D: Role of chemotherapy in oligodendroglial tumors: A review of the experience at the University of Torino (abstract). J Neurooncol 1996;30:153.
63   Mason WP, Krol GS, DeAngelis LM: Low-grade oligodendroglioma responds to chemotherapy. Neurology 1996;46:203–207.
64   Kyritsis AP, Yung WKA, Bruner J, Gleason MJ, Levin VA: The treatment of anaplastic oligodendrogliomas and mixed gliomas. Neurosurgery 1993;32:365–371.
65   Duffau H, Albuquerque L, Ameri A, Sanson M, Poisson M, Delattre JY: Chemotherapy for newly diagnosed and recurrent anaplastic oligodendrogliomas and mixed gliomas: An analysis of 42 cases (abstract). Neurology 1995;45 (suppl 4):A261.
66   Brown M, Cairncross JG, Vick NA, et al: Differential response of recurrent oligodendrogliomas vs. astrocytomas to intravenous melphalan (abstract). Neurology 1990;40(suppl 1):397.
67   Raff MC, Miller RH, Noble M: A glial progenitor cell that develops in vitro into an astrocyte or an oligodendrocyte depending on the culture medium. Nature 1983;303:390–396.
68   Nutt CL, Costello JF, Bambrick LL, et al: O6-methylguanine-DNA methyltransferase in tumors and cells of the oligodendrocyte lineage. Can J Neurol Sci 1995;22:111–115.
69   LeDoux SP, Williams BA, Hollensworth BS, et al: Glial cell-specific differences in repair of O6-methylguanine. Cancer Res 1996;56:5615–5619.
70   Mineura K, Yanagisawa T, Watanabe K, Kowada M, Yasui N: Human brain tumor O6-methylguanine-DNA methyltransferase mRNA and its significance as an indicator of selective chloroethylnitrosourea chemotherapy. Int J Cancer 1996;69:420–425.
71   Silber JR, Mueller BA, Eweres TG, Berger MS: Comparison of O6-methylguanine-DNA methyltransferase activity in brain tumors and in adjacent normal brain. Cancer Res 1993;53:3416–3420.
72   Chamberlain MC, Kormanik PA: Salvage chemotherapy with taxol for recurrent oligodendrogliomas. J Clin Oncol 1997;15:3427–3432.
73   Peterson K, Paleologos N, Forsyth P, Macdonald DR, Cairncross JG: Salvage chemotherapy for oligodendroglioma. J Neurosurg 1996;85:597–601.
74   Fulton D, Urtasun R, Forsyth P: Phase II study of prolonged oral therapy with etoposide (VP16) for patients with recurrent malignant glioma. J Neurooncol 1996;27:149–155.
75   Krouwer HGJ, van Duinen SG, Kamphorst W, van der Valk P, Algra A: Oligoastrocytomas: A clinicopathological study of 52 cases. J Neurooncol 1997;33:223–238.
76   Coons SW, Johnson PC, Scheithauer BW, Yates AJ, Pearl DK: Improving diagnostic accuracy and interobserver concordance in the classification and grading of primary gliomas. Cancer 1997;79: 1381–1391.
77   Maintz D, Fiedler K, Koopmann J, et al: Molecular genetic evidence for subtypes of oligoastrocytomas. J Neuropathol Exp Neurol 1997;56:1098–1104.
78   Wang Y, Hagel C, Hamel W, Kluwe L, Westphal M: Trk family members: Potential lineage markers for glia (abstract). J Neurooncol 1997;35:S47.
79   Luider Th, Van den Bent MJ, Smitt PS, Vecht ChJ, Kros JM: Inventory of proteins in astrocytoma and oligodendroglioma by two-dimensional electrophoresis (abstract). J Neurooncol 1997;35: S28.

80   Golfinos JG, Norman SA, Coons SW, Norman RA, Ballecer C, Scheck AC: Expression of the genes encoding myelin basic protein and protolipid protein in human malignant gliomas. Clin Cancer Res 1997;3:799–804.
81   Florell RC, Macdonald DR, Irish WD, et al: Selection bias, survival, and brachytherapy for glioma (abstract). J Neurosurg 1992;76:179–183.
82   Kirby S, Brothers M, Irish W, et al: Evaluating glioma therapies: Modeling treatments and predicting outcomes (abstract). J Natl Cancer Inst 1995;87:1884–1888.
83   Curran WJ, Scott CB, Weinstein AS, et al: Survival comparison of radiosurgery-eligible and -ineligible malignant glioma patients treated with hyperfractionated radiation therapy and carmustine: A Report of Radiation Therapy Oncology Group 83-02 (abstract). J Clin Oncol 1993;11:857–862.
84   Curran WJ, Scott CB, Horton J, et al: Recursive partitioning analysis of prognostic factors in three Radiation Therapy Oncology Group malignant glioma trials. J Natl Cancer Inst 1993;85:704–710.
85   Stewart DJ, Molepo JM, Green RM, et al: Factors affecting platinum concentrations in human surgical tumour specimens after cisplatin. Br J Cancer 1995;71:598–604.
86   Stewart DJ: A critique of the role of the blood-brain barrier in the chemotherapy of human brain tumors. J Neurooncol 1994;20:121–134.
87   Straathof CSM, Van den Bent MJ, Ma J, et al: The effect of dexamethasone on the uptake of cisplatin in 9L glioma and the area of brain around tumor. J Neurooncol 1998;37:1–8.
88   Walter KA, Tamargo RJ, Olivi A, Burger PC, Brem H: Intratumoral chemotherapy. Neurosurgery 1995;37:1129–1145.
89   Brem H, Piantadosi S, Burger PC, et al: Placebo-controlled trial of safety and efficicacy of intraoperative controlled delivery by biodegradable polymers of chemotherapy for recurrent gliomas. Lancet 1995;345:1008–1012.
90   Gumerlock MK, Belshe BD, Madson R, Watts C: Osmotic blood-brain barrier disruption and chemotherapy in the treatment of high grade glioma patients: Patient series and literature review. J Neurooncol 1992;12:33–46.
91   Neuwelt EA, Barnett PA, Bigner DD, Frenkel EP: Effects of adrenal cortical steroids and osmotic blood-brain barrier opening on methotrexate delivery to gliomas in the rodent: The factor of the blood-brain barrier. Proc Natl Acad Sci USA 1982;79:4420–4423.
92   Groothuis DR, Warnke PC, Molnar P, Lapin GD: Effect of hyperosmotic blood-brain barrier disruption on transcapillary transport in canine brain tumors. J Neurosurg 1990;72:441–449.
93   Warnke PC, Blasberg RG, Groothuis DR: The effect of hyperosmotic blood-brain-barrier disruption on blood-to-tissue transport in ENU-induced gliomas. Ann Neurol 1987;22:300–305.
94   Hiesiger EM, Voorhies RM, Basler GA, Lipschutz LE, Posner JB, Shapiro WR: Opening the blood-brain and blood-tumor barriers in experimental rat brain tumors: The effect of intracarotid hyperosmolar mannitol on capillary permeability and blood flow. Ann Neurol 1986;19:50–59.
95   Black KL, Cloughesy T, Huang SC, et al: Intracarotid infusion of RMP-7, a bradykinin analog, and transport of gallium-68 ethylenediamine tetraacetic acid into human gliomas. J Neurosurg 1997;86:603–609.
96   Gregor A, Lind M, Osborn C: RMP-7 and carboplatin in recurrent malignant glioma (abstract). J Neurooncol 1997;35:S54.
97   Dropcho EJ, Rosenfeld SS, Marawetz RB, et al: Preradiation intracarotid cisplatin treatment of newly diagnosed anaplastic gliomas. J Clin Oncol 1992;10:452–458.
98   Feun LG, Wallace S, Stewart DJ, et al: Intracarotid infusion of cis-diamminedichloroplatinum in the treatment of recurrent malignant brain tumors. Cancer 1984;54:794–799.
99   Rogers LR, Purvis JB, Ledermann RJ, et al: Alternating sequential intracarotid BCNU and cispaltin in recurrent malignant glioma. Cancer 1991;68:15–21.
100 Longee DC, Friedman HS, Albright RE, et al: Treatment of patients with recurrent gliomas with cyclophosphamide and vincristine. J Neurosurg 1990;72:583–588.
101 Nakagawa H, Fujita T, Kubo S, et al: Selective intra-arterial chemotherapy with a combination of etoposide and cisplatin for malignant gliomas: A preliminary report. Surg Neurol 1994;41: 19–27.
102 Feun LG, Lee Y, Yung WA, Savaraj N, Wallace S: Intracarotid VP-16 for malignant brain tumors. J Neurooncol 1987;4:397–401.

103 Shapiro WR, Green SB, Burger PC, et al: A randomized comparison of intra-arterial versus intravenous BCNU, with or without intravenous 5-fluorouracil for newly diagnosed patients with malignant glioma. J Neurosurg 1992;76:772–781.

104 Hiesiger EM, Green SB, Shapiro WR, et al: Results of a randomized trial comparing intra-arterial cisplatin and intravenous PCNU for the treatment of primary brain tumors in adults: Brain Tumor Cooperative Group trial 8420A. J Neurooncol 1995;25:143–154.

105 Cloughesy TF, Gobin YP, Black KL, et al: Intra-arterial carboplatin chemotheapy for brain tumors: A dose escalation study based on cerebral blood flow. J Neurooncol 1998;35:121–131.

106 Finn GP, Souhami RL, Slevin ML, Thomas DGT: High-dose etoposide in the treatment of relapsed primary brain tumors. Cancer Treat Rep 1985;69:603–605.

107 Wolff SN, Phillips GL, Herzig GP: High-dose carmustine with autologous bone marrow transplantation for the adjuvant treatment of high-grade gliomas of the central nervous system. Cancer Treat Rep 1987;71:183–185.

108 Gianonne L, Wolff SN: Phase II treatment of central nervous system gliomas with high-dose etoposide and autologous bone marrow transplantation. Cancer Treat Rep 1987;71:759–761.

109 Phillips GL, Wolff SN, Fay JW, et al: Intensive 1,3-bis(chloroethyl)-1-nitrosourea (BCNU) monochemotherapy and autologous marrow transplantation for malignant glioma. J Clin Oncol 1986;4:639–645.

110 Johnson DB, Thompson JM, Corwin JA, et al: Prolongation of survival for high-grade malignant gliomas with adjuvant high-dose BCNU and autologous bone marrow transplantation. J Clin Oncol 1987;5:783–789.

111 Fernandez-Hidalgo OA, Vanaclocha V, Vieitez JM, et al: High-dose BCNU and autologous progenitor cell transplantation given with intra-arterial cisplatinum and simultaneous radiotherapy in the treatment of high grade gliomas: Benefit for selected patients. Bone Marrow Transplant 1996;18:143–149.

112 Mbidde EK, Selby PJ, Perren TJ, et al: High dose BCNU chemotherapy with autologous bone marrow transplantation and full dose radiotherapy for grade IV astrocytoma. Br J Cancer 1988;58:779–782.

113 Ameri A, Poisson M, Chen QM, Delattre JY: Treatment of recurrent malignant supratentorial gliomas with the association of procarbazine, thiotepa and vincristine: A phase II study. J Neurooncol 1993;17:43–46.

114 Buckner LC, Brown LD, Cascino TL, et al: Phase II evaluation of infusional etoposide and cisplatin in patients with recurrent astrocytoma. J Neurooncol 1990;9:249–254.

115 Ameri A, Poisson M, Chauveinc L, Chen QM, Delattre JY: Treatment of recurrent malignant supratentorial gliomas with the association of carboplatin and etoposide: A phase II study. J Neurooncol 1997;32:155–160.

116 Trojanowski T, Peszynski J, Turowski K, Kaminski S, Goscinski I, Reinfus M, et al: Postoperative radiotherapy and radiotherapy combined with CCNU chemotherapy for treatment of brain gliomas. J Neurooncol 1988;6:285–291.

M.J. van den Bent, Department of Neuro-Oncology, Dr. Daniel den Hoed Cancer Clinic, PO Box 5201, M-3008 AE Rotterdam (The Netherlands)
Tel. +31 10 4391415, Fax 31 10 4845743, E-Mail bent@neuh.azr.nl

Wiegel T, Hinkelbein W, Brock M, Hoell T (eds): Controversies in Neuro-Oncology.
Front Radiat Ther Oncol. Basel, Karger, 1999, vol 33, pp 192–201

....

Indication for Repeat Surgery of Glioblastoma: Influence of Progress of Disease

M. Mühling, J. Krage, S. Hussein, M. Samii

Department of Neurosurgery, Hannover Medical School, Hannover, Germany

Introduction

The short and tragic course of the glioblastoma disease has been widely documented in numerous articles [6, 8, 9, 17, 41, 45, 47]. However, very little has been written on the particular problem regarding recurring glioblastomas which arise in each case of this disease leaving the patient with a poor prognosis [7]. The question remains, if and when a recurring glioblastoma should be surgically removed. This is of high topical interest for neurosurgeons; however, there is much discrepancy whether or not a recurrent glioblastoma should be surgically removed.

The purpose of this study was to determine the influential factors for repeat surgery and the scope of treatment for the multidisciplinary adjuvant therapeutical procedures.

Patients and Methods

Between the years 1990 and 1996, 185 patients underwent surgery for primary glioblas-tomas at the Hannover Medical School. During this time, 35 (23%) patients underwent a second operation with the intention, as with the first operation, to remove the total tumor. The reason for the discrepancy in the number of patients were clinical (inoperable) findings and medical treatment in other departments starting after the first operation. The progress of the disease was evaluated until time of death. The retrospective study with the usual parameters was drawn up, e.g. Karnofsky index for neurological deficiencies associated with tumors, age, sex and localization of the glioblastoma. The survival time following repeat surgery was analyzed using the Kaplan-Meier statistics. A recent aspect, not yet documented in the literature, is the possible connection of blood group O of the ABO system with the genetic predisposition for the cancerous genesis of a glioblastoma. The corresponding parameters were investigated statistically with the χ^2 test.

Results

Distribution of Age and Sex

Twenty of the 35 patients between 20 and 71 years of age were male (57%) and 15 (43%) female. The mean age at the time of the initial operation was 48 years and at the second operation 49 years. The interval between the two operations was less than 12 months in 69% of cases. 80% of patients were more than 40 years of age at the time of the first operation.

Neurological Findings

An assessment of the neurological status with the standardized Karnofsky index was made before and after each surgical procedure, i.e. at the time of admission and discharge. Prior to the initial operation the patients were rated with an average of 64 points (min 30/max 100). 68.6% of patients had 60 points or more. They were able to manage their daily life with some occasional help, however, were incapable of working. Postoperatively, the average neurological status increased to 73 points. The patients were then able to care for themselves without any additional help, but were still unable to work. Prior to the repeat operation, the findings corresponded to the neurological status before the initial operation with 66 points. Postoperatively, the patients were dependent on regular support and medical care with a median of 53 points. The statistical calculation, using the simple linear correlation (Pearson r), resulted in correlation coefficients of $r = 0.51$ and $r = 0.43$ in both the preoperative and postoperative groups. These coefficients and a wide deviation of values outside the 95% confidence interval show clearly the variability of the subjective rating of neurological deficiencies and cannot, therefore, be included as an adequate final assessment.

Tumor Localization and Proliferation

Twenty-five of 35 patients (71.4%) were afflicted with right-sided glioblastomas. These tumors were mainly located in the temporal region, whereas the left-sided glioblastomas mainly occurred in the frontal region. In the operation-free interval, 40% of recurrent cases showed a change in proliferation, compared to the preoperative neuroradiological imaging procedures (CT and MRI), in the form of a growth extending over the lobes, a stem ganglion and a butterfly glioma as a result of contralateral infiltration. 17% of tumors demonstrated an increase of more than double the average size of 3.9 cm prior to the initial operation and 10% of recurring tumors were multilocular.

Table 1. Correlation of survival rate and radicality of first and second surgical procedures in 35 cases

First/second operation	Patients	Survival time months
Total/total	15	10.2
Subtotal/subtotal	11	5.4
Total/subtotal	6	10.8
Subtotal/total	3	4.6

Surgical Radicality and Survival Rate

A total tumor resection was achieved in 69% of cases during the first operation and in 60% of cases during repeat surgery.

Four aspects were indicated when comparing the surgical radicality with the postoperative survival times: (1) A large number of patients underwent both surgical procedures with the same degree of radicality (15 patients both operations total and 11 patients both operations subtotal). (2) The patients who had 2 subtotal operations were found to have a much shorter survival time compared to those patients who had 2 total operations (5.4–10.2 months after the second operation). (3) When comparing the survival times, it is remarkable to note two similar results with regard to the initial operation. In the case of a total operation, the patients survived, on average, 10 months. In a subtotal operation, the survival time amounted to 5 months regardless of the outcome of the second operation. (4) Furthermore, 2 subtotal operations resulted in an average survival time of 5.4 months, whereas on total repeat surgery, the average survival time even was around 4.6 months.

The statistical calculation of the survival time following repeat surgery, according to Kaplan-Meier, gave a median survival time of 6.7 months on the 50th percentile (fig. 1). The patients with right-sided glioblastomas survived, on average, 11.6 months. Those patients with left-sided glioblastomas only survived 5.8 months. The average time from the initial operation until time of death amounted to 15 months.

Adjuvant Therapeutical Procedures: Radiation versus Chemotherapy

Twenty-two of the patients who had a second operation underwent radiation therapy following the first operation and 11 further patients had a combination of both radiation therapy and chemotherapy with BCNU. One patient was treated with BCNU only and another patient did not have any adjuvant therapy (personal wish). Therapy took place mainly in the clinics to where the patients were initially referred and reflected upon the heterogenic

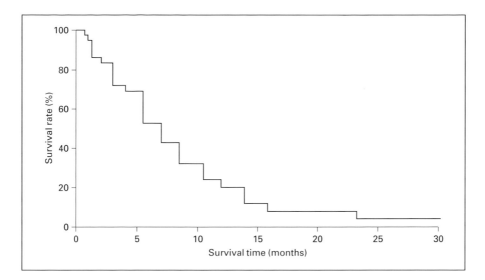

Fig. 1. Statistical calculation (Kaplan-Meier) of the survival time following repeat surgery in 35 cases.

therapeutical approaches. The patients who underwent combination therapy were found to have the longest survival time with 10.1 months followed by the group with radiation only (7.8 months). The survival time of the patient who was treated only with BCNU was 6 months and the patient with no additional therapy only survived for a period of 3 months.

Rate of Complications

Postoperative complications increased from 17.1 to 68.8% on repeat surgery. During the first operation, complications arose only in the head region such as infections, CSF fistula, hydrocephalus or epidural hematoma. Following the second operation, the most frequent complication was a deep venous thrombosis in 7 (20%) patients with pulmonary embolism in 3 cases and pneumonia in 5 (14.3%) cases. Two (5.7%) patients had a cerebrovascular accident (CVA), 3 (8.6%) patients had infections and 2 patients a CSF fistula. In-patient mortality following repeat surgery amounted to 11.4% (4 of 35 patients).

Predisposition of Blood Group O

Compared to the normal blood group classification in Central Europe, this group of patients showed incidence of blood group O of 58% opposed to the statistical rate of 40%. Blood group A showed a low incidence of 31%

opposed to 43% and B corresponded to the normal distribution (11%). Group AB was not present. In the group of 185 patients who underwent surgery for primary glioblastoma, 49% showed an increased incidence of blood group O. This marked incidence was statistically evaluated with the χ^2 test. The number of patients (185) was too low for a significant evaluation. Had the number of patients amounted to more than 300, there would have been a high significance for the predisposition of blood group O.

Discussion

Indication for Repeat Operation

Ray [42] was, in 1964, the first author to publish his views on the potential role of repeat surgery on multiform glioblastomas. Since then, very little has been documented on this specific aspect of the disease and there is, still today, a vast differing of opinions as to the indications for operation even for primary glioblastomas [3, 15, 16, 32, 44, 48, 58]. Influential factors as to the course of the disease are often sought only in a personal working sphere and multidisciplinary aspects are often ignored. This study gives a general insight into a randomized group of patients with recurring glioblastomas in order to clarify the influential factors of all therapeutical procedures and their association with one another.

The patient group corresponded in the distribution of age and sex with data derived from the literature. Men were more frequently afflicted (57%) and 80% were over 40 years old. One aspect not yet discussed in the literature, is the correlation of the prevalence of the glioblastoma with the blood group O.

While blood group A, for example, is widely known as a predisposing factor for stomach cancer, there is no reference made to the classification of tumors of the central nervous system for hematology. 49% of the patients with primary glioblastomas and even 58% with recurrent tumors showed blood group O which means an obvious higher prevalence than the Central European norm of 43%. According to statistical calculation by means of the χ^2 test, the total number of those undergoing investigation was too low to be of significance. In 33 patients, the increased prevalence of blood group O would be of great significance. If the percentage proves to be similar in specimens taken from both large and small groups, further studies are required to clarify this point, the outcome would then be verified. In this case, however, blood group O plays a part in the cancerous genesis of a glioblastoma in association with other endogenic and exogenic cofactors.

The main localization of gliomas has been widely discussed in the literature together with the sex specificity. Numerous authors have reported a large number of temporally situated glioblastomas, followed by tumor located in the frontal region [9, 13, 21, 23, 26–28, 30, 39, 49, 58]. This study also reports on a primary attack of the temporal lobe with a right-sided glioblastoma and of the frontal lobe with a left-sided glioblastoma.

The most significant factor for surgical radicality is the phase between the first and second operation in view of the survival time for the patient: the influence of the radicality on repeat surgery does not appear to play a role in the length of survival time. On total operation the first time, the patients survived for a period of 10 months on average, regardless of whether or not the second operation involved total or subtotal surgery. If the first operation involved a subtotal removal of the tumor, the mean survival time was 5.4 months, also with a subtotal removal and even 4.6 months following a total removal the second time round. In this case too, the second radicality was irrelevant. This raised the question whether it would be more beneficial for the patient to undergo subtotal surgery the second time. Since there is no literature available for any basic form of discussion, the influence of radicality on repeat surgery still remains uncertain.

The adjuvant therapeutical procedures include firstly radiation and the cytostatic treatment with chemotherapy such as BCNU, etc. [29, 34, 56]. 63% of the patients participating in our study were treated postoperatively with radiation and survived, on average, 7.8 months. 31% of the patients underwent a combination therapy of radiation and chemotherapy after the first operation. One patient died 6 months after repeat surgery following chemotherapy for a left-sided frontal glioblastoma. Another patient, with no adjuvant therapy for right-sided frontal glioblastoma, survived for 3 months only. This patient denied adjuvant treatment and used alternative medicine such as herbs. Tönnis and Walter [50] and Weir [54] were of the opinion that radiation alone was significant for a prolonged survival time [30]. This was proved otherwise, thus corresponding to the statement made by Kothe and Phuphanich et al. [cf. 10, 38, 43], who considered a combination therapy to be the decisive factor for prolonged survival. Chang et al. [11], on the other hand, opposed this view and considered chemotherapy alone to be the most effective treatment. Ultimately, the adjuvant forms of therapy also produced different effects (radiation injuries, toxicity of cytostatic agents, etc.) and are still viewed in a controversial way as are the surgical techniques [2, 12, 18–20, 52].

Three patients taking part in our study demonstrated a visible multilocular growth on CT. All other cases revealed a local recurrence (in some cases, extended). In the operation-free interval, 40% of local recurrences showed a change in proliferation on preoperative CT. Two glioblastomas were found to extend over the lobes, 2 had infiltrated the basal ganglia, 3 had spread in a contralateral direction resembling a butterfly glioma and 5 had increased more than double the average size. Just how specific this information is remains a point of contention between the authors. According to Duff, Wallner et al. [53], Harsh et al. [16], Forsting et al. [14] or Kreth et al. [30], CT cannot distinguish between a surgically induced contrast medium concentration and glioblastoma cells administered with contrast medium.

According to Forsting et al. [14], the critical time lies between the 3rd and 4th postoperative day, during which time it is possible to distinguish between the nonneoplastic contrast medium enhancement and the enhancement of the residing glioblastoma cells. An early postoperative imaging during this critical time could produce a more specific prognosis.

The survival time plays an important part in the indication for repeat operation. All authors give, with exception of the so-called 'long-term survivors', a period of less than 1 year with values between 6 months [22, 32, 37, 46, 55, 58, 60] and 12 months [11, 16, 25, 26, 40]. The survival time following repeat operation lies around 6.7 months. The length of time between the final operation until time of death in 26 of 35 cases (74.3%) was between the 10th and the 20th month of the complete course of the disease. It was interesting to note that during this particular time, the survival time curve of the surviving patients showed a drastic fall from 85 to 35%. This may indicate that repeat operation does not necessarily prolong the life span; on the contrary, it could even shorten the survival time. This hypothesis states, as opposed to the results of Bucy [6] and Harsh et al. [16], that repeat operation influences greatly the quality and quantity of the survival time, or Kornblith et al. [25] and Jelsmas and Bucy [23], who stated that surgery plays a vital role in the survival time of the patients. The majority of authors refer only to the initial operation.

A further important parameter for the survival prognosis is the neurological status of the patients using the Karnofsky index. Numerous authors consider the neurological status as highly significant [3, 32, 33, 58]. The Karnofsky status of patients with recurrent glioblastomas showed an average of 64 (range 0–100) prior to the first operation. The patients were, at this stage, unable to work and required occasional supportive care. Postoperatively (at discharge), the patients had an average of 73. This means that they were capable of managing their daily lives. Despite the fact that they were still unable to work, the neurological deficiency of the patients improved.

In the operation-free interval the status fell again to 66 and postoperatively, further to 55 points. Following repeat operation the patients were reliant on extra support and medical care.

The rapid drop in the survival curve during this time indicated a further worsening of the neurological deficiencies. A few authors viewed a status of 60 as a 'satisfactory result' for glioblastoma therapy. Over 60% of patients had a Karnofsky status of 60 or more prior to the initial and repeat operations. The patients with a lower status survived, on average, longer than 8 months, i.e. above the total mean time. Of the 6 patients who had a status of below 60 prior to both operations, 3 survived for 4.8 months and 3 survived for follow-up at the end of the study. These survival times give some doubt as to the correct classification of patients according to the Karnofsky scale.

In their article, 'Should we treat glioblastoma multiforme?', Taveras et al. [49] stress the uncertainty of a neurological statistic with too many variables beginning with the subjective classification of the patients with individual values. An instructive total picture must be formed for the objectivation of indication for operation. An approach towards this is introduced by this study, i.e. to reduce the surgical radicality of repeat operation in relation to lack of influence on the survival rate. The patient would therefore have a better survival rate and the actual perioperative mortality could be reduced [44]. Another approach could be the further improvement of adjuvant therapy, in particular, immunotherapy [1, 4, 5, 24, 25, 31, 35, 36, 51, 57, 59]. A decision as to which form of therapy should be carried out has to be orientated to an interdisciplinary 'quality-of-life concept' which takes into account the individual and situation-specific circumstances.

References

1   Apuzzo MLJ, Mitchell MS: Immunological aspects of intrinsic glial tumors. J Neurosurg 1981;55: 1–18.
2   Bashir R, Hochberg FH, Linggood R, Hottleman K: Preirradiation internal carotid artery BCNU in treatment of glioblastoma multiforme. J Neurosurg 1988;68:917–919.
3   Berger MS, Tucker BA, Spence A, Winn HR: Reoperation for glioma. Clin Neurosurg 1992;39: 172–186.
4   Bosnes V, Hirschberg H: Comparison of in vitro glioma cell cytotoxicity of LAK cells from glioma patients and healthy subjects. J Neurosurg 1988;69:234–238.
5   Brooks WH, Caldwell HD, Mortara RH: Immune responses in patients with gliomas. Surg Neurol 1974;2:419–423.
6   Bucy PC: Glioblastomas. Surg Neurol 1985;24:589–590.
7   Burger PC, Dubois PJ, Schold SC: Computerized tomographic and pathologic studies of the untreated, quiescent, and recurrent glioblastoma multiforme. J Neurosurg 1983;58:159–169.
8   Burger PC, Green SB: Patient age, histologic features, and length of survival in patients with glioblastoma multiforme. Cancer 1987;59:1617–1625.
9   Burger PC, Vogel FS, Green SB, et al: Glioblastoma multiforme and anaplastic astrocytoma. Cancer 1985;56:1106–1111.
10   Chandler KL, Prados MD, Malec M, Wilson CB: Long-term survival in patients with glioblastoma multiforme. Neurosurgery 1993;32:716–720.
11   Chang CH, Horton J, Schoenfeod D: Comparison of postoperative radiotherapy and combined postoperative radiotherapy and chemotherapy in the multidisciplinary management of malignant gliomas. Cancer 1983;52:997–1007.
12   DeVita VT Jr: The relationship between tumor mass and resistance to chemotherapy. Cancer 1983; 51:1209–1220.

13   Diemath HE: The course or glioblastoma multiforme. Neurochirurgia 1960;3:45–59.
14   Forsting M, Albert FK, Kunze S, et al: Extirpation of glioblastomas: MR and CT follow-up of residual tumor and regrowth patterns. Am J Neuroradiol 1993;14:77–87.
15   Fusek I, Vorreith M: Indications for repeat surgery of brain gliomas. Zentralbl Neurochir 1976;37: 45–50.
16   Harsh GR IV, Levin VA, Gutin PH, et al: Reoperation for recurrent glioblastoma and anaplastic astrocytoma. Neurosurgery 1987;21:615–621.
17   Heppner F: The glioblastoma multiforme: A lifelong challenge to the neurosurgeon. Neurochirurgia 1986;29:9–14.
18   Hoshino T: A commentary on the biology and growth kinetics of low-grade and high-grade gliomas. J Neurosurg 1984;61:895–900.
19   Hoshino T, Barker M, Wilson CB: Cell kinetics of human gliomas. J Neurosurg 1972;37:15–26.
20   Hoshino T, Wilson CB, Rosenblum ML, Barker M: Chemotherapeutic implications of growth fraction and cell cycle time in glioblastomas. J Neurosurg 1975;43:127–135.
21   Jellinger K: Glioblastoma multiforme: Morphology and biology. Acta Neurochir 1978;42:5–32.
22   Jellinger K, Volc D, Grisold W, et al: Multimodality treatment of malignant gliomas – Comparison of several adjuvant approaches. Zentralbl Neurochir 1981;42:99–122.
23   Jelsma R, Bucy PC: Glioblastoma multiforme: Its treatment and some factors effecting survival. Arch Neurol 1969;20:161–171.
24   Kornblith PK, Walker M: Chemotherapy for malignant gliomas. J Neurosurg 1988;68:1–17.
25   Kornblith PK, Welch WC, Bradley MK: The future of therapy for glioblastoma. Surg Neurol 1993; 39:538–543.
26   Kothe W, Richter HH: Prognosis and therapy of glioblastoma multiforme. Psychiatr Neurol Med Psychol 1963;15:276–282.
27   Krause G, Zülch KJ: Prevalence of brain gliomas in different regions of the brain. Zentralbl Neurochir 1951;11:221–230.
28   Krayenbühl H: Anamnesis and clinical course of glioblastoma multiforme. Acta Neurochir 1959; 6:31–39.
29   Kreth FW, Berlis A, Scheremet R, Ostertag CB: Heterogeneous treatment effects after surgery and/ or radiotherapy of glioblastoma multiforme. Zentralbl Neurochir 1996;suppl 43.
30   Kreth FW, Warnke PC, Scheremet R, Ostertag CB: Surgical resection and radiation therapy versus biopsy and radiation therapy in the treatment of glioblastoma multiforme. J Neurosurg 1993;78: 762–766.
31   Kuppner MC, Hamou MF, de Tribolet N: Activation and adhesion molecule expression on lymphoid infiltrates in human glioblastomas. J Neuroimmunol 1990;29:229–238.
32   Landy HJ, Feun L, Schwade JG, et al: Retreatment of intracranial gliomas. South Med J 1994;87:2.
33   Leibel SA, Sheline GE: Radiation therapy for neoplasms of the brain. J Neurosurg 1987;66:1–22.
34   Levin VA, Crafts DC, Norman DM, et al: Criteria for evaluating patients undergoing chemotherapy for malignant brain tumors. J Neurosurg 1977;47:329–335.
35   Mahaley MS: Immunotherapy of brain tumors – Is there a future? Clin Neurosurg 1977;25:382–387.
36   Mahaley MS, Brooks WH, Roszman TL, et al: Immunobiology of primary intracranial tumors. J Neurosurg 1977;46:467–472.
37   McLendon RE, Robinson JS, Chambers DB, et al: The glioblastoma multiforme in Georgia, 1977–1981. Cancer 1985;56:894–897.
38   Müller H, Brock M, Ernst H: Long-term survival and recurrence-free interval in combined surgical, radio- and chemotherapy of malignant brain gliomas. Clin Neurol Neurosurg 1985;87:167–171.
39   Neumann J: Actual prognosis of glioblastoma multiforme. Nervenarzt 1983;54:191–193.
40   Ramsey RG, Brand WN: Radiotherapy of glioblastoma multiforme. J Neurosurg 1973;39:197–202.
41   Ransohoff J, Lieberman A: Surgical therapy of primary malignant brain tumors. Clin Neurosurg 1978;25:403–411.
42   Ray BS: Surgery of recurrent intracranial tumors. Clin Neurosurg 1964;10:1–30.
43   Reeves GI, Marks JE: Prognostic significance of lesion size for glioblastoma multiforme. Radiology 1979;132:469–471.
44   Salcman M: Specialty rounds: Glioblastoma multiforme. Am J Med Sci 1980;279:84–94.

45 Salcman M: Survival in glioblastoma: Historical perspective. Neurosurgery 1980;7:435–439.
46 Salcman M, Kaplan RS, Ducker TB, et al: Effect of age and reoperation on survival in the combined modality treatment of malignant astrocytoma. Neurosurgery 1982;10:454–462.
47 Selby R: The surgical treatment of cerebral glioblastoma multiforme: A historical review. J Neurooncol 1994;18:175–182.
48 Strömblad LG, Anderson H, Malmström P, Saford LG: Reoperation for malignant astrocytomas: Personal experience and a review of the literature. Br J Neurosurg 1993;7:623–633.
49 Taveras JM, Thompson HG Jr, Pool JL: Should we treat glioblastoma multiforme? AJR 1962;87:473–479.
50 Tönnis W, Walter W: Glioblastoma multiforme. Acta Neurochir 1959;6:40–61.
51 Trouillas P, Lapras C: Immunothérapie active des tumeurs cérébrales. Neurochirurgie 1970;16:143–170.
52 Ushio Y, Hayakawa T, Hasegawa H, Yamada K, Arita N: Chemotherapy of malignant gliomas. Neurosurg Rev 1984;7:3–12.
53 Wallner KE, Galicich JH, Malkin MG, et al: Inability of computed tomography appearance of recurrent malignant astrocytoma to predict survival following reoperation. J Clin Oncol 1989;7:1492–1496.
54 Weir B: The relative significance of factors affecting postoperative survival in astrocytomas, grades 3 and 4. J Neurosurg 1973;38:448–452.
55 Wilson CB: Glioblastoma: The past, the present, and the future. Clin Neurosurg 1992;38:32–48.
56 Wilson CB, Hoshino T: Current trends in the chemotherapy of brain tumors with special reference to glioblastomas. J Neurosurg 1969;31:589–603.
57 Yasuda K, Alderson T, Phillips J, Sikora K: Detection of lymphocytes in malignant gliomas by monoclonal antibodies. J Neurol Neurosurg Psychiatr 1983;46:734–737.
58 Young B, Oldfield EH, Markesbery WR, et al: Reoperation for glioblastoma. J Neurosurg 1981;15:917–921.
59 Young HF, Sakalas R, Kaplan AM: Inhibition of cell-mediated immunity in patients with brain tumor. Surg Neurol 1976;5:19–23.
60 Zülch KJ: Glioblastoma multiforme: Morphology and biology. Acta Neurochir 1959;6:2–29.

Dr. M. Mühling, Neurochirurgische Klinik, Gesundheitszentrum St. Martin GmbH,
Johannes-Müller-Strasse 7, D–56068 Koblenz und
Medizinische Abteilung Experimentelle Neurochirurgie, Medizinische Hochschule Hannover,
Konstanty-Gutschow-Str. 8, D–30625 Hannover (Germany)

Wiegel T, Hinkelbein W, Brock M, Hoell T (eds): Controversies in Neuro-Oncology.
Front Radiat Ther Oncol. Basel, Karger, 1999, vol 33, pp 202–213

....

Comparison of Coplanar and Non-Coplanar Irradiation Techniques for Malignant Glioma: An Analysis of Dose-Volume Histograms

U. Mock, K. Dieckmann, U. Wolff, R. Pötter

Department of Radiotherapy and Radiobiology, University Hospital, Vienna, Austria

Introduction

Life expectancy of patients with malignant glioma (anaplastic astrocytoma, glioblastoma multiforme) is limited. Without medical intervention a median survival of about 8 weeks was assessed [1, 7]. Surgery is regarded as the most important treatment option [2, 16] and associated with an increase in median survival [13], although resection is not curative because of the infiltrative nature of these tumors [15, 25]. A constellation of poor prognostic indicators such as preoperative performance status, age, percentage of tumor resection, residual tumor volume has a significant impact on time of progression [2, 17, 34].

Postoperative radiotherapy is an established treatment modality, which is mostly administered in form of an external beam irradiation and considerably prolongs recurrence-free survival of these patients [7]. The role of additional chemotherapy, hyperthermia, brachytherapy, stereotactic irradiation, neutron therapy, hyperfractionated irradiation schemes, variable immunotherapies, etc. are still under investigation, even if published results are partly promising [3, 18, 21, 25, 27, 28, 30, 32, 33]. Radiotherapy treatment planning is performed on the basis of CT and/or MRI images [10], which facilitate delineation of tumor extent. Tolerance of surrounding normal brain tissue to radiation doses is influenced by various factors like total radiation dose, fraction size and number, duration of treatment and volume of irradiated brain, etc. [20, 23, 35].

Three-dimensional (3D) conformal radiotherapy offers a way to conform the high-dose volume region closely to the individual tumor configuration, while sparing the surrounding normal tissue, which might provide a decrease in morbidity and an improved therapeutic outcome [24, 29, 31]. Dose-volume histograms (DVH) correlate the volume irradiated with the dose received and have been used to calculate probabilities of tumor control and normal tissue complications [5, 19]. Contrasting two-dimensional (2D) and 3D treatment planning procedures or standardized and individual shielding block configurations for irradiation of malignant glioma, improvements in dose distribution were correlated with more individualized techniques [7]. Thereby, treatment was performed using static coplanar beam arrangements. In order to optimize external beam radiotherapy, non-coplanar beam arrangements have been proposed. The purpose of this study was to investigate if this more complicated non-coplanar technique is indeed superior to coplanar beam arrangements. We compared both techniques for each individual target volume and different structures at risk intending to define the differences in dose distribution as volume and different structures at risk intending to define the differences in dose distribution as a basic for future treatment strategies.

Methods and Materials

Patient's Characteristics
The study was conducted on the basis of 30 patients undergoing external beam irradiation for malignant, supratentorial located brain glioma. There were 20 males and 10 females with a mean age of 57 years (range 26–73) and a median Karnofsky performance status scored of 80% (range 60–100%). The pretreatment evaluation consisted of physical examination with special attention to neurological deficits and CT or MRI scans in all cases. On the basis of these preoperative CT or MRT images, the primary gross tumor volumes (GTV) were evaluated. The initial tumor diagnosis was histologically confirmed by stereotactic biopsy in 10 patients, whereas macroscopic subtotal or total surgical resection was part of the initial treatment in 15 and 5 cases, respectively. All malignancies were graded according to the WHO Classification [36] and anaplastic astrocytoma grade III was revealed in 7 cases and glioblastoma multiforme grade IV in 23 patients. The majority of patients took dexamethasone in individual doses and received additionally chemotherapy, including lomustine (CCNU) in varying schedules and doses.

Treatment Planning
All patients underwent a planning CT as part of the routine treatment planning. Individual plastic masks were used as an immobilization device in order to ensure reproducible beam setting. The planning CT images were transferred to a Helax 3D planning system. Without specific CT-MR image fusion, preoperative MR images were used complementary to CT in order to improve the treatment planning procedure. According to the current policy of our department, treatment planning was performed by defining the CTV equivalent to the initial gross tumor volume including the edema region. Definition of the PTV was accomplished by circumferentially adding a safety margin of 20 mm to account for the infiltrating nature of disease and treatment uncertainties.

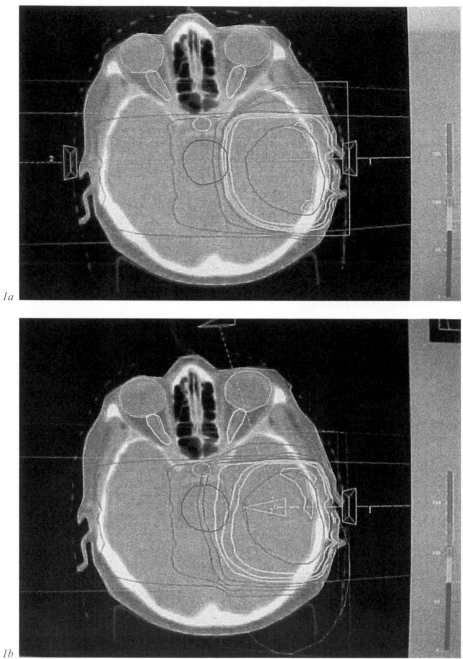

1a

1b

Additionally, the anatomical structures of different organs at risk (whole brain, bulbus occuli, optical nerves, brainstem) were delineated in the corresponding CT slices. Treatment planning was performed by a physicist and a physician, both of them being familiar with the treatment planning procedure of the two irradiation techniques. For each patient two different, conformal treatment plans were designed:

(1) Treatment plan I (TP I): TP I was characterized by a single isocenter and multiple; static, coplanar beam technique. Each beam was individually designed to conform to the specific target and critical structures (fig. 1a).

(2) Treatment plan II (TP II): TP II was generated consisting of a combination of individually shaped coplanar and non-coplanar static beams with one isocenter (fig. 1b). The number of beams used for the different treatment plans depended on the individual tumor configuration. As illustrated in figure 1a and b, the different treatment plans consisted of 2–3 static beams.

Dose Prescription

In all cases, dose was prescribed to the ICRU reference point and the 95% isodose encompassed the PTV including the primary tumor extent, the edema area and a safety margin of 20 mm. Treatment was applied using a high linear accelerator. For TP I and TP II, beam weights and wedge angles were adjusted aiming to achieve a dose homogeneity within the PTV. Fraction size was 2.0 Gy delivered to the 95% isodose line using a daily fractionated schedule with a break at the weekend. The prescription for total target dose was 66 Gy. The majority of patients were irradiated using beam arrangements according to TP II. Radiation doses of the PTV and the defined anatomical structures were determined from the 3D dose distributions.

Data Analysis

Investigations were performed with regard to various predominant tumor localizations in the frontal, parietal, temporal and occipital lobe. Retrospective evaluation was performed by analyzing the DVHs of the defined anatomical structures. Corresponding values resulting from the alternative TP I and TP II were compared by contrasting DVHs of the PTV and the relevant anatomical structures at risk. Analysis of volumes receiving a given dose was thereby accomplished in 10% intervals.

To estimate the differences between the two irradiation techniques, discrepancies between corresponding volumes of TP I and TP II receiving an applied dose were calculated. Differences below 10% were thereby classified as an unchanged result ($\pm$), differences between 10 and 30% were classified as a small change ($+/-$) and discrepancies exceeding 30% were regarded as a definite alteration in dose distribution ($++/--$). '+' was used if an improved dose distribution resulted from TP II when compared with TP I, whereas the worsened dose distribution of TP II was signed with '−'.

Fig. 1. a Dose distribution of TP I: Planning section for a glioblastoma located in the parietal lobe. The different organs at risk and the PTV were outlined. Two beams were used. Compared to the illustrated PTV a larger treated volume is notable, which is caused by an increasing volume of the PTV in the sections above the illustrated region. *b* Dose distribution of TP II: Planning section for a glioblastoma located in the parietal lobe. The different organs at risk and the PTV were outlind. Three beams were used.

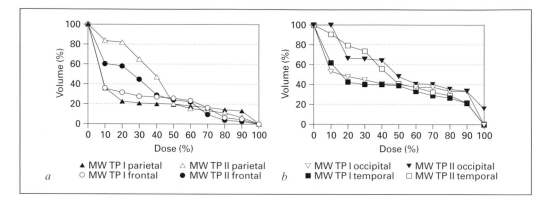

Fig. 2. DVHs concerning the brainstem: *a* Differences between coplanar and non-coplanar beam arrangements concerning irradiation for tumors in the frontal and parietal lobe. *b* Corresponding data for the occipital and temporal lobe are seen. MW = Mean value; TP I = coplanar treatment plan; TP II = non-coplanar treatment plan.

Results

Tumor Localization and Volumes of Interest (*GTV and PTV and Organs at Risk*)

The most common, prevalent tumor localization was the temporal lobe (n = 14) and the frontal lobe (n = 7), followed by the parietal (n = 6) and the occipital region (n = 3). Almost similar results were found as regards tumor manifestation in the right (n = 16) and left (n = 14) hemisphere. The primary GTV ranged from 8 to 216 cm³ (mean extent 96 cm³). The estimated mean size of PTV, including the GTV, surrounding edema and a safety margin of approximately 2 cm, was quoted to be 402 cm³ (range 189–805).

Side Effects

During radiotherapy all patients developed acute grade I or II skin reactions and grade II–III alopecia. No patient failed to complete external beam radiotherapy because of significant side effects or tumor progression.

Dose Distribution

Brainstem. Averaged results of the different groups are illustrated in figures 1–3. With regard to the brainstem, non-coplanar beam arrangements were correlated with increasing doses to the organ at risk in the 0–50% interval. Concerning the dose level exceeding 50%, almost similar results were found for both techniques. Analysis according to the various tumor localizations revealed no difference (fig. 2a, b).

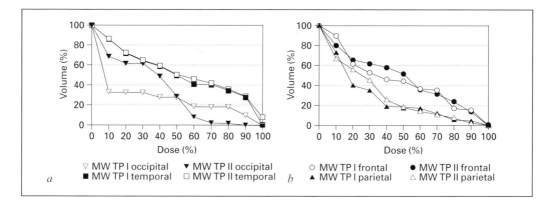

Fig. 3. DVHs concerning the ipsilateral optical nerve. *a* Differences between coplanar and non-coplanar beam arrangements concerning irradiation of the occipital and temporal lobe. *b* Corresponding data for the frontal and parietal lobe are illustrated. MW = Mean value; TP I = coplanar treatment plan; TP II = non-coplanar treatment plan.

Ipsilateral Optical Nerve. With regard to the optical nerve and tumor manifestation in the frontal, parietal and temporal lobe, no significant differences in dose distribution were notable between both techniques (fig. 3a, b). Compared to non-coplanar treatment techniques, coplanar beam irradiation of tumors in the occipital lobe resulted in a decreasing dose level in the low and intermediate dose intervals and an increase in dose in the high-dose region. Dose distribution to the ipsilateral optical nerve is thereby explained by large PTV volumes, which could not be restricted to the occipital lobe alone.

Whole Brain. Comparing both beam arrangements, the non-coplanar technique almost regularly resulted in a decrease in brain volume receiving intermediate or high doses (%) and an increase in volume of normal tissue receiving low doses (%) (fig. 4a, b). Analyzing the dose delivery to different anatomical structures for each individual patient, almost similar results were found for both techniques. In only 2/30 patients the more complicated non-coplanar treatment technique resulted in an improved dose distribution for all the analyzed structures. In all the other cases decreasing dose in one defined structure was correlated with increasing dose levels in another one (table 1).

Discussion

Malignant gliomas (WHO III–IV) are generally treated with radiotherapy after surgical tumor resection [16], but persistence or regrowth of tumor after treatment remains the predominant pattern of failure with conventional radio-

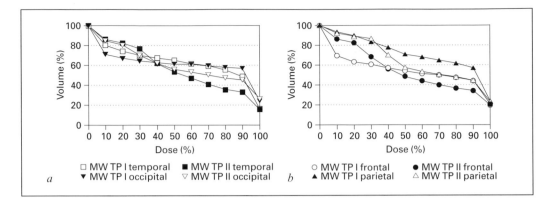

Fig. 4. DVHs concerning the whole brain. *a* Differences between coplanar and non-coplanar beam arrangements concerning all patients receiving irradiation to the frontal and parietal lobe. *b* Corresponding data for the occipital and temporal lobe are seen. MW = Mean value; TP I = coplanar treatment plan; TP II = non-coplanar treatment plan.

therapy [18]. Aiming at an effective local therapy, a high dose has to be applied, while relatively sparing adjacent normal tissue. The concept of CT-based, individualized 3D treatment planning consists of defining tumor volumes equivalent to the CT-enhancing regions, planning target volumes, which include additional safety margins and creating individual treatment plans according to patient anatomy and tumor configuration. Nevertheless, the proper volume for the treatment of supratentorial malignant glioma is still controversial [12, 30]. Burger et al. [4] examined whole-brain sections of autopsied untreated glioblastoma patients and found large extension of tumor cell beyond the CT-enhancing area. Hochberg and Pruitt [11] compared autopsy extension of tumors with CT scans performed within 2 months before death and found gross and microscopic disease to lie within 2 cm of a volume defined by the contrast CT in 80% of cases. Based on these findings, a safety margin of at least 2 cm appears to be necessary for adequate target coverage and was therefore used in the current study.

Choice of treatment modality and technique is dependent on the likelihood of clinically significant treatment-related morbidity. The clinical relevance of normal tissue irradiation is variable. Comparison of alternate plans is generally performed using DVH, which summarize the relationship of volume and dose in a quantitative way.

On the basis of DVH, the current study compared two different commonly used beam arrangements in terms of dose distribution to the PTV and defined anatomical structures. Concerning brain glioma, Grosu et al. [7] analyzed advantages of 3D conformal radiotherapy including coplanar and non-copla-

Table 1. Individual patient data concerning decreasing (+ +), equivalent (±), slightly increasing (−) or significant >30% (− −) increasing dose levels by using the non-coplanar irradiation technique

	PTV size cm³	Brainstem	Optical nerve ipsil.	Optical nerve contral.	Bulbus ipsil.	Bulbus contral.	Brain
Frontal lobe							
	317	±	+ +	+ +	±	±	±
	369	− −	+	+	+	+ +	− −
	298	+	+ +	+ +	±	±	+
	467	− −	±	±	+ +	+ +	+
	420	− −	− −	− −	− −	±	− −
	433	+	− −	+ +	−	+	+
	388	±	+	±	+	±	− −
Temporal lobe							
	466	− −	− −	− −	+ +	±	+
	404	− −	+	+ +	±	±	+ +
	363	− −	+	+ +	+ +	+ +	+ +
	224	− −	+	+ +	+	+	+
	475	±	±	− −	±	±	+
	439	− −	− −	+ +	±	+ +	+
	190	− −	+ +	+ +	±	±	+
	415	− −	−	+ +	+ +	+ +	+
	189	− −	−	+ +	±	±	±
	204	±	+	+ +	±	±	±
	461	±	+ +	+ +	+ +	+ +	+
	290	−	−	+	+ +	±	+
	435	− −	+ +	+ +	±	±	+
	446	− −	− −	+	±	±	+
Parietal lobe							
	484	+ +	+ +	+	+ +	±	+
	467	− −	− −	−	±	±	±
	805	− −	+ +	+	+ +	+	+
	214	±	±	+ +	±	±	±
	282	− −	− −	−	+ +	±	−
	622	− −	− −	+ +	±	±	+ +
Occipital lobe							
	201	− −	±	±	±	±	− −
	521	− −	− −	−	±	±	+
	744	±	+ +	+	+	− −	±

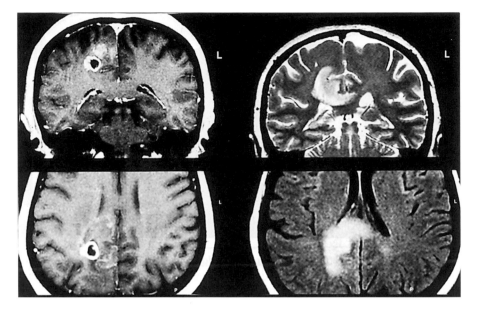

Fig. 3. Axial and coronal MRI of a glioblastoma in T1 with gadolinium enhancement which shows the well-described tumor surrounded by a T2 enhancement which extends already into the corpus callosum, represents the edema and most likely the area of real tumor involvement.

images (fig. 3). It has to be postulated that the area of T2 signal changes in reality already reflects the extent of brain involvement with the tumor. It would thus be desirable to deliver local therapy to this volume and that has been the reasoning for a local drug delivery approach which was named enhanced convection. Cells from gliomas are capable of producing a variety of factors which are involved in the regulation of neovascularization and vascular permeability. Among these factors, VEGF is of major importance in this biology and causes blood vessels to become leaky which is at the basis of the edema associated with glioma. The edema has its own dynamics and with bulk flow, a considerable volume of liquid which is originating in the tumor bed is actually flowing centrifugally into the surrounding tissue where the fluid is eventually taken up and cleared [10]. This bulk flow is an intriguing way to transport large molecules into the T2-weighted zone and it has been found that the tissue around a tumor has actually a capacity to take up more fluid than produced by the tumor, allowing for additional microinfusion into the tumor, thus enhancing the bulk flow. Initial studies were designed to evaluate the clinical feasibility and at the same time the efficacy of therapeutics delivered in this manner [11]. The investigators came to the conclusion that large molecules such as immunotoxins or toxin conjugates which were linked to transferrin could safely be delivered via a stereotactically implanted catheter which is connected to a constant infusion micropump [12]. The transferrin receptor seemed to be a useful target as it is expressed in abundance on proliferating/neoplastic cells, thus providing selectivity and safety within the environment of the brain. The volumes which can be delivered vary individually but are considerable because with tolerated infusion rates of up to 10 µl/min, volumes of 14 ml/day can be achieved which would allow for delivery of a large amount of therapeutic agents to the tumor and its surroundings. This methodology is a very promising addition to the armamentarium of drug administration to brain tumors, in particular as the substances are applied on the other side of the blood-brain barrier and thus circumvent the issue of solubility, permeability and perfusion heterogeneity. Also, by direct application into the intercellular space, some substances may have much longer half-lifes than with intravenous or intra-arterial application.

For the next years it has to be expected that a large number of very different reagents will be explored for their usefulness in this new treatment paradigm. Antibodies, conjugates, liposomes and maybe even viruses seem candidates for this route of application, provided they can be provided in solutions in which they are stable for several days within the reservoir of the infusion pump. The problems with this technique are based on the selection of the right timing and patient subpopulations. In contrast to the other local therapies, like gene therapy or the implantation of biodegradable wafers, the principle on which this whole concept is based, changes when the tumor is removed which usually results in a reversal of bulk flow and resolution of the edema within a short time period. At that point in time, there is just diffusion as with the Gliadel® unless the therapeutic material is physically placed where it is supposed to go as in the trial with intraoperative HSV-Tk gene therapy (see below). Thus in this therapeutic approach, ideal targets would be small tumors which are surgically not accessible but are easily reached by stereotactic infusion. This methodology would also have advantages over focussed irradiation, brachytherapy and photon gun because it might be able to carry therapeutics into the invasion zone (see below) which is out of reach for the other therapies.

Selectivity is an issue with the enhanced convection as with any other therapy. Applying the reagents on the other side of the blood-brain barrier, selectivity would have to come via the targeting or via specific intracellular activation. The molecules which on the cell surface of tumor cells have potential to be used as specific receptors are such which are relevant in the context of a proliferating cell or which are specific to tumors. Of the first description, there are molecules like the afore-mentioned transferrin receptor or the IL-4

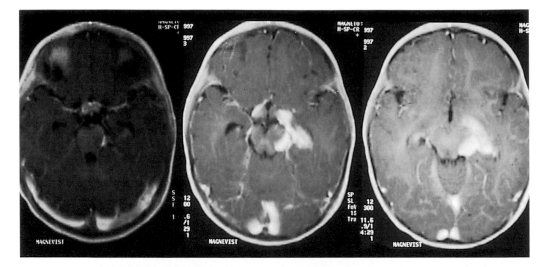

Fig. 5. Axial MRI of a child with neurofibromatosis and an optic nerve glioma which has not yet been histologically confirmed. The extension of the tumor along the optic radiation is clearly seen and illustrates the intrinsic biological capacity of glial cells to migrate along white matter tracts.

trial in primary glioblastoma has just been completed in April 1998, the results from this trial will not be expected before the year 2000.

This kind of gene therapy with the injection of VPCs is strictly local and does reach the infiltrating single cells only to a limited extent. Other local concepts call for application of replication competent viruses or delivery via liposomes. In addition, local as well as systemic gene therapies have been developed which aim to compensate the lack of specificity in their pan-transduction by restricted activity of the gene only in those cells which have a specific defect such as a mutation of the p53 gene [19].

As with the compounds which can possibly be put in the biodegradable polymers or the substances possibly infused with the enhanced convection technology, there is no limitation to the genetic strategies to be delivered with suitable vector systems. VDEPT is only one approach, anti-sense strategies against oncogenes is another, just as replacement of defective tumor suppressor genes or combinations with genetic manipulations of the immune response.

The Invasive Phenotype of the Glioma and Its Implications for Therapy

Everyday clinical experience would support the quest for better local control of malignant gliomas. The highly invasive nature of this disease pre-

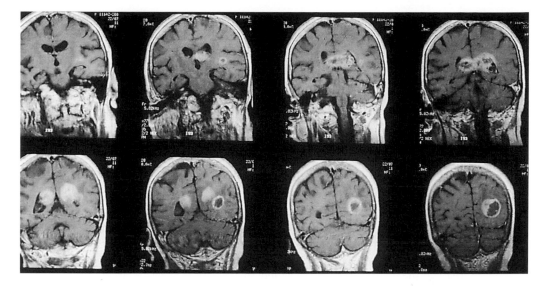

Fig. 6. Coronal gadolinium-enhanced MRI of a glioblastoma which most likely has originated occipital of the corpus callosum and which has made contact with the large commissural tracts along which it has massively infiltrated the splenium and crossed the midline.

cludes rapid success of such strategy in the long term and even in the short term hampers the development of effective local controls because there are no real good models to test the efficacy of a local delivery concept to an infiltrative zone. In particular the invasive behavior is very difficult to model as in most animal models, xenotransplants lack the capacity to infiltrate because the enzymes needed for invading into a rodent brain show a high species specificity.

Despite the present momentum of local therapy development, invasion of human malignant glioma cells will be the limitation and only better understanding of its biological foundations may offer additional options to enhance the efficacy of local strategies. Migration of glioma cells away from the main tumor mass does not seem to be a random process but rather follows certain pathways of pre-existing anatomical and biochemical pathways in the central nervous system. Beyond the edge of a lesion that may appear to be well delineated, invasive glioma cells can be found to follow small blood vessels where perivascular cuff formation may be observed. Also, tumor cells show a high affinity to myelinated fiber tracts, in which single glioma cells show intrafascicular, perifascicular, and interfibillary migration. The consequence of this high affinity to myelinated fiber tracts results in spread of a tumor for example along the optic tract (fig. 5) or through the corpus callosum (fig. 6).

Clinically it is evident that whenever a tumor extends to the ependymal and subependymal layer along the ventricles, very distant spread of the tumor will occur rapidly and satellite lesions may form following the contour of the ventricular system, sometimes even into the contralateral ventricle [20]. Single invasive cells may be found several centimeters away from the macroscopically visible margin of the tumor in the T2-enhancing area which comprises the aforementioned target volume of the enhanced convection. Even biopsies obtained from normal T1 and T2 areas contained tumor cells in a significant number of samples implicating that tumor spread is not only confined to the area of edema [21]. In a series of 100 consecutive untreated glioblastomas there was evidence for histological tumor spread to the contralateral hemisphere in 47% of the cases [22].

Invasive tumor cells are clonogenic. It has been demonstrated that glioma cells from up to 4 cm beyond the visible tumor can be isolated and grown in tissue culture [23]. It is therefore likely that this pool of invasive cells gives rise to the recurrent tumor, which in 96% of the cases arises immediately adjacent to the resection margin or within 3 cm from the resection cavity [24]. The pattern of local treatment failure is most likely due to a high density of remaining tumor cells within the proximity of the removed highly cellular part of the lesion, but may also be due to changes of the extracellular matrix environment after formation of scar tissue following the resection. Along those lines, control of the disease by local treatment strategies could possibly reduce the rate of local failure and may increase the time to local progression which may even translate into prolonged survival time. Considering the distant spread of the disease, however, with frequent extension into the contralateral hemisphere, gliomas can hardly be called a local disease. It is not surprising that with local therapies such as application of Gliadel® or with the current gene therapy protocols, investigators start observing cases of more distant satellite lesions upon recurrence. This changing pattern of recurrence will be a direct consequence of local therapies as the true potential of single glioma cells for migration and invasion remains unaltered.

There is increasing experimental evidence that invasive glioma cells may represent a fraction of tumor cells with a distinct phenotype. Burger and Kleihues [25] suggested that cells identified as single invasive cells most distant from the mass lesion most often are fairly homogenous small dedifferentiated cells, in contrast to the cells within the mass which show a very heterogenous morphology. Such tumor cells can be isolated in vitro and show a highly migratory phenotype but also show decreased proliferation. Analyzing the effects of permissive extracellular matrix proteins as well as soluble motility factors, it can be shown experimentally that glioma cells, when stimulated to migrate, show a marked decrease of their proliferation rate [26]. If an invasive phenotype thus occurs at the expense of a lowered proliferation rate, these invading cells could be more resistant to antiproliferative agents. Invasive glioma cells therefore represent a specific challenge to treatment not only because of their tendency to disseminate but also because of their specific biology.

Identification of genes associated with the invasive phenotype may offer modes to specifically interfere with this cellular behavior. Recently we have identified such a gene overexpressed in highly migratory glioma clones [27].

As attractive as local concepts for the therapy of human gliomas appear to be at the present time, they are doomed to failure in the long term without anti-invasive concepts. In the present situation with rather poor systemic options, local control appears to be a first step – worthwhile taking.

Acknowledgments

The Center for Neuro-Oncology in the Department of Neurosurgery has enjoyed the continuous support of Prof. Hans-Dietrich Herrmann and is indebted to the clinical colleagues within the department and in other departments for their cooperation. Over the years the work has been supported by the Deutsche Forschungsgemeinschaft and the Deutsche Krebshilfe and private foundations.

References

1 Salcman M: The value of cytoreductive surgery. Clin Neurosurg 1994;41:464–488.
2 Dirks P, Bernstein M, Muller PJ, Tucker WS: The value of reoperation for recurrent glioblastoma. Can J Surg 1993;36:271–275.
3 Cairncross JG, Macdonald DR, Ramsay DA: Aggressive oligodendroglioma: A chemosensitive tumor. Neurosurgery 1992;31:78–82.
4 Cristante L, Siepmann G, Westphal M, Hagel C, Hermann HD: Superselective application of cisplatinum in recurrent human glioblastoma. Reg Cancer Treat 1992;4:188–194.
5 Shapiro WR, Green SB, Burger PC, Selker RG, Van Gilder JC, Robertson JT, Mealey J Jr, Ransohff J, Mahaley MS: A randomized comparison of intra-arterial versus intravenous BCNU, with or without intravenous 5-fluorouracil, for newly diagnosed patients with malignant glioma. J Neurosurg 1992;76:772–781.
6 Fross RD, Warnke PC, Groothuis DR: Blood flow and blood to tissue transport in 9L gliosarcomas: The role of the brain tumor model in drug delivery research. J Neurooncol 1991;11:185–197.
7 Brem H, Tamargo RJ, Olivi A, Pinn M, Weingart JD, Wharam M, Epstein JI: Biodegradable polymers for controlled delivery of chemotherapy with and without radiation therapy in the monkey brain. J Neurosurg 1994;80:283–290.
8 Brem H, Piantadosi S, Burger PC, Walker M, Selker R, Vick NA, Black K, Sisti M, Brem S, Mohr G, Muller P, Morawetz R, Clifford Schold S, for the Polymer-Brain Tumor Treatment Group: Placebo-controlled trial of safety and efficacy of intraoperative controlled delivery by biodegradable polymers of chemotherapy for recurrent gliomas. Lancet 1995;345:1008–1012.
9 Valtonen S, Timonen U, Toivanen P, Kalimo H, Kivipelto L, Heiskanen O, Unsgaard G, Kuurne T: Interstitial chemotherapy with carmustine-loaded polymers for high-grade gliomas: A randomized double-blind study. Neurosurgery 1997;41:44–49.

10 Reulen HJ, Graber S, Huber P, Ito U: Factors affecting the extension of peritumoural brain oedema. A CT study. Acta Neurochir 1988;95:19–24.

11 Liebermann DM, Laske DW, Morrison PF, Bankiewicz KS, Oldfield EH: Convection-enhanced distribution of large molecules in gray matter during interstitial drug infusion. J Neurosurg 1995; 82:1021–1029.

12 Laske DW, Youle RJ, Oldfield EH: Tumor regression with regional distribution of the targeted toxin TF-CRM 107 in patients with malignant brain tumors. Nat Med 1997;3:1362–1368.

13 Sugawa N, Ekstrand AJ, James CD, Collins VP: Identical splicing of an aberrant epidermal growth factor receptor transcripts from amplified rearranged genes in human glioblastomas. Proc Natl Acad Sci USA 1990;87:8602–8606.

14 Reist CJ, Archer GE, Kurpad SN, Wikstrand CJ, Vaidyanathan G, Willingham MC, Moscatello DK, Wong AJ, Bigner DD, Zalutsky MR: Tumor-specific anti-epidermal growth factor receptor variant III monoclonal antibodies: Use of a tyramine-cellobiose radioiodination method enhances cellular retention and uptake in tumor xenografts. Cancer Res 1995;55:4375–4382.

15 Kramm CM, Sena-Esteves M, Barnett FH, Rainov NG, Schuback DE, Yu JS, Pechan PA, Paulus W, Chiocca EA, Breakefield XO: Gene therapy for brain tumors. Brain Pathol 1995;5:345–381.

16 Culver KW, Ram Z, Wallbridge S, Ishii H, Oldfield EH, Blaese RM: In vivo gene transfer with retroviral vector producer cells for treatment of experimental brain tumors. Science 1992;256: 1550–1552.

17 Mesnil M, Piccoli C, Tiraby G, Willecke K, Yamasaki H: Bystander killing of cancer cells by herpes simplex virus thymidine kinase gene is mediated by connexins. Proc Natl Acad Sci USA 1996;93: 1831–1835.

18 Ram Z, Culver KW, Oshiro EM, et al: Therapy of malignant brain tumors by intratumoral implantation of retroviral vector-producing cells. Nat Med 1997;3:1354–1361.

19 Köck H, Harris M, Anderson SC, Machemer T, Hancock W, Sutjipto S, Wills KN, Gregory R, Shepard HM, Westphal M, Maneval DC: Adenovirus-mediated p53 gene transfer suppresses growth of human glioblastoma cells in vitro and in vivo. Int J Cancer 1996;67:808–815.

20 Giese A, Westphal M: Glioma invasion in the central nervous system. Neurosurgery 1996;39: 235–252.

21 Kelly PJ, Daumas-Duport C, Kispert DB, Kall BA, Scheithauer BW, Illig JJ: Imaging-based stereotaxic serial biopsies in untreated glial neoplasms. J Neurosurg 1987;66:865–874.

22 Matsukado Y, MacCarty CS, Kernohan JW: The growth of glioblastoma multiforme in neurosurgical practice. J Neurosurg 1961;18:636–644.

23 Silbergeld DL, Madsen CL, Chicoine MR: Isolation and characterization of human malignant glioma cells from histologically normal brain. J Neurosurg 1997;86:525–531.

24 Burger PC, Heinz ER, Shibata T, Kleihues P: Topographic anatomy and CT correlations in the untreated glioblastoma multiforme. J Neurosurg 1988;68:698–704.

25 Burger PC, Kleihues P: Cytologic composition of the untreated glioblastoma with implications for evaluation of needle biopsies. Cancer 1989;63:2014–2023.

26 Giese A, Loo MA, Tran N, Haskett D, Coons SW, Berens ME: Dichotomy of astrocytoma migration and proliferation. Int J Cancer 1996;67:275–282.

27 McDonough W, Tran N, Giese A, Norman S, Berens ME: Altered gene expression in human astrocytoma cells selected for migration: I. Thromboxane synthase. J Neuropathol Exp Neurol 1998;57:449–455.

Dr. Manfred Westphal, Department of Neurological Surgery,
University Hospital Eppendorf, Martinistrasse 52, D–20246 Hamburg (Germany)
Tel +49 40 4717 3751, Fax +49 40 4717 4596, E-Mail westphal@plexus.uke.uni-hamburg.de

Wiegel T, Hinkelbein W, Brock M, Hoell T (eds): Controversies in Neuro-Oncology.
Front Radiat Ther Oncol. Basel, Karger, 1999, vol 33, pp 227–240

....

Intra-Arterial Virus and Nonvirus Vector-Mediated Gene Transfer to Experimental Rat Brain Tumors

Nikolai G. Rainov[a], *Keiro Ikeda*[b], *Nazir Qureshi*[b], *Shivani Grover*[c],
Faith H. Barnett[c,d], *Ulrich Herrlinger*[c], *Ariel Quinones*[a],
E. Antonio Chiocca[b], *Xandra O. Breakefield*[c]

[a] Department of Neurosurgery, Faculty of Medicine, Martin Luther University
Halle-Wittenberg, Halle, Germany; [b] Neuro-Oncology Laboratory,
Neurosurgical Service, Massachusetts General Hospital, Boston, Mass.;
[c] Molecular Neurogenetics Unit, Neuroscience Center, Massachusetts General
Hospital, and Neurology Department, Harvard Medical School, Boston, Mass., and
[d] Neurosurgical Service, Brigham and Women's Hospital, Harvard Medical School,
Boston, Mass., USA

Introduction

A major limitation of all current protocols for gene therapy of brain tumors is the inability to transduce a large enough pool of tumor cells to confer cytotoxicity to the whole tumor [Kramm et al., 1995]. In addition, vector delivery must be tumor-selective to reduce toxicity to normal brain. Finally, choice of vector affects both transduction efficiency and tumor selectivity, as well as the extent and stability of transgene expression, replication of vectors within tumor, immune response to vectors, and toxicity to normal tissues [Chiocca et al., 1994; Schofield and Caskey, 1995]. Three modes of vector delivery to experimental brain tumors have been studied: stereotactic intratumoral inoculation [Boviatsis et al., 1994a; Viola et al., 1995, Eck et al., 1996], intrathecal application [Kramm et al., 1996], and most recently, intra-arterial application [Doran et al., 1995; Neuwelt et al., 1991; Nilaver et al., 1995; Rainov et al., 1995]. Stereotactic intratumoral application has the advantage of a high spatial accuracy with high local vector titers, but suffers from distribution limited to a few millimeters surrounding the injection site, and also depends on the biological properties of the used vectors [Boviatsis et al., 1994b]. Intrathecal delivery of vectors seems to be primarily suited to treating intrathecal and intraventricular neoplasms or to attacking the intrathecal parts of intracerebral tumors, but suffers from significant side effects [Viola et al., 1995; Kramm et al.,1996]. Intra-arterial vector application with or without disruption of the blood-brain barrier (BBB) or the blood-tumor barrier (BTB) seems to offer a solution to the difficulties of vector distribution by employing the well-developed tumor neovasculature for transgene delivery to all vascularized tumor foci. In contrast to the normal BBB, which limits the size of substances entering from the bloodstream into brain cells and brain interstitial space, the brain tumor neovasculature has a somewhat more permeable barrier [Cox et al., 1976; Inamura and Black, 1994]. However, the BTB still limits delivery of high molecular weight substances to tumor tissue and to immediately adjacent, partly tumor-infiltrated areas of the brain [Hoshino, 1984]. The ability to achieve selective pharmacological opening of the BTB using bradykinin (BK) and its derivatives facilitates the selective delivery of cytotoxic drugs and virus vectors to intracerebral neoplasms [Elliot et al., 1996; Rainov et al., 1995], as the BTB is less rigid than the BBB.

The present study was designed to address the efficiency and selectivity of the intra-arterial application of AV vectors and lipoDNA with or without pharmacological modulation of the BTB.

Materials and Methods

Virus Vector. The virus vector used in this study was a recombinant type 2 AV (Ad2) with disruption of the E1A region, where the *Escherichia coli lacZ* cDNA coding for β-galactosidase (β-gal) was inserted under the control of the cytomegalovirus (CMV) promoter (gift of the Genzyme Corp., Cambridge, Mass., USA). Viral stocks were generated in 293 cells, concentrated by ultracentrifugation, titered by plaque assays, and stored at –80 °C. Ten microliters of the virus stock (a total of 1×10^9 pfu) were dissolved in 1 ml of warm (37 °C) 0.9% NaCl and immediately introduced into the carotid artery as a bolus injection.

Liposome-DNA Complexes. The T7T7T7Bgal plasmid (Progenitor, Inc., Menlo Park, Calif., USA) was grown in *E. coli* HMS174 cells (Novagen, Madison, Wisc., USA) and isolated by maxi-prep (Qiagen, S. Clarita, Calif., USA). This plasmid, when 'primed' with a small amount of T7 RNA polymerase, generates more RNA polymerase transcripts as well as large amounts of transgene transcripts, which are then translated using the cell's own machinery [Chen et al., 1995]. For intracarotid injections, 10 μg DNA was incubated with 25 U T7 RNA polymerase (New England Biolabs, Beverly, Mass., USA) and then mixed with 5 μl Lipofect-Amine (Life Technologies, Gaithersburg, Md., USA) in 200 μl OptiMEM (Life Technologies) at room temperature and incubated for 20 min at room temperature before injection.

Animal studies. Twenty adult male Fisher 344 CD rats (Charles River Laboratories, Wilmington, Mass., USA) weighing 200–250 g were used in this study. There were four groups: BK infusion and AV injection (n = 5), vehicle infusion and AV injection (n = 5), BK infusion and lipoDNA injection (n = 5), and vehicle infusion and lipoDNA injection (n = 5).

Procedures and housing of animals were performed in accordance with the guidelines issued by the Massachusetts General Hospital Subcommittee on Animal Care. Intracerebral solitary 9L tumors were produced by stereotactic inoculation of 1×10^5 tumor cells in 5 µl Dulbecco's Modified Eagle's Medium (DMEM; Life Technologies) into the right frontal lobe of the rats. Anesthesia and implantation technique were as described elsewhere [Rainov et al, 1995]. Seven days after tumor implantation, animals were reanesthetized for intracarotid catheterization. The right common carotid artery (CCA) was exposed through a 3-cm midline incision as previously described [Rainov et al., 1995]. Bradykinin acetate (Sigma, St. Louis, Mo., USA) was dissolved in distilled water (25 µg/ml) and kept on ice. Immediately prior to infusion the solution was warmed to 37 °C and infused at a rate of 10 µg/kg/min for 10 min using a microsyringe pump (Medfusion Syst., Norcross, Ga., USA). BK infusion was immediately followed by injection of virus or lipoDNA in 1 ml of vehicle over 5 min.

Fixation, Sectioning and Staining. For histochemical analysis of marker gene expression, rats were sacrificed 48 h after intracarotid infusion by a lethal dose of sodium-pentobarbital (15 mg) and transcardial perfusion with 4% paraformaldehyde in PBS (pH = 7.4). Brain, spinal cord, and internal organs – liver, lung, kidney, heart, testes, and lymph nodes – were placed in 30% sucrose for cryoprotection, frozen 2–4 days later over liquid nitrogen, and stored at –80 °C until further processing (not longer than 6 weeks). Tissue blocks were mounted in OCT compound (Miles, Inc., Elkhart, Ind., USA) and 20-µm thick serial sections were cut on a Jung cryostat (Cryocut 2800 E, Leica, Inc., Deerfield, Ill., USA). Every fifth section in the tumor area and every tenth section in normal brain, cerebellum, and internal organs was mounted on silane-coated slides (Superfrost®, Fisher Sci., Pittsburgh, Pa., USA) and air-dried at room temperature. Tissue sections were stained for *lacZ* expression by histochemistry using the X-gal substrate (Sigma) as previously described [Turner et al., 1990]. After rinsing with water for 5 min, sections were counterstained with Meyer's hematoxylin (Sigma) or Neutral Red (Fisher Sci.), dehydrated in ethanol, immersed for 5 min in xylene, and then mounted under coverslips. Control sections of rat brain not treated in the present study were stained in parallel to assure specificity of the staining process.

Cell Counting and Evaluation of Sections. LacZ-positive and negative cells were counted at a 200-fold magnification using a light microscope (Nikon, Inc., Garden City, N.Y., USA). Evaluation of sections was carried out in a blinded fashion. For the study of lipoDNA gene transfer, 1,000 cells were counted in each of three random visual fields throughout the tumor, since the pattern of distribution was fairly homogeneous. In animals with AV injection, small foci (<0.5 mm) were evaluated by counting total numbers of stained and nonstained cells. In larger tumors (2–5 mm), three random visual fields in the tumor periphery (defined as the part of tumor remaining in the microscopic visual field when normal brain tissue is also visible), and three random fields in the tumor center were counted and values averaged. Normal brain and internal organs were evaluated qualitatively.

Statistical Evaluation. For calculation of mean values and standard error of the mean, as well as for all significance tests, such as F-test and Student's t-test, the SPSS for Windows software package was used.

Results

AV Application. When 1×10^9 pfu of AV were injected into internal carotid artery in the absence of BK, 3–9% (mean 6.2%) of tumor cells in large tumor with or without pharmacological modulation of the BTB. While replication-deficient AV vectors seem to be inferior to lipoDNA in terms of tumor transductions rates, they do, however, possess a higher specificity and selectivity for intracerebral tumors. The relatively high transduction rates of normal brain capillaries and glia seen with lipoDNA did not cause adverse effects in the present marker gene study, and should be offset in future by the spatially regulatable expression of therapeutic toxic transgenes.

Acknowledgements

This study was supported in part by grants from the German Academy of Nature Researchers 'Leopoldina' and from the State Ministry of Culture of Saxony-Anhalt, Germany (FKZ 2794A/0087H), to N.G.R.; by an educational scholarship of the German Research Council (DFG) to U.H., and by NCI grant CA69246 to X.O.B. and E.A.C.

References

Badie B, Drazan KE, Kramar MH, Shaked A, Black KL: Adenovirus-mediated p53 gene delivery inhibits 9L glioma growth in rats. Neurol Res 1995;17:209–216.

Behr TP, Demeneix B, Loeffler JP, Perez-Mutul J: Efficient gene transfer into mammalian primary endocrine cells with lipopolyamine-coated DNA. Proc Natl Acad Sci USA 1989;86:6982–6986.

Berens ME, Rutka JT, Rosenblum ML: Brain tumor epidemiology, growth, and invasion. Neurosurg Clin North Am 1990;1:1–18.

Boucher Y, Leunig M, Jain RK: Tumor angiogenesis and interstitial hypertension. Cancer Res. 1996;56: 4264–4266.

Boviatsis EJ, Chase M, Wei M, Tamiya T, Hurford RK Jr, Kowall NW, Tepper RI, Breakefield XO, Chiocca EA: Gene transfer into experimental brain tumors mediated by adenovirus, herpes simplex virus (HSV), and retrovirus vectors. Hum Gene Therapy 1994a;5:183–191.

Boviatsis EJ, Park JS, Sena-Esteves M, Kramm CM, Chase M, Efird JT, Wei MX, Breakefield XO, Chiocca EA: Long-term survival of rats harboring brain neoplasms treated with ganciclovir and a herpes simplex virus vector that retains an intact thymidine kinase gene. Cancer Res 1994b;54: 5745–5751.

Byrnes AP, MacLaren RE, Charlton HM: Immunological instability of persistent adenovirus vector in the brain: Peripheral exposure to vector leads to renewed inflammation, reduced gene expression and demyelination. J Neurosci 1996;16:3045–3055.

Chen SH, Shine HD, Goodman JC, Grossman RG, Woo SL: Gene therapy for brain tumors: regression of experimental gliomas by adenovirus mediated gene transfer in vivo. Proc Natl Acad Sci USA 1994;91:3054–3057.

Chen X, Li Y, Xiong K, Xie Y, Aizicovici S, Snodgrass R, Wagner TE, Platika D: A novel nonviral cytoplasmic gene expression system and its implications in cancer gene therapy. Cancer Gene Ther 1995;2:281–289.

Chiocca EA, Andersen J, Takamiya Y, Martuza R, Breakefield XO: Virus-mediated genetic treatment of rodent gliomas; in Wolf JA (ed): Gene Therapeutics. Boston, Birkhauser, 1994, pp 245–262.

Cox DJ, Pilkington GJ, Lantos PL: The fine structure of blood vessels in ethylnitrosurea-induced tumours of the rat nervous system: With special reference to the breakdown of the blood-brain barrier. Br J Exp Pathol 1976;57:419–430.

Curiel DT: High efficiency gene transfer mediated by adenovirus-polylysine-DNA complexes. Ann NY Acad Sci 1994;716:36–57.

Doran SE, Dan Ren X, Betz AL, Pagel MA, Neuwelt EA, Roessler BJ, Davidson BL: Gene expression from recombinant viral vectors in the CNS following blood-brain barrier disruption. Neurosurgery 1995;36:965–970.

Eck SL, Alavi JB, Alavi A, Davis A, Hackney D, Judy K, Mollman J, Phillips PC, Wheeldon EB, Wilson JM: Treatment of advanced CNS malignancies with the recombinant adenovirus H5.010RSVTK: A phase I trial. Hum Gene Ther 1996;7:1465–1482.

Elliott PJ, Hayward NJ, Huff MR, Nagle TL, Black KL, Bartus RT: Unlocking the blood-brain barrier: A role for RMP-7 in brain tumor therapy. Exp Neurol 1996;141:214–224.

Felgner JH, Kumar R, Sridhar CN, Wheeler CJ, Tsai YJ, Border R, Ramsey P, Martin M, Felgner PL: Enhanced gene delivery and mechanism studies with a novel series of cationic lipid formulations. J Biol Chem 1994;269:2550–2561.

Felgner PL, Tsai YJ, Sukhu L, Wheeler CJ, Manthorpe M, Marshall J, Cheng H: Improved cationic lipid formulations for in vivo gene therapy. Ann NY Acad Sci 1995;772:126–139.

Fritz JD, Herwejer H, Zhang G, Wolff JA: Gene transfer into mammalian cells using histone-condensed plasmid DNA. Hum Gene Ther 1996;7:1395–1404.

Hess JF, Borkowski JA, Young GS, Strader CD, Ransom RW: Cloning and pharmacological characterization of a human bradykinin (BK-2) receptor. Biochem Biophys Res Commun 1992;184:260–268.

Hoshino T: A commentary on the biology and growth kinetics of low-grade and high-grade gliomas. J Neurosurg 1984;61:895–900.

Huard J, Lochmuller H, Acsadi G, Jani A, Massie B, Karpati G: The route of administration is a major determinant of the transduction efficiency of rat tissues by adenoviral recombinants. Gene Ther 1995;2:107–115.

Hug P, Sleight RG: Liposomes for the transformation of eukaryotic cells. Biochim Biophys Acta 1991; 1097:1–17.

Inamura T, Black KL: Bradykinin selectively opens blood-tumor barrier in experimental brain tumors. J Cereb Blood Flow Metab 1994;14:862–870.

Kramm CM, Rainov NG, Sena-Esteves M, Barnett FH, Chase M, Herrlinger U, Pechan PA, Chiocca EA, Breakefield XO: Long-term survival in a rodent model of disseminated brain tumors by combined intrathecal delivery of herpes vectors and ganciclovir treatment. Hum Gene Ther 1996; 7:1989–1994.

Kramm CM, Sena-Esteves M, Barnett FH, Rainov NG, Schuback DE, Yu JS, Pechan PA, Paulus W, Chiocca EA, Breakefield XO: Gene therapy for brain tumors. Brain Pathol 1995;5:345–381.

Maron A, Gustin T, Le-Roux A, Mottet I, Dedieu JF, Brion JP, Demeure R, Perricaudet M, Octave JN: Gene therapy of rat C6 glioma using adenovirus-mediated transfer of the herpes simplex virus thymidine kinase gene: Long-term follow-up by magnetic resonance imaging. Gene Ther 1996;3: 315–322.

Michael SI, Curiel DT: Strategies to achieve gene delivery via the receptor-mediated endocytosis pathway. Gene Ther 1994;1:223–232.

Neuwelt EA, Pagel MA, Dix RD: Delivery of ultraviolet inactivated ^{35}S-herpesvirus across an osmotically modified blood-brain barrier. J Neurosurg 1991;74:475–479.

Nilaver G, Muldoon LL, Kroll RA, Pagel MA, Breakefield XO, Davidson BL, Neuwelt EA: Delivery of herpesvirus and adenovirus to nude rat intracerebral tumors following osmotic blood-brain barrier disruption. Proc Natl Acad Sci USA 1995;92:9829–9833.

Perez-Cruet MJ, Trask TW, Chen SH, Goodman JC, Woo SL, Grossman RG, Shine HD: Adenovirus-mediated gene therapy of experimental gliomas. J Neurosci Res 1994;39:506–511.

Rainov NG, Dobberstein KU, Heidecke V, Dorant U, Chase M, Kramm CM, Chiocca EA, Breakefield XO: Long-term survival in a rodent brain tumor model by bradykinin-enhanced intra-arterial delivery of a therapeutic herpes simplex virus vector. Cancer Gene Ther 1998;5:158–162.

Rainov NG, Zimmer C, Chase M, Kramm CM, Chiocca EA, Weissleder R, Breakefield XO: Selective uptake of viral and monocrystalline particles delivered intra-arterially to e × perimental brain neoplasms. Hum Gene Ther 1995;6:1543–1552.

San H, Yang ZY, Pompili VJ, Jaffe ML, Plautz GE, Xu L, Felgner JH, Wheeler CJ, Felgner PL, Gao X, et al: Safety and short-term toxicity of a novel cationic lipid formulation for human gene therapy. Hum Gene Ther 1993;4:781–788.

applications of radiobiological concepts and experimental data, generated from radiation myelopathy models, in these settings are discussed.

Clinical Manifestations of Iatrogenic Neurologic Deficits

Radiation myelopathy usually has a subtle onset after a latency of >5–6 months [2]. Objective signs and symptoms include changes in gait (often foot drop), spasticity, paresis, and less frequently Brown-Sequard syndrome (ipsilateral paralysis and loss of discriminatory sensation and contralateral loss of pain and temperature sensation), incontinence, and occasionally pain. Hyperreflexia and Babinski signs are often found on neurological exam. In some cases, the patient may have been asymptomatic until some trauma initiated a progressive neurological deficit. The overall functional repercussion of myelopathy depends on the segment of the spinal cord affected.

The dose-incidence relationship is reasonably well established in adults. A literature review by Schultheiss and Stephens [2] indicates that a total dose of 45 Gy in 22–25 fractions results in ~0.2% incidence of myelopathy. A realistic estimate of the ED_5 (5% complications) for 2-Gy fractions is between 57 and 61 Gy (also see further).

Focal cerebral necrosis is the typical late effect of therapeutic or incidental brain irradiation. The onset is generally between 6 months and 2 years after therapy. Symptoms and signs include site-specific focal deficits (e.g. paresis, paresthesia, aphasia, etc.), seizures, and symptoms of intracranial hypertension. CT scans usually reveal low-density white matter changes with irregular enhancement often associated with surrounding, more diffuse edema and a variable degree of mass effect confined to the high-dose volume. MRI shows similar changes and often identifies more pronounced white matter edema [3]. In patients with brain cancer, differentiation from tumor recurrence or progression may be difficult.

Focal brain necrosis has rarely been observed at radiation doses <60 Gy for conventionally fractionated external beam irradiation given as a single modality treatment [4, 5]. A threshold of 57.6 Gy has been reported for daily irradiation with fraction sizes <2 Gy [6]. The incidence, however, is highly dependent upon fraction size. Most reported necroses following 'incidental' brain irradiation have occurred with fractions of >2.2–2.25 Gy [5].

In patients with brain neoplasms, it is important to recognize the *subacute encephalopathy* syndrome. This syndrome manifests most frequently 2–6 months after therapy as fatigue, somnolence, and the exacerbation of focal neurologic symptoms and signs. It may be difficult to differentiate this usually transient syndrome from tumor progression which could lead to prescription of additional therapy for presumed disease recurrence [3].

Diagnosis and Pathology

Diagnosis of iatrogenic neurotoxicity is generally made by exclusion since there are no pathognomonic symptoms or signs. Factors to be taken into account are spatial and temporal relationship with radiation, radiation dose and absence of other causes of CNS injury. The symptom complex may sometimes be helpful in making the differentiation diagnosis. For example, existence of upper extremity symptoms without lower extremity symptoms is a strong argument against radiation myelopathy as the cause of neurologic deficit. It should also be realized that by far the most common cause for CNS damage in a cancer patient is tumor progression or metastases. The available diagnostic imaging techniques can usually identify tumor progression as the cause of CNS injury. In case of uncertainty, further follow-up generally resolves the differential diagnosis.

Histopathologic study of radiation-induced CNS necrosis in humans is generally restricted to symptomatic patients. As a result, the available clinical material represents only the more advanced injury. Studies on rodent and primate myelopathy models [7, 8] have provided a broader picture of the lesions by affording the opportunity to view milder degrees of injury and address the relationships between the pathologic changes and such factors as dose, time, volume, etc.

Radiation-induced injury to the CNS is typically confined to the white matter. Demyelination and malacia, though not pathognomic, are the dominant morphological features. A highly variable degree of vascular anomaly and proliferative response of glial cells accompany these changes. The gray matter is usually not involved, at least, without accompanying changes in the white matter. Based on morphological features of the lesions, cases of radiation myelopathy can be grouped into three categories based on the structural distribution of tissue damage, i.e. predominantly white matter demyelination and malacia (type I), mainly vascular anomalies (type II), or combination of both components (type III). Vascular changes most often encountered in the type III class are endothelial alterations, telangiectasia, hyalinosis, and fibrinoid necrosis.

In general, latent periods of $<17-18$ months are associated with type I or type III lesions. In contrast, longer latency tends to be associated with type II lesions with significant vascular anomalies such as thrombosis, necrosis, and hemorrhage [9]. Type III lesion is most frequently observed in human cases in a monkey model [7, 10, 11].

In addition to architectural changes described earlier, there are modifications in the cellular composition within the white matter. Generally, the number of microglia and astrocytes increases in the irradiated spinal cord segment.

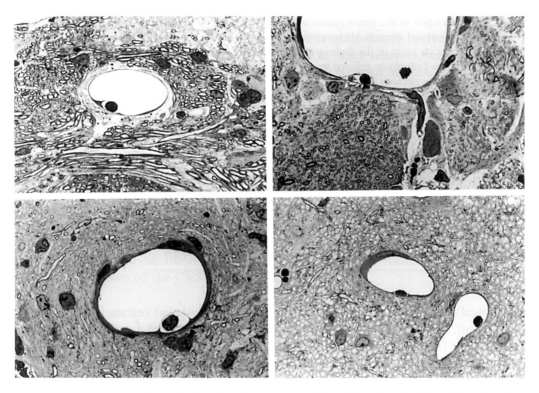

Fig. 1. Examples of white cell adherence to dilated blood vessels, diapedesis and perivascular infiltration, in the fimbria of the hippocampus of rats 52 weeks after irradiation with a single dose of 25.0 Gy [Reyners et al., unpubl. data, with permission].

mena quantified above, are illustrated in figure 2. The starting point is the known increase in vascular permeability or the implied upregulation of adhesion molecules. However, these two possible pathways are clearly interrelated, as discussed in more detail elsewhere [12].

Evidence for the Absence of Involvement of Glial Progenitors

Recent experimental studies have examined the effects of thermal neutron irradiation on the spinal cord of rats [13]. These studies were unique in the fact that they were combined with ^{10}B carriers as part of preclinical study to evaluate normal tissue effects prior to the clinical application of boron neutron capture therapy (BNCT) at Brookhaven National Laboratory (BNL), New York. In these studies the capture agents' *p*-boronophenylalanine (BPA)

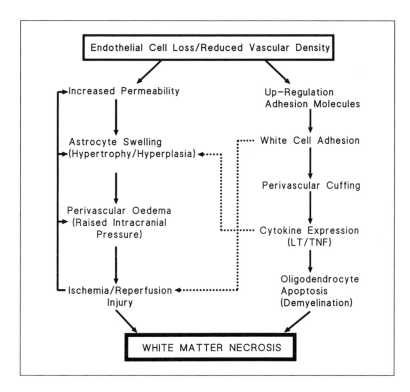

Fig. 2. Schematic representation of possible cascades linking gradual endothelial cell loss to white matter necrosis in the CNS. TNF/LT = Tumour necrosis factors α and β, respectively.

and boracaptate sodium (BSH) were used. These differ by the fact that one [10]B capture agent (BPA) crosses the normal blood-brain barrier, the other (BSH) does not. Despite this major difference, and the associated difference in the distribution of the physical radiation from the [10]B neutron capture reaction, the histological appearance of the lesion in the spinal cord of rats developing paralysis was the same after both types of BNCT-type irradiation [14, 15] and identical to that seen after thermal neutron or photon exposures. This in itself points to a vascular mediated pathogenesis for selective white matter necrosis.

The physical radiation doses to the parenchyma of the spinal cord, associated with the development of a 50% incidence of paralysis in these studies, as a consequence of white matter necrosis, are given in figure 3. This was for irradiation with blood boron levels of 12 and 120 μg/g from BPA and BSH, respectively. The corresponding doses from the thermal reactor beam on the

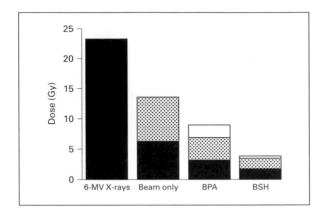

Fig. 3. Total physical radiation dose (Gy) to the parenchyma cells of the spinal cord from γ-rays (■), fast neutrons (▨) and from the ^{10}B(n, α)^{7}Li reaction (□) at the ED_{50} for white matter necrosis after irradiation with 6-MV X-rays, the thermal neutron beam at the BNL Medical Research Reactor and BNCT mediated by BPA or BSH.

Brookhaven Medical Research Reactor alone, a combination of fast neutrons and incident and induced γ-rays was ∼14 Gy [13], and for 6-MV X-rays, ∼23 Gy.

As a consequence of these studies, investigations were undertaken to determine the effects of doses, iso-effective for the production of late damage, on the clonogenic survival of glial O2A progenitor cells in the irradiated rat spinal cord after one week. In order to obtain measurable numbers of cell colonies, total doses approximating to $\frac{1}{3}$ ED_{50} for paralysis were used [16]. Due to the lack of significant dose sparing following fractionated thermal or BNCT-mediated exposure, a dose ∼$\frac{1}{3}$ of the ED_{50} was used. The resulting surviving fractions of O2A progenitor, sampled at 1 week after irradiation, are given in figure 4. Progenitor survival was lowest after uniform irradiation with the thermal neutron beam alone ∼3.2% and highest after BNCT irradiation, mediated with BSH (∼45%). The BPA group produced an intermediate level of cell survival. This indicates that the initial effect of irradiation on glial progenitors was not iso-effective, even though doses approximately iso-effective for late damage had been used. These differences in glial progenitor survival directly reflect the large difference in the parenchymal dose relative to that of the vessel wall.

In another series of experiments, animals were irradiated with the approximate ED_{90} for paralysis with thermal neutrons alone or in combination with BPA or BSH. Groups of animals were killed at 120 or 135 days after irradiation. Glial progenitor survival was assayed and compared with results following

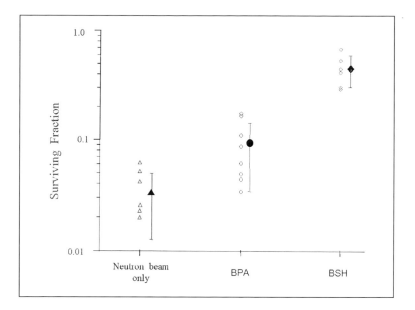

Fig. 4. Mean surviving fraction of glial O2A progenitors (95% confidence interval) in the rat spinal cord 7 days after irradiation with thermal neutrons, alone or with the ^{10}B capture agents BPA and BSH at $\sim\frac{1}{3}ED_{50}$ for early delayed injury (white mater necrosis).

doses of 15 or 25 Gy of 6-MV X-rays (fig. 5). Despite the fact that the assay times selected were approaching to that normally associated with the development of paralysis, marked differences were seen in glial progenitor survival. Following irradiation with BSH-mediated BNCT the surviving fraction was $\sim 80\%$, not dissimilar to that found after 15 Gy of X-rays, a dose that was $\sim 50\%$ of the ED_{50} for white matter necrosis and a dose not associated with the development of paralysis. The surviving fraction after irradiation with the thermal neutron beam alone was low $\leq 3\%$ approaching the lower limit of resolution of this assay. The values obtained after BPA-mediated BNCT was between 10 and 20%, similar to that seen after 23 Gy of 6-MV X-rays, which was also the approximate ED_{90-100}.

Somewhat surprisingly, the mean latent period ($\pm$ SE) asociated with the development of paralysis, as a consequence of white matter necrosis, varied with the exposure conditions. It was longest in animals receiving uniform irradiation of the parenchyma and vasculature, beam-only exposure (166 ± 2 days), and shorter when the dose differential was greatest, BSH-mediated BNCT (137 ± 3 days), a small but significant ($p < 0.001$) difference. Irradiation with BPA-mediated BNCT produced an intermediate latent interval of 153 ± 3 days. The reason for the difference is unknown, however, it is tempting to

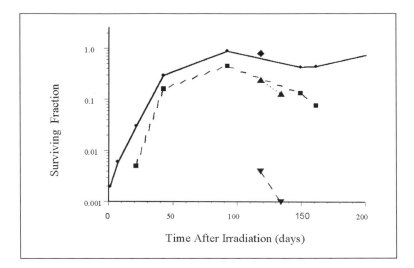

Fig. 5. Time-related changes in the surviving fraction of O2A glial progenitor cells in the rat spinal cord after irradiation with doses of thermal neutrons (▼), BPA-mediated BNCT (▲) and BSH-mediated BNCT (♦) at doses equivalent to the ∼ED$_{90}$ for white matter necrosis. The time-related response after 23 Gy (■) and 15 Gy (●) of 6-MV X-rays is given for comparison.

suggest that initiation of the reactive cascade initiated by vascular damage is impaired by the higher radiation dose to the parenchyma.

Indirect Evidence of Vascular Involvement

Despite continued uncertainty about the true role of vascular damage in the pathogenesis of late radiation damage to the CNS, this has not inhibited a number of investigators from initiating attempts, in this and other tissue, to ameliorate the development of late damage after exposure.

The hypothesis formulated by Hornsey et al. [11] was that increased capillary permeability led to oedema, reduced blood flow, ischaemia infarction and necrosis, a mechanism not dissimilar to one of those outlined in figure 2. The problem was thought to be exacerbated by an evolving chronic reperfusion problem, whereby H_2O_2 or superoxide radicals were converted to damaging hydroxyl radicals [17]. Since this process is catalysed by the presence of Fe^{2+} ions, attempts at reducing reperfusion injury were considered worthy of further investigation. Animals were locally irradiated to the spinal cord with doses known to produce ataxia or paresis due to white matter necrosis. These rats were then fed a low iron diet from 12 weeks after irradiation and they were also administered desferrioxamine (30 mg, subcutaneously, 3 times weekly). Desferrioxamine administration was started 120 days after irradiation, a time at which vascular permeability was first found to be impaired. In treated animals the time of appearance of ataxia was delayed when compared with those receiving radiation alone. The change in response represents a small, but significant, dose modification factor of ~ 1.1.

In an alternative approach, an attempt was made to correct for the known development in an imbalance in the key eicosanoids for vascular function, prostacyclin and thromboxane [10]. This was achieved by the administration of an oil So-5407 or So-1100 which contain $\sim 7\%$ and $\sim 9\%$ of the essential fatty acid, γ-linolenic acid (GLA), respectively. High intakes of GLA will preferentially increase exogenous levels of prostaglandin E_1 (PGE$_1$) in the monenoic prostanoid cascade, with the subsequent blocking of the dienoic prostinoid pathway. This includes the two eicosanoids believed to be in imbalance. PGE$_1$ has many desirable actions including being a potent vasodilator. The match thromboxane (TXA$_1$) has few of the damage side effects of raised levels of TXA$_2$ [18]. Pigs administered So-5407 orally, daily (12 ml/day), starting the day after irradiation with 22 Gy, showed a reduced incidence of paralysis compared with a similar group of pigs receiving a placebo oil. This difference was highly significant ($p < 0.001$) [19]. Rats receiving So-1100, again daily from the day after irradiation (1 or 2 ml), showed a significant delay in the onset of paralysis after doses well above those received to produce a 100% incidence of paralysis [20]. Post-irradiation treatment with oils containing GLA have been shown to reduce the incidence and severity of radiation damage in a number of animal models after both single and fractionated doses [21]. Comparable results have been obtained in patients [22].

Conclusions

The results presented indicate that there is both direct and indirect evidence that the vasculature is a primary target, damage to which results in a cascade of changes leading to the development of white matter necrosis. This cascade does involve an interaction with parenchymal elements. While the studies to examine the effects of different irradiation modalities in the short- and long-term survival of glial progenitors infer no direct involvement in the development of early delayed damage, clearly parenchymal dose does have an effect on the latency for this effect.

The indirect evidence for vasculature involvement is also encouraging since it suggests that intervention after irradiation can, in a still unclear way, influence the incidence of early delayed lesions. Since it seems reasonable to suggest that this interference in the tissues' response to injury may be normal tissue-specific, it offers a possible opportunity for a safe escalation of the radiation dose with the potential for an improvement in the therapeutic ratio for radiotherapy treatment.

Acknowledgements

The authors are grateful to Mrs. Margaret Staff for typing the manuscript and to colleagues for their contribution to the ideas and information included in the manuscript, specifically Dr. G.M. Morris, Dr. M. Rezvani and Dr. H. Reyners.

References

1 Van der Kogel AJ: The nervous system: Radiobiology and experimental pathology; in Scherer E, Streffer L, Trott KR (eds): Radiopathology of Organs and Tissues. Berlin, Springer, 1991, pp 191–212.
2 Roman DD, Sporduto PW: Neuropsychological effects of cranial irradiation; current knowledge and future direction. Int J Radiat Oncol Biol Phys 1995;31:983–998.
3 Hopewell JW: Late radiation damage to the central nervous system: A radiobiological interpretation. Neuropathol Appl Neurobiol 1979;5:329–343.
4 Calvo W, Hopewell JW, Reinhold HS, Yeung TK: Time- and dose-related changes in the white matter of the rat brain after single doses of X-rays. Br J Biol 1988;61:1043–1052.
5 Hubbard BM, Hopewell JW: Changes in the neuroglial cell population of the rat spinal cord after local X-irradiation. Br J Radiol 1979;52:816–821.
6 Hopewell JW, Morris AD, Dixon-Brown A: The influence of field size on the late tolerance of the rat spinal cord to single doses of X-rays. Br J Radiol 1987;60:1099–1108.
7 Hopewell JW: Models of CNS radiation damage during space flight. Adv Space Res 1994;14: 433–442.
8 Jaenke RS, Robbins MEC, Bywaters T, Whitehouse E, Rezvani M, Hopewell JW: Capillary endothelium: Target site of renal radiation injury. Lab Invest 1993;68:396–405.
9 Hopewell JW, Calvo W, Jaenke R, Reinhold RS, Robbins MEC, Whitehouse EM: Microvasculature and radiation damage. Recent Adv Cancer Res 1993;130:1–16.
10 Siegel T, Pfeffer R: Radiation-induced changes in the profile of spinal cord serotonin, prostaglandin synthesis and vascular permeability. Int J Radiat Oncol Biol Phys 1994;31:57–64.
11 Hornsey S, Meyer R, Jenkinson T: The reduction of radiation damage in the spinal cord by post-irradiation administration of vasoactive drugs. Int J Radiat Oncol Biol Phys 1990;18:1437–1442.
12 Hopewell JW: Radiation injury to the central nervous system. Med Pediatr Oncol 1998;suppl 1: 1–9.
13 Morris GM, Coderre JA, Hopewell JW, Micca PL, Nawrocky MM, Liu HB, Bywaters A: Responses of the central nervous system to boron neutron capture irradiation: Evaluation in the rat spinal cord. Radiother Oncol 1994;32:249–255.
14 Morris GM, Coderre JA, Whitehouse EM, Micca P, Hopewell JW: Boron neutron capture therapy: A guide to the understanding of the pathogenesis of late radiation damage to the rat spinal cord. Int J Radiat Oncol Biol Phys 1994;28:1107–1112.
15 Morris GM, Coderre JA, Bywaters A, Whitehouse E, Hopewell JW: Boron neutron capture irradiation of the rat spinal cord: Histopathological evidence of a vascular-mediated pathogenesis. Radiat Res 1996;146:313–320.

16   Van der Kogel AJ, Kleiboer BJ, Verhagen I, Morris GM, Hopewell JW, Coderre JA: White matter necrosis of the spinal cord: Studies on glial progenitor survival and selective vascular irradiation; in Hagen V, Harder D, Jung H, Streffer C (eds): Radiation Research 1895–1995. Würzburg, 1995, vol 2, pp 769–772.

17   Weisfeldt ML: Reperfusion and reperfusion injury. Clin Res 1987;35:13–20.

18   Horrobin DF: Prostaglandin E_1: Physiological significance and clinical use. Wien Klin Wochenschr 1988;10:471–477.

19   Hopewell JW, van den Aardweg GJMJ, Morris GM, Rezvani M, Robbins MEC, Ross GA, Whitehouse EM: Unsaturated lipids as modulators of radiation damage in normal tissue; in Horrobin DF (ed): New Approach to Cancer Treatment. London, Churchill Communications, 1994, pp 88–106.

20   El-Agamawi AY, Hopewell JW, Plowman PN, Rezvani M, Wilding D: Modulation of normal tissue responses to radiation. Br J Radiol 1996;69:374–375.

21   Hopewell JW, van den Aardweg GJMJ, Morris GM, Rezvani M, Robbins MEC, Ross GA, Whitehouse EM, Scott CA, Horrobin DF: Amelioration of both early and late radiation-induced damage to pig skin by essential fatty acids. Int J Radiat Oncol Biol Phys 1994;30:1119–1125.

22   Hopewell JW: Modifying radiation injury to normal tissues: New opportunitities; in Meyer JL, Vaeth JM (eds): Front Radiat Ther Oncol. Basel, Karger, 1999, pp 9–20.

J.W. Hopewell, Normal Tissue Radiobiology Group, Research Institute University of Oxford, The Churchill Hospital, Headington, Oxford OX3 7LJ (UK)

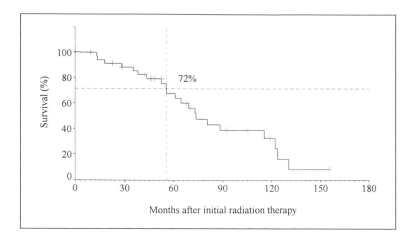

Fig. 2. Overall survival after initial radiotherapy of 36 patients treated for brain tumors. Dashes represent censored patients.

patients after completion of reirradiation. In none of the patients was chemotherapy applied concurrent to the initial radiation or the retreatment course.

The median follow-up time after reirradiation was 9 months (range 0.6–46). Clinical examinations and MRI/CT imaging were performed. Endpoints of this retrospective analysis were overall survival and progression-free interval. These endpoints were evaluated using Kaplan-Meier statistics. Log-rank test and Cox proportional hazards model were used for univariate und multivariate analysis (SPSS for Windows Release 6.1.2). Source parameters for the analysis of prognostic factors were age ($</$ median), sex, histology (glioblastoma, non-glioblastoma, no histological diagnosis), grade (from G1 to G4, GX) of primary and recurrent tumor, and residual tumor burden after surgical resection (R1, R2, biopsy). No corrections for multiple tests were performed.

Results

Overall survival at 5 years after initial radiotherapy was 72% (standard error $\pm 8\%$; fig. 2). Grading of the primary tumor was the only significant prognostic factor for overall survival (log-rank test: $p = 0.03$).

In 27 patients the recurrent tumor was located within the treatment volume of the first radiation course, in 8 patients recurrences occurred at the field margins, and only in 1 patient the tumor recurred outside the initial treatment volume. A shift of tumor histology towards high-grade glioma was observed in 12 out of 17 patients who prior to reirradiation received second surgery after initially low-grade glioma.

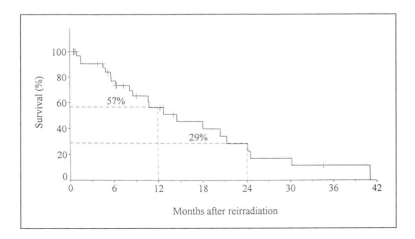

Fig. 3. Survival after reirradiation of 36 patients with recurrent brain tumors. Dashes represent censored patients.

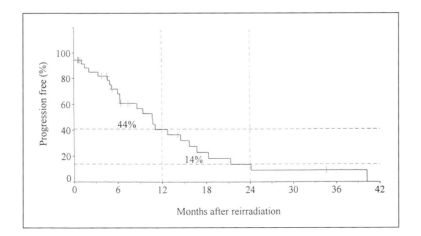

Fig. 4. Progression-free interval after reirradiation of 36 patients with recurrent brain tumors. Dashes represent censored patients.

Survival after retreatment was 57% ($\pm 10\%$) at 1 year and 29% ($\pm 10\%$) at 2 years (fig. 3). The last patient died 3.7 years after retreatment. Tumor progression, based on clinical symptoms and/or imaging (CT/MRI), was the cause of death in all cases. Forty-four percent ($\pm 10\%$) of the patients were free of progression 1 year after reirradiation and 14% ($\pm 7\%$) at 2 years (fig. 4). Uni- and multivariate analysis revealed no significant parameters for survival

Table 1. Details of treatment and follow-up

Patient No.	Gender	Age years	First course dose/ dose per fraction, Gy	Gap days	Second course dose/ dose per fraction, Gy	Cumulative dose[1], Gy	BED[2] Gy$_{2Gy}$	Sight pre-RT[3]	Follow-up time[4], months	Visual changes post-RT[5]
1	f	63	50.0/2.0	114	30.0/2.0	80.0	63.5	1	113	0
2	m	48	49.5/1.5	142	15.0/1.5	64.5	56.2	1	63	0
3	f	73	60.0/2.0	–	–	60.0	59.9	1	19	1
4	m	61	60.0/2.0	195	20.0/2.0	80.0	70.1	1	10	3
5	f	70	49.5/1.5	226	30.0/1.5	79.5	55.1	1	20	0
6	f	44	60.0/1.5	–	–	60.0	55.2	Blind	8	–
7	m	59	60.0/2.0	77	20.0/2.0	80.0	75.2	1	12	0
8	f	37	49.5/1.5	301	10.5/1.5	60.0	52.3	1	135	0
9	m	46	60.0/2.0	–	–	60.0	42.9	0	159	0
10	m	40	60.0/2.0	82	20.0/2.0	80.0	73.3	1	44	0
11	m	34	60.0/2.0	–	–	60.0	33.9	1	100	2
12	m	42	37.5/1.5	–	–	60.0	56.0	1	186	0
13	m	51	60.0/2.0	–	–	60.0	47.7	1	4	0
14	f	68	50.0/2.0	70	30.0/2.0	80.0	53.5	1	67	0
15	m	45	60.0/2.0	175	20.0/2.0	80.0	79.6	1	121	0
16	m	57	80.0/2.0	–	–	80.0	79.9	0	120	0
17	m	57	60.0/2.0	–	–	60.0	51.9	1	79	0
18	f	36	50.0/1.5	265	19.5/1.5	69.5	60.3	1	186	2
19	f	21	60.0/2.0	–	–	60.0	60.0	0	90	0
20	f	44	59.4/1.8	–	–	59.4	54.1	1	147	0
21	m	32	80.0/2.0	–	–	80.0	78.0	0	130	0
22	m	61	66.0/2.0	–	–	66.0	81.4	1	83	0
23	f	50	59.4/1.8	–	–	59.4	55.1	1	64	0
24	f	47	80.0/2.0	–	–	80.0	79.4	0	129	0
25	m	60	28.0/2.0	68	40.0/2.0	68.0	65.7	1	93	0

[1] Phys. cumulative dose to the maximum (reference dose).
[2] Max. biol. equivalent dose to 2-Gy fractions to the optic chiasm.
[3] 0 = Normal vision; 1 = visual impairment.
[4] 0 = No change; 1 = deterioration due to tumor progression; 2 = deterioration due to surgery or hypertension; 3 = deterioration due to radiation or cerebrovascular disease.
[5] Follow-up for visual assessment.

In none of these cases was death caused by the pituitary tumor (heart and lung diseases, $n = 5$; cerebrovascular disease, $n = 2$; tumor of the adrenals, $n = 1$). The actuarial overall survival was 80% (standard error $\pm 8\%$) and 65% ($\pm 11\%$) after 5 and 10 years, respectively (fig. 1a).

Local control was evaluated using CT and/or MRI. The median follow-up time for this endpoint was 49 months (4–162). Tumor progression was observed in 4 patients after 10, 25, 27 and 59 months. The actuarial progression-free survival was 79% ($\pm 9.3\%$) after 5 and 10 years (fig. 1b).

Table 1 lists the retrospectively estimated doses to the optic chiasm for all individual patients. The median physical dose to the chiasm was 61 Gy (40–80), the median BED_{2Gy} was 60 Gy_{2Gy} (33–82). Median follow-up for information on visual acuity of the patients was 90 months (4–186). Before start of radiotherapy, visual assessment was performed by an ophthalmologist in 9 patients and by a radiation oncologist in the remaining 16 patients. All 17 patients who were alive could be re-examined at our institution between April 1997 and January 1998. Fourteen of these patients consented to an ophthalmologic examination including perimetry of visual fields and fundoscopy. For the 8 patients who died intercurrently, information was obtained from records of our institution and the primary care physicians. The results of the examinations are also summarized in table 1.

Before start of radiotherapy, 14 patients (56%) showed signs of chiasmatic syndrome with visual field deficits of one or both eyes. One patient was blind on both eyes. Three other patients were blind on one eye, one of them with poor vision (only dark-light discrimination) on the other eye. Two additional patients developed unilateral palsy of the oculomotorius nerve after surgery, 1 of these patients additionally had abducens nerve palsy.

Only in 2 patients the vision improved after radiotherapy while in 18 patients vision was found unchanged. A deterioration of vision was found in 4 patients. In *patient 3*, deterioration was caused most likely by tumor progression that was confirmed by CT imaging. In *patient 11* the cause of visual deterioration was postoperative oculomotorius nerve palsy resulting in a dry eye syndrome without any signs of optic neuropathy, confirmed by the ophthalmologist. *Patient 18* developed ablation of the retina and severe neovascularization in both eyes 2 years after radiation. This patient suffered from hypertension that was treated only after the development of the eye symptoms. Five years after radiotherapy this patient was repeatedly treated with laser. No signs of optic neuropathy were found by the ophthalmologist. After laser therapy and pharmacological treatment of the high blood pressure, the visual acuity of this patient remained stable. Radiotherapy in this case was given in a split course with 50 and 19.5 Gy separated by 265 days. The dose calculated retrospectively for the retina was 9–12 Gy, which is not sufficient to explain

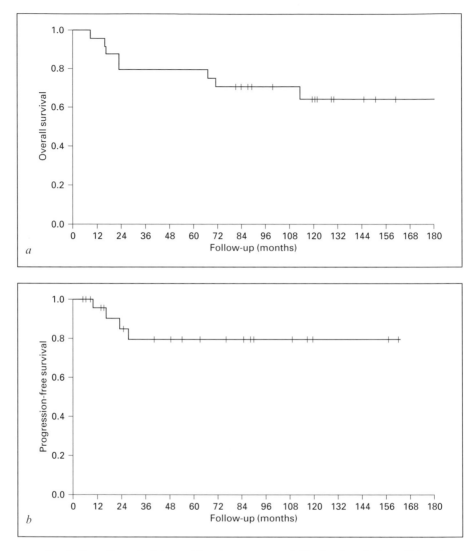

Fig. 1. Overall survival (*a*) and local tumor control (*b*) after irradiation of 25 patients with pituitary tumors to high doses between 60 and 80 Gy. Dashes represent patients censored for the respective endpoint.

the retinal disease of this patient [7]. *Patient 4* complained about visual deterioration 295 days after start of treatment. Radiation in this case was given as a split course to 60 Gy plus 20 Gy, separated by 195 days. The estimated biological effective dose to the chiasm was 70.1 Gy_{2Gy}. CT images obtained at the same time showed no evidence of tumor progression. Shortly after onset

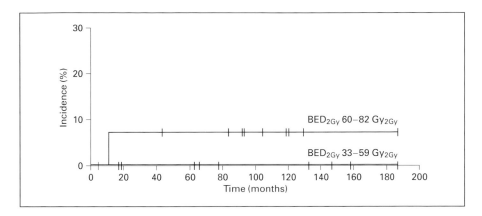

Fig. 2. Actuarial incidence of radiation damage of the optic chiasm in 24 patients at risk. Only 1 patient developed symptoms consistent with radiation injury 295 days after application of a biological effective dose to the chiasm of 70.1 Gy_{2Gy}. Alternatively the symptoms in this patient may have been caused by cerebrovascular disease. Dashes represent censored patients.

of visual deterioration the patient suffered from a cerebrovascular stroke and died 4 months later. No ophthalmologic examination of the visual symptoms of this patient is available.

For calculation of the actuarial incidence of radiation-induced chiasm damage, *patient 6* was excluded because she was blind on both eyes already before radiotherapy. If one assumes that *patient 4* suffered from radiation damage to the chiasm, the risk at 10 years is 8.3% ($\pm 8.9\%$) for 12 eligible patients who received doses to the optic chiasm of 60–81.4 Gy_{2Gy} (fig. 2). None of the 12 patients who received doses lower than 60 Gy_{2Gy} developed visual deterioration due to radiation. The actuarial incidence of chiasm injury for all 24 patients at risk was 4.4% ($\pm 4.3\%$), or, if the symptoms in *patient 4* were caused by cerebrovascular disease, 0%.

Discussion

The radiation tolerance of optic chiasm and optic nerves is frequently dose-limiting in radiation therapy of tumors close to the base of skull. In many centers the tolerance dose$_{5/5}$ (TD$_{5/5}$, i.e. the dose that results in 5% complications within 5 years from treatment) of the chiasm is assumed to be 50 Gy at 2-Gy fractions [8]. The data presented here on 25 patients – of whom 24 were elegible for visual analysis – who were treated to unusual high doses

Table 6. α/β values taken from literature

Authors	α/β, Gy	Comment
Amols et al. [cited in 30]	2.3–2.9	
Ang et al. [20]	1.5–2.0	Cervical
Ang et al. [32]	1.7	Complete repair
Ang et al. [32]	4.3	Incomplete repair
Hall [33]	1.7–4.9	All regions
Leith et al. [30]	3.8–4.1	
Reinhold et al. [31]	1.7–1.9	Necrosis
Reinhold et al. [31]	2.8	Vessel injury
Thames et al. [36]	2.2–3.0	Cervical
Van der Kogel [1]	1.8–2.7	Cervical
Van der Kogel [1]	3.7–4.5	Lumbal
Van der Kogel [35]	1.5–2.5	Cervical, necrosis
Van der Kogel [35]	3–5	Lumbal, necrosis
Van der Kogel [35]	2.8	Vessel injury
Van der Kogel et al. [37]	1.0–1.4	Cervical
Van der Kogel et al. [37]	2.5–2.6	Lumbal
White and Hornsey [34]	1.6–1.9	Cervical
White and Hornsey [34]	4.1–4.9	Lumbal
Own results	1.54	Cervical

of 53.6 Gy using hyperfractionation can be applied safely. In fact, the true tolerance dose of spinal cord may be far higher. This could not be examined using our clinical data because of the limited dose to spinal cord. Here we had to analyze the world literature.

There it was rather difficult to derive exact BED values from the data published. It sometimes was not stated clearly whether the doses were applied to the ICRU reference point or the spinal cord itself. There was a great variety of techniques, beam qualities and dosages. In summary, in only 48 out of 68 papers did we succeed in computing a BED of any reliability.

The main problem evaluating literature data was, however, whether the tolerance data were based on the complete avoidance of myelopathy (e.g. the tolerance dose 0% over 5 years, TD 0/5) or whether a frequency of 5% was accepted as tolerable (e.g. the tolerance dose 5% over 5 years, TD 5/5).

Table 7 shows a selection of important literature data with – to our knowledge – the highest BEDs *yielding no myelopathy.* In our opinion, these data allow the conclusion that a BED of 115 Gy seems to be safe. This fits with a total dose of 50 Gy given in 25 single doses of 2.0 Gy once daily or, alternatively, to a total dose of 64. 8 Gy given in 54 single doses of 1.2 Gy

Table 7. TD 0/5 data taken from literature

Author(s)	Total/single dose, Gy	BED (Gy, $\alpha/\beta = 1.54$ Gy)
Dische et al. [25]	30/5	127
Orecchia et al. [38]	46/2	106
Petrovich et al. [39]	50/2	115
Wong et al. [40]	50/2	115

Table 8. TD 5/5 data taken from literature

Author(s)	Total/single dose, Gy	BED (Gy, $\alpha/\beta = 1.54$ Gy)	Incidence of myelopathy, %
Abramson et al. [41]	40/4	144	1.5
Glanzmann et al. [42]	42.5–61.5/1.68–2.25	95–151	2.1
Macbeth et al. [28]	39/3	115	2.5
Schultheiss and Stephens [43]	60/2	140	5
Simpson et al. [44]	36/6	176	1.9
Van Harskamp et al. [45]	48/3	142	2.7

twice daily (interval between the doses at least 6 hours). The results of some authors (e.g. Dische et al. [25]) indicate that this value might be even higher.

There were a few author groups [26–29] that reported a myelopathy frequency in the range of 1.1–12.5% after a BED of 110–115 Gy. It must be pointed out, however, that two of them [27, 28] applied a single dose of 2.7–3.0 Gy. The important influence of the single dose (see experimental data) might explain these differences. Furthermore, Fossa et al. [26] report lumbar myelopathy, while the paper published by Locksmith and Powers [27] is rather old (1968) so that influences of dose distribution and beam qualities cannot be excluded. Despite these results, a total dose of 50 Gy (probably even a higher dose) seems nowadays to be recommendable.

Accepting a 5% risk of myelopathy as the highest tolerable frequency, the dose values taken from the literature are far higher. Table 8 shows a selection of important literature data with doses yielding frequencies of myelopathy in the range of 1.5–5%. In our opinion, these data allow the conclusion that – taking into account a myelopathy rate of 5% – a BED of 140–150 Gy seems to be tolerable. This fits with a total dose of 60–65 Gy in single doses of 2.0 Gy once daily or, alternatively, with a total dose of 78–84 Gy given in single doses of 1.2 Gy twice daily.

Conclusions

The animal experiments resulted in the significant probability that using hyperfractionation a 28% higher dose (at the 50% level of damage) or a 39% higher dose (at the 5% level of damage) could be applied compared to using conventional fractionation.

The α/β value was 1.54 Gy at the 50% level of damage and 0.17 Gy at the 5% level of damage; however this last value is rather uncertain due to the sparse data in this part of the dose-effect curve.

Data taken from the literature and the own clinical experience suggest that a total dose of 50 Gy in daily single doses of 2.0 or 64.8 Gy in twice-daily single doses of 1.2 Gy seems to be safely applicable to human cervical spinal cord.

Acknowledgment

The authors acknowledge Mr. A.G. Page for his meticulous repeated corrections of the manuscript.

References

1 Van der Kogel AJ: Late Effects of Radiation on the Spinal Cord. Amsterdam, University of Amsterdam, 1979.
2 Niewald M, Feldmann U, Feiden W, Niedermayer I, Kiessling M, Lehmann W, Abel U, Berberich W, Staut W, Büscher E, Walter K, Nieder C, Nestle U, Deinzer M, Schnabel K: Multivariate logistic analysis of dose-effect relationship and latency of radiomyelopathy after hyperfractionated and conventionally fractionated radiotherapy in animal experiments. Int J Radiat Oncol Biol Phys 1998; 41:681–688.
3 Van der Kogel AJ: Radiation tolerance of the rat spinal cord: Time-dose relationships. Radiology 1977;122:505–509.
4 Goffinet DR, Marsa GW, Brown JM: The effects of single and multifraction radiation courses on the mouse spinal cord. Radiology 1976;119:709–713.
5 Hopewell JW, Morris AD, Dixon Brown A: The influence of field size on the late tolerance of the rat spinal cord to single doses of X-rays. Br J Radiol 1987;60:1099–1108.
6 Hosmer DW, Lemeshow S: Applied Logistic Regression. New York, Wiley, 1989.
7 SAS/STAT User's Giude. Cary, SAS Institute Inc, 1989.
8 Rubin P, Whitaker JN, Ceckler TL, Nelson D, Gregory PK, Baggs RB, Constine LS, Herman PK: Myelin basic protein and magnetic resonance imaging for diagnosing radiation myelopathy. Int J Radiat Oncol Biol Phys 1988;15:1371–1381.
9 Schultheiss TE, Stephens LC, Jiang GL, Ang KK, Peters LJ: Radiation myelopathy in primates treated with conventional fractionation. Int J Radiat Oncol Biol Phys 1990;19:935–940.
10 Schultheiss TE, Stephens LC, Ang KK, Jardine JH, Peters LJ: Neutron RBE for primate spinal cord treated with clinical regimens. Radiat Res 1992;129:212–217.
11 Schultheiss TE, Stephens LC, Ang KK, Price RE, Peters LJ: Volume effects in rhesus monkey spinal cord. Int J Radiat Oncol Biol Phys 1994;29:67–72.
12 Mason KA, Withers HR, Chiang CS: Late effects of radiation on the lumbar spinal cord of guinea pigs: Re-treatment tolerance. Int J Radiat Oncol Biol Phys 1993;26:643–648.

13   Van den Aardweg GJ, Hopewell JW, Whitehouse EM, Calvo W: A new model of radiation-induced myelopathy: A comparison of the response of mature and immature pigs. Int J Radiat Oncol Biol Phys 1994;29:763–770.

14   Lavey RS, Johnstone AK, Taylor JM, McBride WH: The effect of hyperfractionation on spinal cord response to radiation. Int J Radiat Oncol Biol Phys 1992;24:681–686.

15   Lelieveld P, Brown JM, Goffinet DR, Schoeppel SL, Scoles M: The effect of BCNU on mouse skin and spinal cord in single drug and radiation exposures. Int J Radiat Oncol Biol Phys 1979;5: 1565–1568.

16   Habermalz HJ, Valley B, Habermalz E: Radiation myelopathy of the mouse spinal cord – Isoeffect correlations after fractionated radiation. Strahlenther Onkol 1987;163:626–632.

17   Hornsey S, White A: Isoeffect curve for radiation myelopathy. Br J Radiol 1980;53:168–169.

18   Melki PS, Halimi P, Wibault P, Masnou P, Doyon D: MRI in chronic progressive radiation myelopathy. J Comput Assist Tomogr 1994;18:1–6.

19   Masuda K, Reid BO, Withers HR: Dose-effect relationship for epilation and late effects on spinal cord in rats exposed to gamma rays. Radiology 1977;122:239–242.

20   Ang KK, van der Kogel AJ, van der Schueren E: The effect of small radiation doses on the rat spinal cord: The concept of partial tolerance. Int J Radiat Oncol Biol Phys 1983;9:1487–1491.

21   Van der Kogel AJ, Barendsen GW: Late effects of spinal cord irradiation with 300 kV X-rays and 15 MeV neutrons. Br J Radiol 1974;47:393–398.

22   Van der Schueren E, Landuyt W, Ang KK, van der Kogel AJ: From 2 Gy to 1 Gy per fraction: Sparing effect in rat spinal cord? Int J Radiat Oncol Biol Phys 1988;14:297–300.

23   Ang KK, van der Kogel AJ, van der Schueren E: Lack of evidence for increased tolerance of rat spinal cord with decreasing fraction doses below 2 Gy. Int J Radiat Oncol Biol Phys 1985;11:105–110.

24   Powers BE, Beck ER, Gillette EL, Gould DH, LeCouter RA: Pathology of radiation injury to the canine spinal cord. Int J Radiat Oncol Biol Phys 1992;23:539–549.

25   Dische S, Warburton MF, Saunders MI: Radiation myelitis and survival in the radiotherapy of lung cancer. Int J Radiat Oncol Biol Phys 1988;15:75–81.

26   Fossa SD, Aass N, Kaalhus O: Long-term morbidity after infradiaphragmatic radiotherapy in young men with testicular cancer. Cancer 1989;64:404–408.

27   Locksmith JP, Powers WE: Permanent radiation myelopathy. Am J Roentgenol Radium Ther Nucl Med 1968;102:916–926.

28   Macbeth FR, Wheldon TE, Girling DJ, Stephens RJ, Machin D, Bleehen NM, Lamont A, Radstone DJ, Reed NS: Radiation myelopathy: Estimates of risk in 1,048 patients in three randomized trials of palliative radiotherapy for non-small cell lung cancer. The Medical Research Council Lung Cancer Working Party. Clin Oncol R Coll Radiol 1996;8:176–181.

29   Macbeth FR, Bolger JJ, Hopwood P, Bleehen NM, Cartmell J, Girling DJ, Machin D, Stephens RJ, Bailey AJ: Randomized trial of palliative two-fraction versus more intensive 13-fraction radiotherapy for patients with inoperable non-small cell lung cancer and good performance status. Medical Research Council Lung Cancer Working Party. Clin Oncol R Coll Radiol 1996;8:167–175.

30   Leith JT, DeWyngaert JK, Glicksman AS: Radiation myelopathy in the rat: An interpretation of dose effect relationships. Int J Radiat Oncol Biol Phys 1981;7:1673–1677.

31   Reinhold HS, van Putten WL, Hopewell JW, van der Kogel AJ: The latent period in clinical radiation myelopathy (editorial). Int J Radiat Oncol Biol Phys 1984;10:2385–2387.

32   Ang KK, Thames HD, van der Kogel AJ, van der Schueren E: Is the rate of repair of radiation-induced sublethal damage in rat spinal cord dependent on the size of dose per fraction? Int J Radiat Oncol Biol Phys 1987;13:557–562.

33   Hall EJ: Radiobiology for the Radiologist. Philadelphia, Lippincott, 1994.

34   White A, Hornsey S: Radiation damage to the rat spinal cord: The effect of single and fractionated doses of X-rays. Br J Radiol 1978;51:515–523.

35   Van der Kogel AJ: Radiation-induced damage in the central nervous system: An interpretation of target-cell reponses. Br J Cancer 1986;53(suppl VII):207–217.

36   Thames HD, Ang KK, Stewarts FA, van der Schueren E: Does incomplete repair explain the apparent failure of the basic LQ model to predict spinal cord and kidney responses to low doses per fraction? Int J Radiat Biol Relat Stud Phys Chem Med 1988;54:13–19.

37   Van der Kogel AJ, Gutin PH, Leibel SA, Sheline GE (eds): Radiation Injury to the Nervous System, chapter 6: Central Nervous System Radiation Injury in Small Animal Models. New York, Raven Press, 1991, pp 91–111.
38   Orecchia R, Airoldi M, Sola B, Ragona R, Bussi M, Bongioannini G, Cavalot A, Valente G: Results of chemotherapy plus external reirradiation in the treatment of locally advanced recurrences of nasopharyngeal carcinoma. Eur J Cancer B Oral Oncol 1992;28B:109–111.
39   Petrovich Z, Stanley K, Cox JD, Paig C: Radiotherapy in the management of locally advanced lung cancer of all cell types: Final report of randomized trial. Cancer 1981;48:1335–1340.
40   Wong CS, Van Dyk J, Milosevic M, Laperriere NJ: Radiation myelopathy following single courses of radiotherapy and retreatment (see comments). Int J Radiat Oncol Biol Phys 1994;30:575–581.
41   Abramson N, Cavanaugh PJ: Short-course radiation therapy in carcinoma of the lung. A second look. Radiology 1973;108:685–687.
42   Glanzmann C, Aberle HG, Horst W: The risk of chronic progressive radiation myelopathy. Strahlentherapie 1976;152:363–372.
43   Schultheiss TE, Stephens LC: Invited review: Permanent radiation myelopathy. Br J Radiol 1992; 65:737–753.
44   Simpson JR, Perez CA, Phillips TL, Concannon JP, Carella RJ: Large fraction radiotherapy plus misonidazole for treatment of advanced lung cancer: Report of a phase I/II trial. Int J Radiat Oncol Biol Phys 1982;8:303–308.
45   Van Harskamp G, Boven E, Vermorken JB, van Deutekom H, Stam J, Njo KH, Karim AB, Tierie AH, Golding RP, Pinedo HM: Phase II trial of combined radiotherapy and daily low-dose cisplatin for inoperable, locally advanced non-small cell lung cancer (NSCLC). Int J Radiat Oncol Biol Phys 1987;13:1735–1738.

Marcus Niewald, MD, Department of Radiotherapy, University Hospital of Saarland,
D–66421 Homburg (Germany)
Tel. +49 6841 164626, Fax +49 6841 164673, E-Mail ramnie@med-rz.uni-sb.de

Wiegel T, Hinkelbein W, Brock M, Hoell T (eds): Controversies in Neuro-Oncology.
Front Radiat Ther Oncol. Basel, Karger, 1999, vol 33, pp 305–314

....

Dose-Volume Tolerance of the Brainstem after High-Dose Radiotherapy

J. Debus [a], *E.B. Hug* [b], *N.J. Liebsch* [b], *D. O'Farrel* [b], *D. Finkelstein* [b],
J. Efird [b], *J.E. Munzenrider* [b]

[a] Department of Radiation Oncology, University of Heidelberg, Germany
[b] Department of Radiation Oncology, Massachusetts General Hospital, Boston, Mass.
    and Harvard Cyclotron Laboratory, Cambridge, Mass., USA, and

Introduction

Radiotherapy of head and neck tumors and skull base tumors may be associated with significant radiation to the unaffected brainstem. Permanent injury to the brainstem or spinal cord can be a devastating complication of patients treated by radiotherapy [28]. In 1950, Boden [4, 5] described 6/24 patients with brainstem necrosis after treatment with orthovoltage radiation for tumors of the middle ear and nasopharynx. He concluded that the brainstem is more radiosensitive than the cerebrum. Since that time several published reports have attempted to define radiation tolerance of the cervical spinal cord [2, 6, 14, 15, 22]. Only a few however have analyzed systematically tolerance of brainstem to homogeneous radiation of the whole brainstem and there are no published reports of brainstem tolerance to inhomogeneous radiation. Optimized conformal radiotherapy requires accurate data on tumor control and tolerance of critical nontarget structures such as brainstem or spinal cord to inhomogeneous radiotherapy.

There are different tools available to evaluate treatment plans and dose distributions in conformal radiotherapy. Dose-volume histograms are used to reduce the information of a three-dimensional dose distribution. The value of dose-volume histograms has not yet been examined for clinical decisions regarding radiotolerance of brainstem.

Parts of this paper have been published before.

Wiegel T, Hinkelbein W, Brock M, Hoell T (eds): Controversies in Neuro-Oncology.
Front Radiat Ther Oncol. Basel, Karger, 1999, vol 33, pp 318–326

....

A Status of Radiotherapy for Cerebral Metastases

R. Engenhart-Cabillic

Department of Radiotherapy, Philipps University, Marburg, Germany

Introduction

For the last two decades the number of patients with diagnosed brain metastases has increased clearly. Responsible for the increased frequency are, among others, improved radiological imaging, effective therapeutical control of primary cancer with the prolongation of median survival time as well as changes in the age pyramid resulting in increasing affection to tumor disease.

Up to 20% of patients with malignancies develop symptomatic brain metastases. For most of these patients, progress of neurologic deficits is a dominant symptom limiting the prognosis. Untreated patients have a median survival of about 1 month, treatment with corticosteroids results in a median survival of 2 months, whereas patients treated with whole-brain radiotherapy have a median survival of 3–6 months [3, 10, 13, 16]. The median survival increases from 6 to 12 months in patients who received craniotomy and postoperative irradiation to the brain [20–22]. The optimal therapy, however, for patients with metastatic disease depends on the tumor type, spread and the clinical setting. Whatever the modalities of treatment are, median survival of >12 months are only reported in superselective prognostically favorable groups of patients. However, for most patients, palliation of neurological symptoms remains the primary therapeutic goal. Short treatment time with an immediate improvement or at least maintenance of quality of life is of great importance. Consequently, numerous clinical trials have investigated different dose fractionation schemes. The overall poor prognosis of these patients has complicated the evaluation of treatment effectiveness. However, a group of patients was identified for which an aggressive schedule showed a clear benefit in quality of life and length of survival [6, 9, 19].

Radiosurgery as a minimally invasive therapy modality enables the local application of a high single dosis, while the tolerance dose of the normal brain tissue is not exceeded. In this article the author reviews the experience of different time-dose fractionation schemes under the special consideration of prognostically referable characteristics in patients with brain metastases.

Prognostic Factors

The prognosis of patients with brain metastases which have been reported from different treatment modalities might be biased by selecting factors as to quality of life and survival is influenced by tumor- and patient-related factors. Based on multivariate analysis of the survival data from large RTOG studies, only few independent favorable factors were defined [6]. The following independent factors were identified for their prognostic value on survival of brain metastases patients: Performance status, extracranial tumor activity (stable vs. progressive and metastatic exstent) and age. Independent prognostic characteristics are: KPS 70:100, patients without extracranial metastases and with controlled primary tumors, patients of age <60 years and younger; lesions with the highest predicted ability of surviving assess all favorable characteristics (52% of patients survive >6 months; 30%/year). Conversely the most unfavorable surviving rates are defined with patients having uncontrolled extracerebral tumor manifestation [6]. Therefore, patients with good performance status, controlled or absent extracranial tumor activity, age <60 years, should be treated with an aggressive modality [9, 20]. Especially for patients with single brain metastases, radiosurgery or surgery combined with radiotherapy should be used.

Treatment Technique

WBRT: For patients with multiple brain metastases the primary option is whole-brain irradiation [3, 11, 14]. The choice of treatment, total dose and dose per fraction should be based on prognostic value [6]. For patients with progressive extracranial disease, rapid accelerated regimes should be considered. More protracted schedules (40 Gy in 4 weeks) should be used for patients in a good performance status without extracerebral disease to avoid neurocognitive deficits seen in patients with higher single dose. WBRT contains the entire intracranial contents, through opposing lateral fields. Under simulation the inferior field border should be inferior to the cribriforme plate, the middle cranial fossa and the foramen magnum. Treatment should be considered with of radiosurgery and whole-brain radiotherapy resulted in a superior local control rate with 92 and 86% at 1 and 2 years after treatment. For radiosurgery alone, the 1- and 2-year actual local control rates were 89 and 72%. Overall actual median survival was 5.5 months (range 0.5–91) for the whole series. The 1-year survival rate was 19.2% in the group of patients treated with radiosurgery alone and 30.4% after combined modality treatment (p = 0.75). Independent prognostic factor for survival (p < 0.001) was low evidence of extracranial progression at the time of treatment (median survival 12.5 vs. 4.4 months) in patients without extracranial disease. A trend of superior survival after combination of radiosurgery with whole-brain radiotherapy was found with a median survival of 15.4 months instead of 8.3 months. For patients with active extracranial disease at the time of radiosurgery there was no difference in survival between both treatment modalities. Flickinger et al. [11] reported improved local control after combination of radiosurgery and whole-brain radiotherapy, but no improvement in survival. In the Heidelberg group, the subgroup of patients without extracranial disease survival equals the data reported in randomized and nonrandomized trials comparing surgery alone with the combination of whole-brain radiotherapy.

Conclusions

Patients undergoing surgery and radiotherapy have significantly fewer recurrences at the initial metastatic sight compared to those receiving radiotherapy alone. They also have significant increased survival and improved quality of life. The biological and physical characteristics of metastases, the lack of invasion, < 3 cm in diameter and spherical, appear to make them ideal radiosurgery targets. SRS is now an established treatment modality for solitary brain metastases. Theoretically, multiple sites of diseases can even be treated in a high palliative manner without hair loss or increase in neurologic morbidity. In general, SRS is not recommended as first-line treatment of multiple brain metastases, but may represent a reasonable option for recurrent metastases.

Potential advantages of radiosurgery over surgery are reduced morbidity and reduced health-care costs. With similar results, cost-effectiveness issues may ultimately become significant in deciding the choice of treatment [2]. Metha et al. [18] published cost-utility studies comparing SRS vs. resection for single brain metastases. This as other modeling studies indicate that overall SRS may produce superior cost-effectiveness. Without compromising survival and local control it is reasonable to postulate that SRS may be able to replace neurosurgical resection as the treatment of choice in most patients with solitary brain metastases.

References

1 Alexander E III, Moriarity TM, Davis RB, et al: Stereotactic radiosurgery for the definitive noninvasive treatment of brain metastases. J Natl Cancer Inst 1995;87:34–40.

2 Auchter RM, Lamond JP, Alexander E III, et al: A multi-institutional outcome and prognostic factor analysis of radiosurgery for resectable single brain metastases. Int J Radiat Oncol Biol Phys 1996;35:27–35.

3 Borgelt B, Gelber R, Kramer S, et al: The palliation of brain metastases: Final results of the first two studies by the Radiation Therapy Oncology Group. Int J Radiat Oncol Biol Phys 1980;6:1–9.

4 Borgelt B, Gelber R, Larson M, et al: Ultra-rapid dose irradiation schedules for the palliation of brain metastases: Final results of the first two studies by the Radiation Therapy Oncology Group. Int J Radiat Oncol Biol Phys 1981;7:1633–1638.

5 Brenemann JC, Warnick RE, Albright RE Jr, et al: Stereotactic surgery for the treatment of brain metastases. Cancer 1997;79:551–557.

6 Diener-West M, Dobbins TW, Philips TL, Nelson DF: Identification of an optimal subgroup for treatment evaluation of patients with brain metastases using RTOG study 7916. Int J Radiat Oncol Biol Phys 1989;16:669–673.

7 Engenhart R, Kimmig BN, Hover K, et al: Long-term follow-up for brain metastases treated by percutaneous single high dose radiation. Cancer 1993;71:1353–1361.

8 Engenhart R, Wowra B, Kimmig B, et al: Stereotaktische Konvergenzbestrahlung: Aktuelle Perspektiven auf der Grundlage klinischer Ergebnisse. Strahlenther Onkol 1992;168:245–259.

9 Epstein BE, Scott CB, Sause WT, et al: Improved survival duration in patients with unresected solitary brain metastases using accelerated hyperfractionated radiation therapy at total doses of 54.4 Gy and greater. Cancer 1993;71:1362–1367.

10 Flentje M, Kober B, Kohlmann H, Schneider G, Kimmig B: Ergebnisse der Strahlentherapie bei Hirnmetastasen unter Berücksichtigung der Computertomographie. Strahlentherapie 1987;163:148–153.

11 Flickinger JC, Kondziolka D, Lunsford LD, et al: A multi-institutional experience with stereotactic radiosurgery for solitary brain metastases. Int J Radiat Oncol Biol Phys 1994;28:797–802.

12 Fuller BG, Kaplan ID, Adler J, et al: Stereotactic radiosurgery for brain metastases: The importance of adjuvant whole brain irradiation. Int J Radiat Oncol Biol Phys 1992;23:413–418.

13 Glanzmann C: Palliative Radiotherapie von Hirnmetastasen solider Tumoren: Erfahrungen mit hohen Dosen. Strahlenther Onkol 1990;166:119–124.

14 Hendrickson F: The optimum schedule for palliative radiotherapy for metastatic brain cancer. Int J Radiat Oncol Biol Phys 1977;2:165–168.

15 Kocher M, Voges J, Müller RP, Sturm V, Müller J, Staar S, Lehrke R: Linac radiosurgery for patients with a limited number of brain metastases. J Radiosurg 1998;1:9–15.

16 Komarnicky L, Phillips T, Marth K, et al: A randomized phase III trial for the evaluation of misonidazole combined with radiation in the treatment of patients with brain metastases (RTOG-7916). Int J Radiat Oncol Biol Phys 1991;20:53–58.

17 Loeffler JS, Alexander E: Radiosurgery for the treatment of intracranial metastases; in Alexander E, Loeffler JS, Lunsford D (eds): Stereotactic Radiosurgery. New York, McGraw-Hill, 1993.

18 Mehta MP, Boyd TS, Sinha P: The status of stereotactic radiosurgery for cerebral metastases in 1998. J Radiosurg 1998;1:17–30.

19 Nieder C, Berberich W, Nestle U, Niewald M, Walter K, Schnabel K, et al: Relation between local result and total dose of radiotherapy for brain metastases. Int J Radiat Oncol Biol Phys 1995;33:349–355.

20 Noordijk EM, Vecht CJ, Haaxma-Reiche H, et al: The choice of treatment of single brain metastases should be made based on extracranial tumor activity and age. Int J Radiat Oncol Biol Phys 1994;29:711–717.

21 Nussbaum ES, Djalilian HR, Cho KH, et al: Brain metastases: Histology, multiplicity, surgery and survival. Cancer 1996;78:1781–1788.

22 Patchell RA, Tibbs PA, Walsh JW, et al: Randomized trial of surgery in the treatment of single metastases to the brain. N Engl J Med 1990;322:494–500

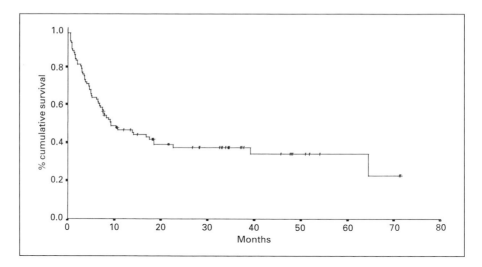

Fig. 1. Cumulative survival curves of 111 patients with single or multiple brain metastases after complete resection of all lesions. Median overall survival and median independent survival – defined as length of survival with a KPS >80 – are 9.2 and 5.5 months, respectively. Causes of death were defined as neurological in 18%, systemic in 49% and as mixed (neur./ syst.) in 33%, if decisions were arbitrary.

score at time of discharge had dropped to a median of 60 ranging from 20 to 90. After 3 months the KPS score had reached 80 (40–100) again. Local control rate, defined as no recurrence of metastases at operative site, was 85% according to serial imaging. According to the questionnaires, 87% of survivors responded in a positive manner to questions related to their surgery, hospitalization and follow-up period.

Actuarial median survival for the whole group of patients was 9.2 months irrespective of operation for single or multiple lesions. Overall median independent survival, defined as length of survival with KPS score >80, was 5.5 months. Cause of death was neurological in 18%, mixed in 33% and systemic in 49% (fig. 1).

A highly significant difference in median survival was related to preoperative performance regardless of age. The cut-off line in KPS score was calculated as high as 80. Survival periods were 22.6 vs. 4.6 months in the respective groups with 40% long-term survivors (>4 years) in the former (fig. 2). Significant neurological deficits accounted for severely depressed preoperative performance in the majority of patients (see inclusion criteria). Extent of systemic disease, however, did not reach statistical significance in difference between median survival (16.8 vs. 7.9 months) with still 25% long-term survivors in the latter group (fig. 3).

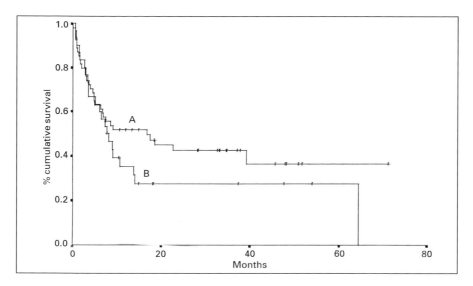

Fig. 2. Cumulative survival dependent on extent of systemic disease, defined as presence of at least one extracerebral metastasis. Although no statistically significant difference could be calculated (p=0.22, log-rank test), median survival was 16.8 months in patients without (line A) and 7.9 months in those with extracerebral metastases (line B).

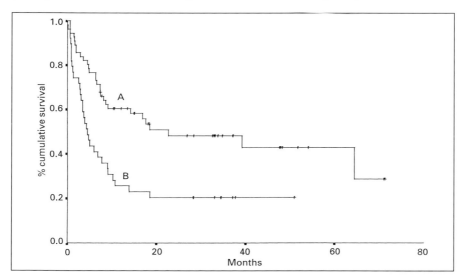

Fig. 3. Highly significant difference in cumulative survival dependent on preoperative performance (p=0.0009 log-rank test). Cut-off KPS was calculated as 80. A Karnofsky index ≥80, independent of age and status of systemic disease proved to be the single most important factor for long and independent survival. Median survival in patients with a preoperative KPS ≥80 (line A) was 22.6 months as opposed to 4.6 months in those with a preoperative KPS <80 (line B).

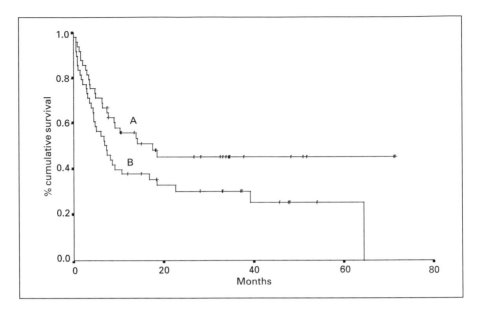

Fig. 4. Survival related to eloquency of tumor site reached a difference close to statistical significance (0.055 log-rank test), but was no independent variable, since eloquency correlated closely with postoperative morbidity (see fig. 5). Median survival in patients with metastases in noneloquent locations (line A) was 17.7 and 7.0 months with eloquent lesions (line B).

A statistical difference close to significance was found in median survival related to eloquency of tumor site. Median survival after resection of metastases in noneloquent brain areas was 17.7 vs. 7.0 months after resection in eloquent regions (fig. 4). The reason behind this was a 2.5-fold increased risk for operative morbidity in patients with lesions in eloquent regions of the brain. Survival related to the occurrence of postoperative complications showed a highly significant difference (16.8 vs. 3.2 months; fig. 5) with no long-term survivors in the latter group. Consequently, a significant dependency of length of survival on immediate postoperative KPS score (cut-off line 80) was also observed (18.6 vs. 5.1 months; fig. 6).

Discussion

In this paper the results from a database of a prospective study on neurosurgical treatment of single and multiple CNS metastases were in part presented. Several other possible calculations and correlations between variables were omitted either for reasons of irrelevance to the defined subject of inquiry

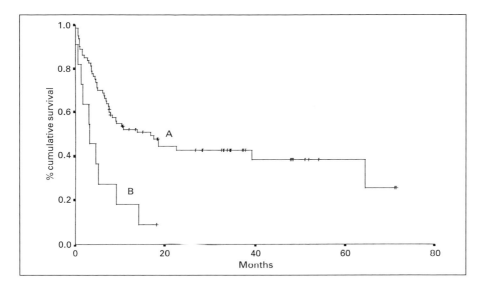

Fig. 5. Occurrence of postoperative complications correlated highly significant (0.015 log-rank test) with short median survival (3.2 months, line B), with no long-term survivors and no independent survival. Patients without postoperative complications had a median survival of 16.8 months (line A).

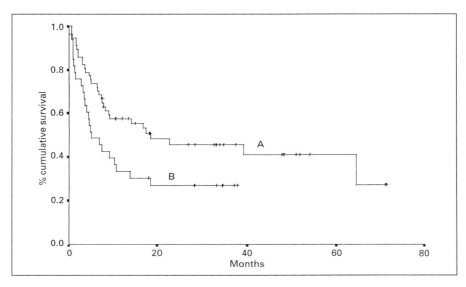

Fig. 6. As a consequence of the close dependency of survival on the occurrence of operative morbidity (see fig. 5) outcome depended also significantly (0.029 log-rank test) on immediate postoperative KPS. Patients with an immediate postoperative KPS ≥ 80 survived a median of 18.6 months (line A) and those with a postoperative KPS < 80 for 5.1 months (line B).

14 Rosner D, Nemoto T, Lane WW: Chemotherapy induces regression of brain metastases in breast carcinoma. Cancer 1986;58:832–839.

15 Cocconi G, Lottici R, Bisagni G, Bacchi M, Tonato M, Passalacqua R, Boni C, Belsanti V, Bassi P: Combination therapy with platinum and etoposide of brain metastases from breast carcinoma. Cancer Invest 1990;8:327–334.

16 Boogerd W, Dalesio O, Bais EM, van der Sande JJ: Response of brain metastases from breast cancer to systemic chemotherapy. Cancer 1992;69:972–980.

17 Rustin GJS, Newlands ES, Bagshawe KD, Begent RHJ, Crawford SM: Successful management of metastatic and primary germ cell tumors in the brain. Cancer 1986;57:2108–2113.

18 Rustin GJS, Newlands ES, Begent RHJ, Dent J, Bagshawe KD: Weekly alternating etoposide, methotrexate, and actinomycin/vincristine and cyclophosphamide chemotherapy for the treatment of CNS metastases of choriocarcinoma. J Clin Oncol 1989;7:900–903.

19 Ardizzoni A, Hansen H, Dombernowsky P, Gamucci T, Kaplan S, Postmus P, Schaefer B, Wanders J: Topotecan, a new active drug in the second-line treatment of small-cell lung cancer: A phase II study in patients with refractory and sensitive disease. J Clin Oncol 1997;15:2090–2096.

20 Bokemayer C, Nowak P, Haupt A, Metzner B, Köhne H, Hartman JT, Kanz L, Schmoll HJ: Treatment of brain metastases in patients with testicular cancer. J Clin Oncol 1997;15:1449–1454.

A. Korfel, Department of Hematology, Oncology and Transfusion Medicine, University Hospital Benjamin Franklin, Freie Universität Berlin, Hindenburgdamm 30, D–12200 Berlin (Germany)

Wiegel T, Hinkelbein W, Brock M, Hoell T (eds): Controversies in Neuro-Oncology.
Front Radiat Ther Oncol. Basel, Karger, 1999, vol 33, pp 349–353

....

Primary CNS Lymphoma: Chemotherapy followed by Radiotherapy or Chemotherapy Alone? A Randomized Multicentric Study

E. Thiel, A. Korfel, W. Hinkelbein

Department of Hematology, Oncology and Transfusion Medicine, University
Hospital Benjamin Franklin, Freie Universität Berlin, Germany

Introduction

Primary CNS lymphoma (PCNSL), initially considered to account for
less than 2% of all non-Hodgkin's lymphomas, is becoming a more frequent
tumor. The increasing incidence is not only due to the increasing number of
immunodeficient patients, but is also seen in immunocompetent individuals
[1]. PCNSL are usually large B-cell, infiltrative tumors with no spread outside
the CNS. Molecular and phenotypic profile of PCNSL correspond to that of
germinal center B cells [2]. In contrast to AIDS patients, no Epstein-Barr virus
genomic DNA could be found within the lymphoma cells in immunocompetent
patients. Recently, there is some evidence for a pathogenetic contribution of
human herpesvirus 8 in both HIV-positive and HIV-negative patients [3].

Therapy of PCNSL

Whole-brain radiotherapy (WBRT) has been the standard treatment for
PCNSL in the last 20 years. Retrospective reviews showed an increase in
survival from 3 to 4 months without any treatment to 12–16 months with
WBRT. The radiation dose-response relationship suggested by retrospective
analyses could not be confirmed in the phase II trial of high-dose radiotherapy
conducted by the Radiation Therapy Oncology Group (RTOG) [4]. The con-

Table 1. BMPD and idarubicin/ifosfamide chemotherapy regimens

BMPD			
BCNU	80 mg/m^2	Intravenously (IV)	Day 1
Methotrexate	15 mg	Intrathecally	Day 1[a]
Methotrexate	1,500 mg/m^2	IV (over 24 h)	Day 2
Procarbazine	100 mg/m^2	Orally	Days 1–8
Dexamethasone	3 × 8 mg	Orally	Days 1–14[b]
	Retreatment after 21 days		
Idarubicin/ifosfamide			
Idarubicin	12 mg/m^2	IV	Days 1–2
Ifosfamide	3 g/m^2	IV (over 24 h)	Day 1
Dexamethasone	3 × 8 mg[b]	Orally	Days 1–14
	Retreatment after 21 days		

[a] Repeated in patients with meningeal involvement.
[b] In course 1 only.

tinued downward trend in survival in this trial and the 92% local failure rate show the limits of radiation alone for treatment of PCNSL.

The effectivity of chemotherapy to treat PCNSL was first demonstrated in 1977 using high-dose methotrexate and leucovorin rescue [5]. Since that time many reports of chemotherapy-induced remissions and survival prolongations up to >30 months have been published. The majority of these reports were retrospective reviews of small and heterogeneously treated collectives. Chemotherapy was usually combined with radiotherapy in these studies. The most encouraging results have been reported by DeAngelis et al. [6] who used WBRT 'sandwiched' between systemic and intrathecal methotrexate and high-dose cytarabine, resulting in a median survival of 42.5 months. In two recent reviews of many published series comprising 792 and 1,408 immunocompetent patients with PCNSL, respectively, the median survival of patients treated with radiotherapy alone was 16.6 versus 29.1 months in patients treated with radiotherapy and chemotherapy in one review, and 16 versus 27 months in the other [7, 8]. Although the optimal chemotherapy protocol is not known, the results of the studies published suggest that high-dose methotrexate is the most efficacious drug in the treatment of PCNSL. Also, the drugs chosen should penetrate the intact blood-brain barrier (BBB), since no survival prolongation as compared to WBRT alone could be reached, when cytostatics unable to cross the BBB were used [9, 10].

As survival of patients with PCNSL after the combined treatment increases, the problem of late neurotoxicity is gaining interest. In two recently

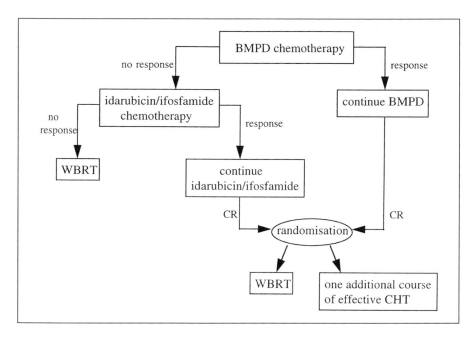

Fig. 1. Study design. CHT = Chemotherapy; CR = complete remission.

published analyses the incidence of leukoencephalopathy in long-term survivors was estimated to be 37 and 26%, respectively [11, 12]. The major risk factors for developing leukoencephalopathy were the age and the sequence radiotherapy before chemotherapy, respectively. Sustained responses following chemotherapy without subsequent WBRT to reduce the risk of late neurotoxicity have been seen [13–15]. However, the survival duration and the incidence of leukoencephalopathy after chemotherapy alone and chemotherapy followed by radiotherapy, have never been compared in a prospective randomized study.

Response-Adjusted Primary Chemotherapy of PCNSL in HIV-Negative Patients with BCNU, Methotrexate, Procarbazine and Dexamethasone (BMPD) and Idarubicin, Ifosfamide with Randomized WBRT

The aim of our recently initiated multicenter randomized trial is to compare the median survival and the late neurotoxicity after chemotherapy alone versus chemotherapy with subsequent WBRT. Eligible are HIV-negative patients with newly diagnosed and histologically confirmed PCNSL. The study protocol is based on exclusively BBB-penetrating drugs. The initial treatment consists of the BMPD chemotherapy (table 1). In a pilot study the BMPD regimen has been shown to be effective and nontoxic [16]. Responding patients are treated with up to 3 cycles of this protocol. Nonresponders receive another chemotherapy protocol composed of idarubicin and ifosfamide (table 1). All complete responders are randomized into subsequent WBRT with 45 Gy or an additional course of the effective chemotherapy regimen (fig. 1). WBRT is performed in all patients who do not reach complete remission after chemotherapy. The study includes the diagnostic of meningeal involvement by the means of polymerase chain reaction and immunocytochemical analysis on poly-L-lysine-coated slides [17, 18].

References

1   Eby NL, Grufferman S, Flannely CM: Increasing incidence of primary brain lymphoma in the US. Cancer 1988;62:2461–2465.
2   Gaidano G, Capello D, Maggiano N, Cingolani A, Rinelli A, Gloghini A: Molecular and phenotypic profile of primary central nervous system lymphoma segregates distinct biologic categories and suggests derivation from germinal center B-cells ASH. ASH Meeting, 1997, abstr 1505.
3   Corboy JR, Garl PJ, Kleinschmidt-DeMasters BK: Human herpesvirus 8 DNA in CNS lymphomas from patients with and without AIDS. Neurology 1998;50:335–340.
4   Nelson DF, Martz KL, Bonner H, Nelson JS, Newall J, Kerman HD: Non-Hodgkin's lymphoma of the brain: Can high dose, large volume radiation therapy improve survival? Report on a prospective trial by the Radiation Therapy Oncology Group (RTOG): RTOG 8315. Int J Radiat Oncol Biol Phys 1992;23:9–17.
5   Skarin AT, Zuckerman KS, Pitman SW, Rosenthal DS, Moloney W, Frei E: High-dose methotrexate with folinic acid in the treatment of advanced non-Hodgkin's lymphoma including CNS involvement. Blood 1977;50:1039–1047.
6   DeAngelis LM, Yahalom J, Thaler HT, Kher U: Combined modality therapy for primary CNS lymphoma. J Clin Oncol 1992;10:635–643.
7   Fine HA, Mayer RJ: Primary central nervous system lymphoma. Ann Intern Med 1993;119:1093–1104.
8   Reni M, Ferreri AJM, Garanzini MP, Villa E: Therapeutic management of primary central nervous system lymphoma in immunocompetent patients. Results of a critical review of the literature. Ann Oncol 1997;8:227–234.
9   Brada M, Dearnaley D, Horwich A: Management of primary cerebral lymphoma with initial chemotherapy: Preliminary results and comparison with patients treated with radiotherapy alone. Int J Radiat Oncol Biol Phys 1990;18:787–792.
10   Schultz C, Scott C, Sherman W, Donahue B, Fields J, Murray K, et al: Preirradiation chemotherapy with cyclophosphamide, doxorubicin, vincristine, and dexamethasone for primary CNS lymphoma: Initial Report of Radiation Therapy Oncology Group Protocol 88-06. J Clin Oncol 1996;14:556–564.
11   Abrey LE, DeAngelis LM, Yahalom J: Long-term survival in primary CNS lymphoma. J Clin Oncol 1998;16:859–863.
12   Blay JY, Conray T, Chevreau C, Thyss A, Quesnel N, Eghbali H, Bouabdallah R, Coiffier B, Wagner JP, LeMevel A, et al: High-dose methotrexate for the treatment of primary cerebral lymphomas: Analysis of survival and late neurologic toxicity in a retrospective series. J Clin Oncol 1998;16:864–871.
13   Neuwelt EA, Goldman DL, Dahlborg SA: Primary CNS lymphoma treated with osmotic blood-brain barrier disruption: Prolonged survival and preservation of cognitive function. J Clin Oncol 1991;9:1580–1590.

14   Cher L, Glass J, Harsh GR, Hochberg FH: Therapy of primary CNS lymphoma with methotrexate-based chemotherapy and deferred radiotherapy: Preliminary results. Neurology 1996;46:1757–1759.

15   Freilich RJ, Delattre JY, Monjour A, DeAngelis LM: Chemotherapy without radiation therapy as initial treatment for primary CNS lymphoma in older patients. Neurology 1996;46:435–439.

16   Thiel E, Korfel A: Successful treatment of non-Hodgkin's lymphoma of the CNS with the BMPD chemotherapy protocol followed by radiotherapy. Exp Hematol 1997;25:846.

17   Rhodes CH, Glantz MJ, Lekos A, Sorenson GD, Hosinger C, et al: A comparison of polymerase chain reaction examination of cerebrospinal fluid and conventional cytology in the diagnosis of lymphomatous meningitis. Cancer 1996;77:543–548.

18   Kranz BR, Thiel E, Thierfelder S: Immunocytochemical identification of meningeal leukemia and lymphoma: Poly-*L*-lysine-coated slides permit multimarker analysis even with minute cerebrospinal fluid cell specimens. Blood 1989;7:1942–1949.

Prof. Dr. E. Thiel, Department of Hematology, Oncology and Transfusion Medicine,
University Hospital Benjamin Franklin, Freie Universität Berlin,
Hindenburgdamm 30, D–12200 Berlin, Germany

Wiegel T, Hinkelbein W, Brock M, Hoell T (eds): Controversies in Neuro-Oncology.
Front Radiat Ther Oncol. Basel, Karger, 1999, vol 33, pp 364–368

....

Topotecan as a 21-Day Continuous Infusion with Accelerated 3D-Conformal Radiation Therapy for Patients with Glioblastoma

Gerhard G. Grabenbauer [a], *Michael Buchfelder* [b], *Ulrich Schrell* [b],
Rudolf Fahlbusch [b], *Rolf Sauer* [a], *Hans-Jürgen Staab* [c]

Departments of [a] Radiation Oncology and [b] Neurosurgery, University Hospitals of
Erlangen, and [c] SmithKline Beecham, München, Germany

Introduction

Despite innovations in imaging, surgery and radiation therapy (RT), local failure remains the principal clinical problem in glioblastoma multiforme (GBM) and highly anaplastic astrocytoma (AA). To date, chemotherapy has no major impact in the treatment of most adult central nervous system (CNS) tumors. The inroads made by chemotherapy in pediatric CNS malignancies suggest that novel drugs, or drug combinations may improve treatment results.

Preclinical studies with the topoisomerase-1 inhibitor topotecan (Tpt) demonstrated unexpected radiosenistizing properties in the human glioma cell line D 54 [Lamond et al., 1996]. In pharmacokinetic and pharmacodynamic investigations within a phase II study it was detected that during a 24- and 72-hour continuous intravenous infusion (CIV) the median CSF penetration of Tpt lactone was 0.29 and 0.42, respectively [Baker et al., 1996].

These features, including the good CNS penetration particularly when the CIV regimen was used prompted us to test CIV together with concurrent RT in a clinical setting (Sauer et al. 1997).

Patients and Methods

Since October 1997, a total of 20 patients was entered into the trial. The median age was 55 years (range 18–73). Fifteen patients had the histologic diagnosis of GBM, 4 were

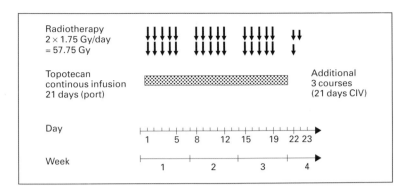

Fig. 1. Treatment protocol of accelerated RT with continuous-infusion Tpt.

diagnosed with recurrent AA and 1 patient with gliosarcoma. The ECOG performance status was required to be between 0 and 2. Before entering the study all patients had given their informed consent and the protocol had been approved by the local ethics committee.

After surgery or stereotactic biopsy, accelerated RT using single fractions of 175 cGy bid was given until a total dose of 5,775 cGy was reached in 3.5 weeks. The minimum interfraction interval was 6 h. All patients were subjected to a 3-d treatment planning process. The contrast enhancing area including edema and a safety margin of 2 cm were treated up to a total dose of 5,075 cGy. An additional local boost of 700 cGy to the macroscopic tumor region was applied resulting in a total dose of 5,775 cGy.

Simultaneous Tpt treatment was given as CIV via port. Tpt doses were increased from 0.3 to 0.8 mg/m^2/day. A minimum of 3 patients per dose level were treated. Chemotherapy was completed with 3 additional cycles at a dose level of 0.5 mg/m^2/day given in 28-day intervals. The protocol is outlined in figure 1. Contrast-enhanced CT or MRI scans were performed after the second and fourth cycle to assess the tumor response.

Results

The 20 patients were given 76 cycles of Tpt. Using the CIV application, toxicity was low and the maximally tolerated dose was not yet reached. Grade 4 hematological toxicity (neutropenia) was seen in 1 patient only at a dose level of 0.5 mg/m^2/day. Grade 3 hematological toxicity was seen in 11/76 cycles, at ≥ 0.7 mg/m^2/day hemotoxicity reached 38% (3/8 cycles). Among the 12 grade 3 and 4 toxicities, 9 were WBC-, 2 Hb- and 1 platelet-related. Toxicity was not increased during the first cycle with concurrent RT. No significant treatment-related toxicity was observed and there was no grade 3 and 4 non-hematological toxicity.

Table 1 summarizes grade 3 and 4 toxicities in this phase I/II trial according to Tpt dose level and number of applied cycles.

Table 1. Grade 3 and 4 hematological toxicities according to Tpt level, dose in mg/m²/day given as a continuous 21-day infusion via port, toxicity was graded according to NCIC CTG toxicity criteria

Tpt level	Anemia	Neutopenia	Thrombocytopenia
0.3	0/10	0/10	0/10
0.4	2/10	0/10	0/10
0.5	0/37	5/37	1/37
0.6	0/11	1/11	0/11
0.7	0/6	2/6	0/6
0.8	0/2	1/2	0/2

Tpt in combination with RT showed an arrest of tumor progression in 15/20 (75%) patients with a median time to progression of 6 months. One patient achieved an objective partial remission. Overall and progression-free survival rates were 39 and 12% at 12 months. The Kaplan–Meier curves for progression-free survival and overall survival rates are outlined in figures 2 and 3.

Discussion

Tpt and its analogues reversibly inhibit the DNA religation step of the reaction catalyzed by the nuclear enzyme topoisomerase-1 (topo-1). This inhibition increases the number of covalent topo-1-DNA complexes within cells, and interaction of these complexes with replication forks results in the formation of small numbers of irreversible double-strand DNA breaks eventually leading to cell death [Kaufmann et al., 1996].

When combined with ionizing radiation in a preclinical setting, cells exposed to Tpt immediately after RT showed a dose-dependent radiosensitization. This effect increased both with exposure time and drug dose and was not seen when cells were treated with the drug before irradiation [Kim et al., 1992].

A recent phase II study tested Tpt alone (1.5 mg/m² daily every 3 weeks) in 31 patients with recurrent and preirradiated malignant glioma. The results with a response rate of 6%, a stable disease in 68% and a median time to progression of 19 weeks seemed promising [Macdonald et al., 1996]. On the other hand, the toxicity of this regimen included grade 4 neutropenia in 58% and grade 4 thrombocytopenia in 10% of the patients. This appears to be a rather inappropriate toxicity for a palliative treatment.

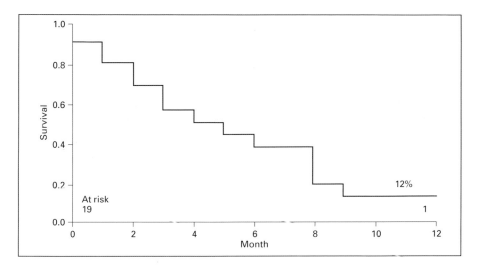

Fig. 2. Progression-free survival in 20 patients with glioblastoma and recurrent AA after accelerated RT with continuous-infusion Tpt.

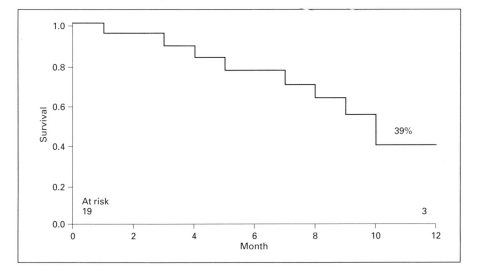

Fig. 3. Overall survival in 20 patients with glioblastoma and recurrent AA after accelerated RT with continuous-infusion Tpt.

Tpt administered as a 21-day continuous infusion (0.5 mg/m^2/day) to patients with colorectal and non-small cell lung cancer [Creemers et al., 1996; Herben et al., 1998] was associated with less hematologic toxicity and seemed therefore preferable in the context of simultaneous radiation in a clinical setting.

Recently, Grant et al. [1997] showed interesting data on the predictive value of 'imaging response' after chemotherapy in malignant glioma. The authors found no difference in survival rates between patients having partial remission, minor remission or stable disease. Only patients with clear disease progression had a significantly reduced survival ($p < 0.001$).

In this phase I/II trial we have seen a response rate of 5% and a stable tumor situation in 75% of the patients at the end of chemotherapy. Given the fact that dose escalation is still ongoing, this combination of radiation and a single-agent chemotherapy deserves further evaluation.

References

Baker SD, Heideman RL, Crom WR, Kuttesch JF, Gajjar A, Steward CF: Cerebrospinal fluid pharmacokinetics and penetration of continuous infusion topotecan in children with central nervous system tumors. Cancer Chemother Pharmacol 1996;37:195–202.

Creemers GJ, Gerrits CJ, Schellens JH, Planting AS, van den Burg ME, van Beurden VM, de Boer-Dennert M, Harteveld M, Loos W, Hudson I, Stoter G, Verweij J: Phase II and pharmacologic study of topotecan administered as a 21-day continuous infusion to patients with colorectal cancer. J Clin Oncol 1996;14:2540–2545.

Grant R, Liang BC, Slattery J, Greenberg HS, Junck L: Chemotherapy response criteria in malignant glioma. Neurology 1997;48:1336–1340.

Herben VM, ten Bokkel-Huinink WW, Schot ME, Hudson I, Beijnen JH: Continuous infusion of low-dose topotecan: Pharmacokinetics and pharmacodynamics during a phase II study in patients with small cell lung cancer. Anticancer Drugs 1998;9:411–418.

Kaufmann SH, Peereboom D, Buckwalter CA, Svingen PA, Grochow LB, Donehower RC, Rowinsky EK: Cytotoxic effects of topotecan combined with various anticancer agents in human cancer cell lines. J Natl Cancer Inst 1996;88:734–741.

Kim JH, Kim HS, Kolozvary A, Khil MS: Potentiation of radiation response in human carcinoma cells in vitro and murine fibrosarcoma in vivo by topotecan, an inhibitor of DNA topoisomerase 1. Int J Radiat Oncol Biol Phys 1992;22:515–518.

Lamond JP, Mehta MP, Boothman DA: The potential of topoisomerase 1 inhibitors in the treatment of CNS malignancies: Report of a synergistic effect between topotecan and radiation. J Neurooncol 1996;30:1–6.

Macdonald D, Cairncross G, Steward D, Forsyth P, Sawka C, Wainman N, Eisenhauer E: Phase II study of topotecan in patients with recurrent malignant glioma. Ann Oncol 1996;7:205–207.

Sauer R, Heuser A: Topoisomerase-1-Inhibitor mit potentiell strahlensensibilisierender Wirkung. Strahlenther Onkol 1997;173:125–130.

G.G. Grabenbauer, MD, Department of Radiation Oncology,
University Hospitals of Erlangen, D–91054 Erlangen (Germany)
Tel. +49 9131 8534086, Fax +49 9131 8539335
E-Mail gerd.grabenbauer@strahlen.med.uni-erlangen.de

Author Index

Subject Index

Ki-67
  grading of gliomas 130–132
  labeling index in anaplastic
    oligodendroglioma 125

Language, *see* Cortical mapping
Liposome-DNA vector, *see* Gene therapy

Magnetic resonance imaging, *see also*
  Functional magnetic resonance imaging,
  Magnetic source imaging
  angiography data superimposition
    88, 93
  correlation with single-photon emission
    computed tomography 36–41
  edema in gliomas 217, 218
  fiberoptic image transmission system for
    movement correction 89, 92
  gene therapy of glioblastoma multiforme,
    findings 248, 249
  segmentation software 88–91, 93
  spatial resolution 10
Magnetic source imaging
  auditory evoked fields 80, 84, 85
  intraoperative procedures 82, 83
  magnetic resonance imaging data
    acquisition and neuronavigation
    81, 82
  magnetoencephalography recording and
    data analysis 80, 81
  motor evoked fields 80, 85
  patient selection 79
  principle 78, 79, 86
  somatosensory evoked fields 80, 83
  time requirements 84
  validation 83–85
Magnetoencephalography, *see* Magnetic
  source imaging
Malignant glioma
  astrocytoma, diagnosis in children
    127–129
  blood group O predisposition in recurrent
    disease 195, 196
  boron neutron capture therapy
    blood-brain barrier disruption with
      mannitol 46
    boronated compound selection 44–46

dose escalation 48
dose prescription 46, 47
fractionation 47, 48, 144
rationale and theory 43, 44
safety of borosulfhydryl
  administration 46
thermal neutron flux 44
chemotherapy
  adverse effect on survival 171
  anaplastic astrocytoma 177, 178, 180,
    183, 186
  dosis intensification
    blood-brain barrier modification or
      circumvention 183, 184
    high-dose chemotherapy with
      autologous bone marrow rescue
      185
    intra-arterial administration
      184, 185
    intratumoral chemotherapy 185
    overview 183
  local chemotherapy
    biodegradable polymers 215–217
    enhanced convection 217–220
  MGMT expression and chemosensitivity
    to BCNU 177, 179, 180
  oligodendroglioma chemosensitivity
    181, 182, 186
  prognostic factors 176, 177, 186
  rationale 174, 175
  recurrent glioma, phase II trials
    cytostatic drug combinations
      179, 180
    fotemustine 179
    interpretation 178
    temozolomide 178, 179
  salvage therapy 156
  survival curves 175
  topotecan 21-day continuous infusion
    with conformal radiotherapy
    cerebrospinal fluid penetration 364
    outcome 365, 366, 368
    study design 364, 365
    toxicity 367
epidemiology 244
epidermal growth factor receptor splice
  variant 220